COMPLEMENTARY, ALTERNATIVE, & TRADITIONAL MEDICINE

COMPLEMENTARY, ALTERNATIVE, & TRADITIONAL MEDICINE

Prospects and Challenges for Women's Reproductive Health

EDITED BY COSTANZA TORRI
AND JENNIE M. HORNOSTY

WOMEN'S PRESS
Toronto | Vancouver

Complementary, Alternative, and Traditional Medicine: Prospects and Challenges for Women's Reproductive Health
Edited by Maria Costanza Torri and Jennie M. Hornosty

First published in 2017 by
Women's Press, an imprint of Canadian Scholars
425 Adelaide Street West, Suite 200
Toronto, Ontario
M5V 3C1

www.womenspress.ca

Library and Archives Canada Cataloguing in Publication

Complementary, alternative, & traditional medicine
: prospects and challenges for women's reproductive health
/ edited by Constanza Torri and Jennie M. Hornosty.
Includes bibliographical references and index.
Issued in print and electronic formats.
ISBN 978-1-55130-918-7 (softcover).--ISBN 978-1-55130-919-4
(PDF).--ISBN 978-1-55130-920-0 (EPUB)
1. Women--Health and hygiene. 2. Reproductive health.
3. Reproductive health services. 4. Maternal health services.
5. Alternative medicine. 6. Integrative medicine.
I. Hornosty, Jennie Mary, 1944-, editor II. Torri, Maria
Costanza, editor
RG125.C65 2017 618'.046 C2017-901097-2
C2017-901098-0
Cover and type design by Elisabeth Springate

17 18 19 20 21 5 4 3 2 1

Canada

Costanza:
To my parents
To Lavinia
In memory of my uncle Marcello

Jennie:
With love for my sons—Jason and Justin

CONTENTS

Acknowledgements

This book would not have been possible without the assistance, guidance, and encouragement of many people in many places. Special thanks are due to Andrea Gill, Acquisitions Editor at CPSI/Women's Press; Keriann McGoogan, former Acquisitions Editor at the Press; Laura Godsoe, Managing Editor; Natalie Garriga, Developmental Editor; Wendy Yano, Copy Editor; and Karri Yano, Production Editor for their enthusiasm and help at every stage of the publication process. We are also grateful to the anonymous reviewers for their thoughtful comments and feedback on the draft version of the manuscript.

Our colleagues in the Department of Sociology at the University of New Brunswick have been a great source of inspiration, friendship, and moral support throughout this process. We also wish to thank Katherine Liong for her perceptive and efficient editorial assistance, without which this book could not have been completed.

It is also a pleasure to acknowledge the kindness and support of our families and friends during this venture. Costanza Torri thanks the women who shared their ideas and experiences with her and all the people who helped her during fieldwork in Ecuador and Bolivia. She also thanks her parents and family in Italy, and especially her wonderful niece Lavinia, whose presence and smile are a constant source of joy. Special thanks are due to her friends in Canada and beyond, for their friendship and unfailing encouragement and reassurance in this and all of her endeavours.

Jennie Hornosty thanks many friends in Fredericton for their ongoing friendship, encouragement, and moral support from a distance, as well as Luda in Ottawa, and dear long-time friends, Susan and John in Montreal. She also acknowledges her family, including her two sons, Jason and Justin, for their unceasing love and support, and her wonderful stepchildren: Michael Richardson, his partner, Meaghan Charlebois, and son, Liam; and Rebecca Richardson, her partner, Phil Allen, and daughters, Gemma and Mika. She also acknowledges her late partner, C. James (Jim) Richardson, for his important and enduring role in her academic life.

Introduction

Costanza Torri, PhD
Department of Sociology, University of New Brunswick, Canada

This volume is about women's reproductive health, traditional medicine (TM), and complementary and alternative medicine (CAM). By adopting a perspective drawn from different social sciences (including sociology, history, and health studies), it aims to explore the uses and values attributed to CAM/TM for women's reproductive health from the point of view of patients, CAM/TM practitioners, and other health care providers.

Women's reproductive health has been defined as encompassing maternal health, family planning, infertility, sexually transmitted diseases, and post-natal health-related concerns (Dudgeon & Inhorn, 2004). Topics discussed in this book include fertility, menopause, birth, post-natal care, breast feeding, and cancer.

Traditional medicine (TM) refers to therapies and health practices that developed over time within particular cultures, such as traditional Chinese medicine (TCM) in China or Ayurveda in India; such practices are also typically informed by specific belief systems. The World Health Organization (WHO) describes TM as the "health practices, approaches, knowledge and beliefs incorporating plant, animal and mineral based medicines, spiritual therapies, manual techniques and exercises, applied singularly or in combination to treat, diagnose and prevent illnesses or maintain well-being," and complementary and alternative medicine (CAM) as adaptations of TM that are used in industrialized countries (World Health Organization [WHO], 2003). In other words, CAM practices are "complementary" and "alternative" when they are not part of the conventional medicine of a specific country and are not fully integrated into the dominant local health care system.

As will be seen in chapter 1, the challenge to define CAM and TM is symbolic of the fact that CAM and TM include diverse practices, therapies, and modalities that differ greatly from one another. Attempts have been made to sub-categorize CAM in western countries in order to overcome this challenge. For example, the National Center for Complementary and Integrative Medicine (NCCIM) in the United States recognizes five domains of CAM:

- Whole medical systems: These include Ayurveda, homeopathic medicine, naturopathic medicine, and traditional Chinese medicine (TCM).
- Mind-body medicines: These include meditation, prayer, and mental healing as well as creative therapies using artistic outlets (e.g., dance).

- Biologically based practices: These include herbs, foods, vitamins, and dietary supplements.
- Manipulative and body-based practices: These include chiropractic and osteopathic manipulation, shiatsu, and massage.
- Energy medicines: These include biofield therapies, *qi gong*, reiki, therapeutic touch, and bioelectromagnetic-based therapies (e.g., pulsed fields, magnetic fields, and current fields).

Thus, CAM and TM comprise an extensive variety of practices, systems, and beliefs. Due to their holistic approach to health and well-being, CAM and TM attempt to address the emotional and psychological needs of individuals as well as their physical sphere. Unlike biomedicine, which operates with an assumption that illnesses are primarily biological, holism maintains that strong interconnections exist between mind, body, and spirit as well as between individuals, communities, and local ecosystems (Chan, Ho & Chow, 2002). According to this view, health not only includes biophysical elements but is the product of the complex interactions of biological, social, and psychological factors. As a consequence, health is maintained and re-established through different therapeutic modalities that promote the capacity of the body to heal itself, and through which a balance between the physical, psychological, social, and spiritual aspects is restored.

In the western world, biomedicine has a dominant role in relation to CAM and TM. The hegemonic position of biomedicine is reflected in the language we use to define the concepts of health, illness, and healing, and mirrors the social power operating in the fields of medicine and healing (Gale, 2014). According to Gale (2014), the acceptance of the terms "alternative," "complementary," or anything other than "biomedicine" can be seen as a form of symbolic violence à la Bourdieu, who suggests that individuals consider the domination they are exposed to is acceptable and inescapable—in this case, the domination of biomedicine over CAM/TM practices.

Prominence of CAM/TM and Reasons for Their Increased Popularity

According to the World Health Organization, 80 percent of the population in Africa still relies on TM, while approximately half of the population in industrialized countries uses CAM (WHO, 2003). TM therapies are also fast gaining acceptance in industrialized countries around the world, both among health care providers and patients. In Europe, more than 100 million people currently use CAM, one-fifth of these on a regular basis, which indicates a distinct preference for health care that incorporates CAM therapies (WHO, 2013). In Canada, CAM therapies have gained popularity in the last few years (Metcalfe et al., 2010). According to the Canadian Community Health Survey (CCHS), a national cross-sectional survey, 12.4 percent of the general population reported consulting a CAM practitioner in the past 12 months (Canadian Community Health Survey, 2015). The most common types of CAM used by individuals are massage therapy (62.9%), acupuncture (18.3%), homeopathy (18.2%), chiropractic care (11.3%), herbalism (5.2%), reflexology (2.4%), and spiritual healing (1.0%). CAM services are generally used in conjunction with standard medical care (Andrews and Boon, 2005; Foltz et al., 2005), although their use is not often disclosed to biomedical health care practitioners (Busse et al., 2005).

The importance of CAM has been highlighted by WHO and other international organizations active in the health care arena, and CAM has become progressively acknowledged as important for global health. The Alma-Ata Declaration in 1978 emphasized the utilization of TM systems as a significant way to make health for all a reality. Approaches to and visions of health and population have changed during the past decades, mainly as a result of global debate at the Cairo (1994) and Beijing (1995) conferences following the Ottawa Charter on Health Promotion (1986). This has generated greater concern for understanding patients' health problems from different viewpoints. One essential perspective concerns the social and cultural aspects that affect people's lives and their health conditions.

In the past two decades, there have been a growing number of both quantitative and qualitative studies investigating patterns of CAM/TM use and patients' experiences of using CAM/TM. Numerous studies have tried to explain the increasing popularity of CAM, especially in western countries. The most recurring explanations pertain to the following:

1. Dissatisfaction with the health outcomes of biomedicine and distrust of biomedical practitioners and chemical drugs that are considered to be unsafe (Gaffney & Smith, 2004; Holst, Wright, Nordeng & Haavik, 2009; Pedersen, 2013; Westfall, 2003).
2. Dissatisfaction with the relationship between biomedical health care providers and patients, and preference for the way in which CAM practitioners treat their patients (de Lacey, Smith & Paterson, 2009; Low Dog, 2009; Nabukera et al., 2006; Rayner, McLachlan, Forster & Cramer, 2009; Ried & Alfred, 2013; Steel et al., 2014).
3. Increased sense of autonomy and control over their health, therapies, and lives (Hall, Griffiths & McKenna, 2011; Nissen, 2013; Sirois, 2008; Sointu, 2006; Steen & Calvert, 2007; Warriner, Bryan & Brown, 2014).

4. The capacity of CAM therapies to fulfill the spiritual and psychological needs of women, and to provide an alternative framework for making sense of their lives (Hall, Griffiths & McKenna, 2011; Nissen, 2013).

According to several scholars, the change in cultural values arising from post-modern values is an important factor that may have facilitated the growing popularity of CAM practices (McQuaide, 2005; O'Callaghan & Jordan 2003; Winnick, 2005). This shift reduces the emphasis on rationality and science by rejecting the notion of one universal truth (McQuaide, 2005). According to Boon et al., (2004), the role and responsibility of the patient for his or her own health are pivotal in CAM practices, since the patient directs the healing relationship with the health care practitioner. Stratton and McGivern-Snofsky (2008) highlight how the emphasis of post-modernism on cultural diversity and subjective experience is in line with neoliberal discourse, which emphasizes individual choice, self-management, and personal responsibility for health. This notion of personal responsibility and active agency for health reflects neoliberal ideals that provide individuals with an incentive to empower themselves by taking control of their physical and psychological health and well-being through CAM therapies (Barrett et al. 2004; Fries 2008).

In the Global South, including Central and South America, Africa, and developing Asia, varying factors play a role in determining the therapeutic choices of local women, and make them more interested in choosing TM. These are higher costs of access to biomedical health care services (Ensor & Cooper, 2004; Ensor & Ronoh, 2005; Somanathan, 2005), geographic obstacles (distance, poor road conditions, transport problems, etc.) (Gohou, Ronsmans & Kacou, 2004; Graham et al., 2006), quality of care (poor facilities, lack of essential drugs, poor treatment by health care professionals in biomedical hospitals and clinics, etc.) (Kunst & Houweling, 2001; Lawn, Cousens & Bhutta, 2004), and socio-cultural and norms (Kyomuhendo, 2003; Larsen et al., 2004).

Integrative Medicine

This volume also addresses a third category, which is often confused with biomedicine and CAM: integrative medicine. Integrative medicine can be defined as "a form of health care that brings together CAM treatments that have been scientifically proven safe and effective with conventional medicine" (Segall & Fries, 2011, p. 329).

Fries (2008) considers integrative medicine in Foucauldian terms "as an expansion of medical rationality into all domains of human life: biological, sociological, and spiritual" (p. 354). Following the so-called "evidence-based" medicine, therapies are accepted and adopted as part of the clinical practices—or rather rejected and dismissed based on the scientific evidence of the effectiveness of their therapeutic outcomes. In this process of acceptance, values and therapeutic paradigms of CAM/TM are lost or neglected. For instance, after randomized clinical trials (RCTs) demonstrated the efficacy and safety of acupuncture for the treatment of back pain, it started to be practised by physicians and other biomedical health care professionals without any connection to Chinese spirituality (Frank & Stollberg, 2004).

According to Collyer (2004), the integration of CAM and biomedicine can mainly be explained by the fact that the marketplace has exploited the demand of the consumer. As Northcott (2009) emphasizes, "the blending of CAM and conventional medicine may also be seen as a manifestation of a globalizing, corporatist, and capitalist agenda that attempts to commodify health care, to exploit existing markets, and to create new markets" (p. 164).

In western countries, the integration of CAM with biomedicine may also be interpreted as a phenomenon that reflects the growing process of medicalization (Northcott, 2009), a process by which all aspects of human life come to be defined and treated as medical conditions, and a strategy used by biomedicine to maintain its dominant role. As Northcott (2009) notes: "in a very sophisticated version of 'if you can't beat them, join them' mainstream scientific medicine has responded to the threat of alternative medicine by redefining the adversary as complementary, and repositioning and redefining itself as integrated, blended, and pluralistic" (p. 164).

Challenges of Integrative Medicine

The increasing popularity of the concept of integrative or "intercultural" medicine may demonstrate concerted efforts by biomedical practitioners to work collaboratively with other health care providers. Nevertheless, the creation of integrative health care systems has received a number of criticisms, the main one being that despite the discourse of integration and inclusion of different therapeutic systems, biomedicine continues to maintain a dominant role vis-à-vis CAM/TM practices (Baer & Coulter, 2008). According to Baer (2004), "despite the best efforts on the part of proponents of holistic health to develop an alternative biomedicine, what in reality has been in large part the co-optation of alternative medicine under the rubrics of CAM and integrative medicine or integrative health care" (p. 149). Willis and White (2004) discuss how therapeutic practices could receive clinical legitimation or political-legal legitimation, the latter based on support from consumers' behaviours, regulatory legislation, state-supported education programs, and state-funded health care insurance.

Scholars such as Garvey (2011), Kim (2006), Sagli (2010), and Zhan (2009) have analyzed the process of cross-cultural translation of medical concepts and the ways through which transfers of knowledge happen between different medical systems. Reddy (2002) examines how Ayurveda has been translated into American biomedical culture and the ways it has been incorporated by New Age and practices of spiritual healing. Zhan's (2009) analysis of traditional Chinese medicine (TCM) in the western world illustrates how this system of medicine has become untraditional and deeply subject to influences that are neither Chinese nor originating in China. She examines the changing dynamics of expertise in TCM, as competency and care are differentially valued by practitioners and patients, and valued differently based on the context in which they are deployed.

Challenges and critiques of integrating CAM/TM with biomedicine are discussed by many contributors to the chapters in this book. The important distinction of integration as incorporation (with asymmetric power toward biomedicine) from integration as mutual transformation (with more complementarity between the two health care systems) is not always acknowledged in the debates surrounding integrative medicine.

The Use of CAM among Women

Although both men and women use CAM, holistic health is presently dominated by women as both clients and practitioners (Doel & Segrott, 2003; Heelas & Woodhead, 2005; Ruggie, 2004; Thomas, Nicholl & Coleman, 2001). For instance, Zhang and colleagues (2015) examined US National Health Interview Survey (NHIS) data from 2012 to understand how American adult CAM users differ by gender in terms of their socio-demographic characteristics. This study, which involved 34,525 participants, showed that women represented the majority of CAM users (60 percent) and were three times more likely to use CAM than men. This is in line with previous NHIS reports on CAM use in 2002 and 2007 (Barnes et al., 2008), as well as recent findings from studies carried out in Europe and Australia (Eardley et al., 2012; Steinsbekk et al., 2008; Xue et al., 2007). A study conducted by Lunny and Fraser (2010) on a sample of 423 menopausal women in Canada found high user rates of CAM therapy; the most common treatments were vitamins (61.5 percent), relaxation techniques (57.0 percent), yoga/meditation (37.6 percent), soy products (37.4 percent), and prayer (35.7 percent).

A growing number of women use CAM for their reproductive health for menstrual disorders, menopause, pregnancy, and childbirth (Smith & Cochrane, 2009; Thomas & Coleman, 2004; Tiran, 2006). CAM use seems to be more prevalent among middle class and educated women (Bishop, Northstone, Green & Thompson, 2011) apparently because access to CAM therapies is influenced by income as well as a mindset that seems to be more prevalent among the middle class (Skeggs, 2004).

Feminist scholars have defined the practice of biomedicine as a place for the production and reproduction of social power relations, arguing that most biomedical health care practices have transformed a diseased person into a diseased body (Davis-Floyd 1990; Oakley 1980).

According to feminist scholars, women are also medically constructed as more prone to disease as well as both physically and emotionally inferior, characteristics that create conditions that medicine defines as biological problems, while making women passive recipients of medical care (Martin, 1984). The use of CAM by women, then, can be interpreted as a way to listen to women's self-knowledge of their own body and bodily experiences, and to resist biomedicine. The act of accepting and using CAM, which encourages women to foster their self-nurturing side, can represent a symbolic refusal by women of the exclusive role of caregivers for others (Sointu & Woodhead, 2008). Moreover, in promoting women's self-care and self-nourishment, CAM confirms the importance of the embodiment of physical and emotional sensations. It also motivates women to value themselves and recognize their uniqueness and individuality (Nissen, 2011). According to Nissen (2011, p. 199), by promoting experiences of embodiment and making the body a central component of the therapy, CAM practices offer space for self-fulfillment and pleasure beyond the male gaze and women's traditional role of caring for others.

Women's interest in CAM therapies can also be explained by growing disappointment with their relationships with biomedical practitioners, which often lack meaningful interaction and effective communication. CAM practices seem to support a model oriented around a partnership between practitioner and patient. In this model, health and illness are explored within networks of relationships and responsibilities where the patient plays an active role. Women's use of CAM practices may illustrate their commitment to participatory and egalitarian relationships, together with approaches to their practice that are influenced by women's shared life experiences and values (Nissen, 2011).

Nevertheless, substantial gaps in our understanding of CAM use among women remain. Few studies in the social sciences have examined cultural and ethnic variability in CAM/TM use for reproductive health among women living in different socio-cultural contexts and geographic settings. The therapeutic and cultural relevance of CAM/TM in many different socio-cultural and geographic contexts calls for a better understanding of the relevance of these therapeutic practices in reproductive health.

Book Organization and Content

This volume is about women's health, in particular reproductive health broadly defined, and adopts a perspective drawn from different social sciences (sociology, history, and health studies). Women's reproductive health has been defined as encompassing maternal health, family planning, infertility, sexually transmitted diseases, and post-natal health-related concerns (Dudgeon & Inhorn, 2004). However, there is a propensity to frame the discussion of women's reproductive health in terms of the female reproductive organs. Women's health issues are often presented as universal and, as a consequence, are assumed to be understood, interpreted, and experienced by all women in the same way. This book challenges these assumptions, locating women's reproductive health within global, national, regional, and local contexts. It reminds us that bodies can only be understood within specific spaces and relations.

Topics discussed in this book include fertility, menopause, birth, post-natal care, breast feeding, and cancer. The outlooks of the patients and CAM/TM health care providers described in these studies have been shaped by socio-cultural and religious beliefs that significantly influence how they interpret and experience health conditions, in the domains of both CAM/TM and biomedicine (i.e., western medicine). These studies illustrate how the efficacy of CAM/TM for reproductive health care has been and is perceived in a wide variety of times and places, from pre-European Canada and colonial America to contemporary Africa, Asia, Australia, Europe, and North and South America. The following chapters illuminate important issues affecting access to CAM/TM services for reproductive health, including women's motivations for seeking out CAM/TM therapies, and the impact of ongoing tensions between the western biomedical model of care versus traditional, community-based medicine.

We explore the following main questions:

1. How is reproductive health understood by patients and health care providers?
2. How does this understanding shape the perception of CAM/TM practices and their relevance for women's reproductive health?
3. How does the availability of biomedical versus CAM/TM health care services affect decisions about treatment for reproductive health concerns?

The book is divided into three parts. Part I provides a general and historical overview of CAM/TM practices and reproductive health, and presents the initial debate on the different interpretations and uses of CAM/TM for women's reproductive health. Part II presents the use of TM for women's reproductive health in the Global South and illustrates how women perceive and use TM for their reproductive health.

Several voices from the field, including those of women, traditional midwives, spiritual healers, herbalists, and other TM practitioners, are presented. Part III analyzes the relevance of CAM in Global North for women and the different processes of translation and transfer of therapeutic concepts from CAM into this socio-cultural setting. The impact of ongoing tensions between biomedical versus traditional models of health care and the challenges facing the implementation of an integrative model are also highlighted.

Through this collection of chapters, this book aims to explore perceptions of the role and value of CAM and TM for women's reproductive health from the point of view of patients, CAM/TM practitioners, and other health care providers. By taking into account cultural and ethnic differences in CAM/TM use, it attempts to provide important insights into not only women's perceptions but also those of traditional practitioners such as traditional birth attendants, and into the effectiveness of CAM and other forms of traditional medicine used for reproductive health both in the Global South and North.

References

Andrews, G., & Boon, H. (2005). CAM in Canada: Places, practices, research. *Complementary Therapies in Clinical Practice, 11*(1), 21–27.

Baer, H. (2004). *Toward an integrative medicine: Merging alternative therapies with biomedicine.* Walnut Creek, CA: Alta Mira Press.

Baer, H., & Coulter, I. (2008). Taking stock of integrative medicine: Broadening biomedicine or co-optation of complementary and alternative medicine. *Heath Sociology Review, 17*, 331–341.

Barnes, P.M., Bloom, B., & Nahin, R.L. (2008). *Complementary and alternative medicine use among adults and children: United States, 2007* (National health statistics reports, no. 12). Hyattsville, MD: National Centre for Health Statistics.

Barrett, B., Marchand, L., Scheder, J., Appelbaum, D., Plane, M.B., Blustein, J., & Capperino, C. (2004). What complementary and alternative medicine practitioners say about health and health care. *Annals of Family Medicine, 2*(3), 253–259.

Bishop, J., Northstone, K., Green, J., & Thompson, E. (2011). The use of complementary and alternative medicine in pregnancy: Data from the Avon Longitudinal Study of Parents and Children (ALSPAC). *Complementary Therapies in Medicine, 1*(9), 303–310.

Boon, H., Verhoef, D., O'Hara, B., Findlay, B., & Majid, N. (2004). Integrative healthcare: Arriving at a working definition. *Alternative Therapies in Health Medicine, 5*, 49–56.

Busse, J., Heaton, G., Wu, P., Wilson, K., & Mills, E. (2005). Disclosure of natural product use to primary care physicians: A cross-sectional survey of naturopathic clinic attendees. *Mayo Clinic Proceedings, 80*(5), 616–623.

Canadian Community Health Survey. (2015). *Annual component*. Retrieved 20 July 2016 from www23.statcan.gc.ca/imdb/p2SV.pl?Function=getSurvey&SDDS=3226&lang=en&db=imdb&adm=8&dis=2

Chan, C., Ho, P., & Chow, E. (2002). A body-mind-spirit model in health. *Social Work in Health Care, 34*(3–4), 261–282.

Collyer, F. (2004). The corporatization and commercialization of CAM. In P. Tovey, G., Easthope, & J. Adams (Eds), *The mainstreaming of complementary and alternative medicine: Studies in social context* (pp. 81–99). London: Routledge.

Davis-Floyd, R.E. (1990). The role of obstetrical rituals in the resolution of cultural anomaly. *Social Science and Medicine, 31*(2), 175–189.

de Lacey, S., Smith, C.A., & Paterson, C. (2009). Building resilience: A preliminary exploration of women's perceptions of the use of acupuncture as an adjunct to in vitro fertilisation. *BMC Complementary and Alternative Medicine, 9*, 50.

Doel, M.A., & Segrott, J. (2003). Self, health, and gender: Complementary and alternative medicine in the British mass media. *Gender, Place & Culture: A Journal of Feminist Geography, 10*(2), 131–144.

Dudgeon, M.R., & Inhorn, M.C. (2004). Men's influences on women's reproductive health: Medical anthropological perspectives. *Social Science & Medicine, 59*(7), 1379–1395.

Eardley, S., Bishop, F.L., Prescott, P., Cardini, F., Brinkhaus, B., Santos-Rey, K., ... Lewith, G. (2012). A systematic literature review of complementary and alternative medicine prevalence in EU. *Forschende Komplementarmedizin, 19*(Suppl. 2), 18–28.

Ensor, T., & Cooper, S. (2004). Overcoming barriers to health service access: Influencing the demand side. *Health Policy Plan, 1*(9), 69–79.

Ensor, T., & Ronoh, J. (2005). Effective financing of maternal health services: A review of the literature. *Health Policy, 7*(5): 49–58.

Foltz, V., St Pierre, Y., Rozenberg, S., Rossignol, M., Bourgeois, P., Joseph, L., ... Fautrel, B. (2005). Use of complementary and alternative therapies by patients with self-reported chronic back pain: A nationwide survey in Canada. *Joint Bone Spine, 72*(6), 571–577.

Frank, R., & Stollberg, G. (2004). Medical acupuncture in Germany: Patterns of consumerism among physicians and patients. *Sociology of Health and Illness, 26*, 351–372.

Fries, C. (2008). Governing health of the hybrid self: Integrative medicine, neoliberalism, and the shifting biopolitics of subjectivity. *Health Sociology Review, 17*, 353–367.

Gaffney, L., & Smith, C. (2004). The views of pregnant women towards the use of complementary therapies and medicines. *Birth Issues, 13*(2), 43–50.

Gale, N. (2014). The sociology of traditional, complementary and alternative medicine. *Sociology Compass, 8*(6), 805–822.

Garvey, M. (2011). The transmission of Chinese medicine in Australia. *PORTAL Journal of Multidisciplinary International Studies, 8*(2), 1–13.

Gohou, V., Ronsmans, C., & Kacou, L. (2004). Responsiveness to life-threatening obstetric emergencies in two hospitals in Abidjan, Cote d'Ivoire. *Tropical Medicine International Health*, *9*(2), 406–415.

Graham, W.J., Cairns, J., Bhattacharya, S., Bullough, C., Quayyum, Z., & Khama, R. (2006). Maternal and perinatal conditions. In D.T. Jamison, J.G. Breman & A.R. Measham (Eds), *Disease control priorities for developing countries* (pp. 499–530). New York & Washington, DC: Oxford University Press & World Bank.

Hall, H., Griffiths, D., & McKenna, L. (2011). The use of complementary and alternative medicine by pregnant women: A literature review. *Midwifery*, *27*(6), 817–824.

Heelas, P. & Woodhead, L. (2005). *The spiritual revolution: Why religion is giving way to spirituality.* Oxford: Blackwell.

Holst, L., Wright, D., Nordeng, H., & Haavik, S. (2009). Use of herbal preparations during pregnancy: Focus group discussion among expectant mothers attending a hospital antenatal clinic in Norwich, UK. *Complementary Therapies in Clinical Practice*, *15*, 225–229.

Kim, J. (2006). Beyond paradigm: Making transcultural connections in a scientific translation of acupuncture. *Social Science & Medicine*, *62*(12), 2960–2972.

Kunst, A.E., & Houweling, T. (2001). Inequalities in the utilisation of delivery care and other maternal health services. *Studies in Health Services Organization and Policy*, *1*(7), 297–315.

Kyomuhendo, G.B. (2003). Low use of rural maternity services in Uganda: Impact of women's status, traditional beliefs and limited resources. *Reproductive Health Matters*, *11*(3), 16–26.

Larsen, G.L., Lupiwa, S., Kave, H.P., Gillieatt, S., & Alpers, M.P. (2004). Antenatal care in Goroka: Issues and perceptions Papua New Guinea. *Medical Journal*, *47*(4), 202–214.

Lawn, J.E., Cousens, S., & Bhutta, Z.A. (2004). Why are 4 million newborn babies dying each year? *Lancet*, *364*, 399–401.

Low Dog, T. (2009). The use of botanicals during pregnancy and lactation. *Alternative Therapies in Health and Medicine*, *15*(1), 54–58.

Lunny, C., & Fraser, S. (2010). The use of complementary and alternative medicines among a sample of Canadian menopausal-aged women. *Journal of Midwifery and Women's Health*, *55*(4), 335–343.

Martin, E. (1984). Pregnancy, labor and body image in the United States. *Social Science and Medicine*, *19*(11), 1201–1206.

McQuaide, M.M. (2005). The rise in alternative health care: A sociological account. *Social Theory and Health*, *3*, 286–301.

Metcalfe, A., Williams, J., McChesney, J., Patten, S., & Jetté, N. (2010). Use of complementary and alternative medicine by those with a chronic disease and the general population—results of a national population-based survey. *BMC Complementary and Alternative Medicine*, *10*, 58.

Nabukera, S.K., Witte, K., Muchunguzi, C., Bajunirwe, F., Batwala, V.K., & Mulogo, E.M. (2006). Use of postpartum health services in rural Uganda: Knowledge, attitudes, and barriers. *Journal of Community Health*, *31*(2), 84–93.

Nissen, N. (2011). Challenging perspectives: Women, complementary and alternative medicine, and social change. *Interface, 3*(2): 187–212.

Nissen, N. (2013). Women's bodies and women's lives in western herbal medicine in the UK. *Medical Anthropology, 32*(1), 75–91.

Northcott, H. (2009). Complementary and alternative medicine in Canada: From marginal to mainstream. In S. Bolaria & H. Dickinson (Eds), *Health, illness, and health care in Canada* (pp. 152–165). Toronto: Nelson Education.

Oakley, A. (1980). *Women confined: Towards a sociology of childbirth.* Oxford: Martin Robertson.

O'Callaghan, F.V., & Jordan, N. (2003). Postmodern values, attitudes and the use of complementary medicine. *Complementary Therapies in Medicine, 11*(1), 28–32.

Pedersen, I.K. (2013). "It can do no harm": Body maintenance and modification in alternative medicine acknowledged as a non-risk health regime. *Social Science & Medicine, 90*, 56–62.

Rayner, J., McLachlan, H.L., Forster, D.A., & Cramer, R. (2009). Australian women's use of complementary and alternative medicines to enhance fertility: Exploring the experiences of women and practitioners. *BMC Complementary and Alternative Medicine, 9*, 52.

Reddy, S. (2002). Asian medicine in America: The Ayurvedic case. *The Annals of the American Academy of Political and Social Science, 583*(1), 97–121.

Ried, K., & Alfred, A. (2013). Quality of life, coping strategies and support needs of women seeking traditional Chinese medicine for infertility and viable pregnancy in Australia: A mixed methods approach. *BMC Women's Health, 13*, 17.

Ruggie, M. (2004). *Marginal to mainstream: Alternative medicine in America.* Cambridge: Cambridge University Press.

Sagli, G. (2010). The establishing of Chinese medical concepts in Norwegian acupuncture schools: The cultural translation of Jingluo ("Circulation Tracts"). *Anthropology and Medicine, 17*(3), 315–326.

Segall, A., & Fries, C. (2011). *Pursuing health and wellness: Healthy societies, healthy people.* Don Mills, ON: Oxford University Press Canada.

Sirois, F.S. (2008). Motivations for consulting complementary and alternative medicine practitioners: A comparison of consumers from 1997–8 and 2005. *BMC Complementary and Alternative Medicine, 8*, 16.

Skeggs, B. (2004). *Class, self, culture.* London: Routledge.

Smith, C., & Cochrane S. (2009). Does acupuncture have a place as an adjunct treatment during pregnancy? A review of randomized controlled trials and systematic reviews. *Birth, 36*(3), 246–253.

Sointu, E. (2006). The search for wellbeing in alternative and complementary health practices. *Sociology of Health & Illness, 28*(3), 330–349.

Sointu, E., & Woodhead, L. (2008). Spirituality, gender, and expressive selfhood. *Journal for the Scientific Study of Religion, 4*(7), 259–276.

Somanathan, A. (2005). *Critical assessment of the extent and mechanisms by which maternal and newborn health care expenditure requirements exacerbate poverty.* Geneva: World Health Organization.

Steel, A., Adams, J., Sibbritt, D., Broom, A., Gallios, C., & Frawley, J. (2014). Determinants of women consulting with a complementary and alternative medicine practitioner for pregnancy related conditions. *Women & Health, 54*(2), 127–144.

Steen, M., & Calvert, J. (2007). Self-administered homeopathy part two: A follow-up study. *British Journal of Midwifery, 15*(6), 359–365.

Steinsbekk, A., Adams, J., Sibbritt, D., Jacobsen, G., & Johnsen, R. (2008). Socio-demographic characteristics and health perceptions among male and female visitors to CAM practitioners in a total population study. *Forschende Komplementarmedizin, 15*(3), 146–151.

Stratton, D., & McGivern-Snofsky, J.L. (2008). Towards a sociological understanding of complementary and alternative medicine use. *Journal of Alternative and Complementary Medicine, 14*(6), 777–783.

Thomas, K., & Coleman, P. (2004). Use of complementary or alternative medicine in a general population in Great Britain. *Journal of Public Health, 26*, 152–157.

Thomas, K.J., Nicholl, J.P., & Coleman, P. (2001). Use and expenditure on complementary medicine in England: A population based survey. *Complementary Therapies in Medicine, 9*(1), 2–11.

Tiran, D. (2006). Complementary therapies in pregnancy: Midwives' and obstetricians' appreciation of risk. *Complementary Therapies in Clinical Practice, 12*, 126–131.

Warriner, S., Bryan, K., & Brown, A.M. (2014). Women's attitude towards the use of complementary and alternative medicines (CAM) in pregnancy. *Midwifery, 30*(1), 138–143.

Westfall, R.E. (2003). Herbal healing in pregnancy: Women's experiences. *Journal of Herbal Pharmacotherapy, 3*(4), 17–39.

Winnick, T.A. (2005). From quackery to "complementary" medicine: The American medical profession confronts alternative therapies. *Social Problems, 52*(1), 38–61.

World Health Organization (WHO). (2003). *Traditional medicine* (Fact sheet no. 134). Retrieved from www.who.int/mediacentre/factsheets/2003/fs134/en/

WHO. (2013). *WHO traditional medicine strategy 2014–2023.* Geneva, Switzerland: Author. Retrieved from http://apps.who.int/iris/bitstream/10665/92455/1/9789241506090_eng.pdf

Willis, E., & White, K. (2004). Evidence-based medicine and CAM. In P. Tovey, G. Easthope & J. Adams (Eds), *The mainstreaming of complementary and alternative medicine: Studies in social context* (pp. 49–63). London: Routledge.

Xue, C.C., Zhang, A.L., Lin, V., Da Costa, C., & Story, D.F. (2007). Complementary and alternative medicine use in Australia: A national population-based survey. *Journal of Alternative and Complementary Medicine, 13*(6), 643–650.

Zhan, M. (2009). *Other-worldly: Making Chinese medicine through transnational frames.* Durham, NC & London: Duke University Press.

Zhang, Y., Leach, M., Hall, H., Sundberg, T., Ward, L., Sibbritt, D., & Adams, J. (2015). Differences between male and female consumers of complementary and alternative medicine in a national US population: A secondary analysis of 2012 NIHS data. *Evidence-based Complementary and Alternative Medicine, 2015*. http://dx.doi.org/10.1155/2015/413173

PART I

KEY ISSUES AND HISTORICAL PERSPECTIVE

The first part of this book discusses the definitions, interpretations, and uses of CAM/TM for women's reproductive health, and provides a general and historical overview of CAM/TM practices for reproductive health.

An analysis of the historical and political circumstances surrounding the relationship between CAM/TM and biomedicine provides a lens through which an historical understanding of the forces that produced the socio-cultural marginalization of CAM/TM can be gained. These chapters show how CAM and TM embody the complexity of cultural adaptation to changing socio-cultural contexts in an historical perspective.

Chapter 1 introduces the major arguments about CAM and TM in reproductive health, and shows how CAM and TM cannot be seen as unified entities but, on the contrary, are used to signify a range of healing practices. The chapter illustrates the distinction between alternative medicine and conventional medicine, and provides an explanation of the increasing popularity of alternative medicine, paying particular attention to women and female reproductive health issues.

The remaining three chapters situate CAM and TM practices for reproductive health within broader historical trends, contextualizing the encounters between CAM/TM and biomedicine as well as the resulting transformations that have arisen in each system, respectively.

Chapter 2 studies the historical marginalization of women as healers, illustrating how—despite women's traditional roles as carers within the family—patriarchal and state preference for the exclusive professionalization and power of male-led biomedical forms of medicine and health care practices have restricted women's ability to practise their skills formally. Chapter 3 investigates the wealth of botanical remedies used by colonial North Americans to treat infertility and other gynecological problems, and discusses how these practices gradually fell out of favour with the rise of modern pharmacology and the increasing power and authority of the medical profession. Lastly, chapter 4 creates a space for midwives to be acknowledged as historical actors in their own right and midwifery as a profession with a much more diverse history than is commonly portrayed. The chapter includes an overview of the history and new developments of midwifery in Canadian Indigenous communities prior to European contact as well as the organization of midwifery in early settler communities.

CHAPTER 1

Introducing Complementary and Alternative Medicine, Traditional Medicine, and Gender

Daniel Hollenberg, PhD
Ontario Health Human Resources Research Network, University of Ottawa, Canada

Costanza Torri, PhD
Department of Sociology, University of New Brunswick, Canada

Learning Objectives

1. To gain an understanding of complementary, alternative and traditional medicine (CAM/TM), and their breadth of medical therapies and treatments.
2. To gain awareness of how gender influences women's decisions about using CAM/TM.

Introduction

Complementary and alternative medicine (CAM) and traditional medicine (TM) are now recognized, global health care phenomena (World Health Organization [WHO], 2013). They occur in nearly all WHO member states, encompassing specific therapies or treatments, healing systems, and health care professions. CAM/TM is also a vehicle of and for primary health care (PHC) for millions of the world's population. In nations that identify with what is commonly thought of as "western" culture, and are often identified by social scientists as "richer" than other nations due to industrialization and related colonial practices, these types of non-biomedical practices are referred to as CAM. Although there are exceptions due to the inherent nature of definitions, and the complexities of shifting health care landscapes, the majority of CAM scholars agree that the term CAM is a western label for non-biomedical healing practices occurring in western health care systems.

It is only recently, however, that CAM's similarities, differences, and link to traditional or Indigenous medicine have begun to be acknowledged (Hollenberg, Zakus, Cook & Xu, 2008). Traditional medicine (TM), while also having varied definitions, is known to be those health care practices from longstanding Indigenous systems of health care usually found in non-western countries (Hollenberg, Zakus, Cook & Xu, 2008), which are often "poorer" than or at a disadvantage to western nations. As with CAM, TM includes specific therapies, healing systems, and health care professions, and is an integral—if not fundamental—component of PHC (Hollenberg, Zakus, Cook & Xu, 2008). The main link between CAM and TM is that forms of TM, when entering and occurring in western health care systems, become labelled as CAM (e.g., Chinese and Ayurvedic medical systems), despite remaining fully developed TM systems in their country of origin. One of the main differences between CAM and TM is that not all types of CAM have an Indigenous link to TM (e.g., naturopathy, homeopathy). The major exception to CAM/TM definitions and boundaries occurs with Indigenous populations within western countries (e.g., First Nations in Canada), which also practice their own medicine. In this case, these Indigenous health care practices would exclusively be referred to as TM, not CAM, due to their Indigenous history, despite occurring in a western health care system.

CAM/TM is the product of diverse cultural, historical, and, arguably, political developments and movements. Although historically CAM/TM has been viewed as the direct opposite of conventional biomedicine (western medicine), the boundaries between biomedicine and CAM/TM are, in fact, constantly in flux. As CAM/TM therapies become more mainstream, biomedicine and health care generally is arguably undergoing a process of global transformation.

As Kelner and Welman (2000) state:

> The definition of CAM is open to many interpretations making it difficult to ensure a common understanding. This lack of consistency is not surprising in a field that has such diverse cultural and historical roots, and is evolving so rapidly. There is confusion about which therapies to include or exclude from the definition, and how to classify the multitude of therapies in some coherent way. There is confusion even about what such therapies should be called—alternative, complementary, holistic, unorthodox, unconventional, non-scientific, and marginal are only some

> of the many descriptors in the literature. Indeed, the borders between orthodox biomedicine and CAM are themselves unclear. (pp. 3–4)

For instance, what was long disparaged historically as unorthodox and "irregular" medicine has now found global recognition as CAM/TM, distinct from conventional biomedicine. This development reflects changing socio-cultural and even political attitudes toward what would previously have been polarized as mainstream (i.e., biomedical) and non-mainstream (i.e., CAM/TM) healing modalities. These shifting boundaries can be seen historically in the context of women's health. For example, social prejudices in 19th-century Europe and North America resulted in female midwives being supplanted by biomedically trained male midwives, despite women's traditional role as midwives and birth assistants (Mitchinson, 1991). Conversely, the emergence of the professional practice of osteopathy in the United States (a non-biomedical form of manual healing with similarities to chiropractic) in the early 20th century showed that there was ample scope for certain alternative therapies to maintain professional autonomy alongside biomedical medicine. In the United States, osteopathic practice and educational institutions are today considered on par with leading medical schools, thus showing the level of professional autonomy achieved by this profession. Similarly, the profession of chiropractic rose from humble beginnings in the early 20th century to become one of the most widely accepted CAM modalities in the western world today. Nevertheless, many other forms of what would now be called CAM did not survive historical marginalization, and ultimately were eliminated by biomedical professional dominance in the early 20th century (Hollenberg, 1999). Despite some advances in Canada and in many other countries, CAM/TM remains marginalized, clearly outside of the dominant biomedical system.

Deconstructing CAM/TM

It must be acknowledged that the perceived divide between conventional biomedicine and CAM/TM is, in sociological terms, a "social construction" (i.e., based on social norms and values). Many practices that are now labelled as CAM/TM were—and still remain—mainstream medicine for many people in the world. As noted, one prominent example is acupuncture, a therapy originating from traditional Chinese medicine (TCM) (although its practice was significantly adulterated by Maoist socio-political movements in the 1950s). In North America and other western countries, acupuncture is perceived as a form of CAM, whereas in Asian countries it is part of mainstream health care derived from traditional or indigenous socio-cultural roots.

Kelner and Wellman have suggested that there must exist some group of concepts that collectively express "the essential nature of CAM" (2000, p. 4). They (2000) propose that CAM definitions should encompass many different kinds of CAM therapies, yet at the same time not be too broad or too narrow. The World Health Organization's most recent definition of CAM notes that "the terms 'complementary medicine' or 'alternative medicine' are used interchangeably with traditional medicine in some countries" but that CAM in westernized health care systems is a "broad set of health care practices that are not part of that country's own tradition … and are not fully integrated into the dominant health care system" (WHO, 2013, p. 15). Thus, as noted, the label CAM is used primarily within the context of western health care systems. Here, we will use the term CAM when referring to non-biomedical health care practices in North American or westernized health care systems, and TM when referring to non-biomedical health care practices in non-westernized health care systems outside of North America, with the exception of Indigenous medicine noted earlier.

Clarke's (2004) definition of CAM offers a good starting point: broadly speaking, CAM is "all those health-care practices that defer from **allopathic medicine**" and which "tend not to be taught at allopathic medical schools and are generally unavailable in North American hospitals" (p. 349). A more technical definition was proposed in 1995 by the American Office of Alternative Medicine, the pre-cursor to the United States' National Center for Complementary and Alternative Medicine and recently renamed the National Center for Complementary and Integrative Health (NCCIH):

> Complementary and alternative medicine (CAM) is a broad domain of healing resources that encompasses all health systems, modalities, and practices, and their accompanying theories and beliefs, other than those intrinsic to the politically dominant health system of a particular society or culture in a given historical period. CAM includes all such practices and ideas self-defined by their users as preventing or treating illness or promoting well-being. Boundaries between CAM and the CAM domain and the domain of the dominant system are not always sharp or fixed. (O'Connor et al., 1997)

Note how this definition draws attention to the political nature of health care systems and professional autonomy in deciding which healing modalities are CAM/TM versus conventional ones. Yet other parameters are also needed in order to attempt to capture exactly what CAM/TM means.

In addition to types of therapies, attitudes toward health provide another site of differentiation. For instance, it has been noted that CAM/TM practices include and generally emphasize the uniqueness of each individual; the integration of body, mind, and spirit; the flow of energy as a source of healing; and disease as having multiple dimensions beyond the purely biological (Berliner & Salmon, 1979). The concept of "life force" has also been found to be an essential element of the healing process within CAM/TM modalities, and emphasis has often been placed on the role of the environment, the subjective experience of patients, the healing power of nature, and the idea of health as a positive "state of being" (Goldstein, 1999). As Vincent, Furnham & Richardson (1998) have described extensively, CAM/TM therapies often share an underlying theory, philosophy, and approach to illness. They point out that many CAM/TM systems include some aspect of vitalism whereby "the body and emotions, mental and spiritual life, are all maintained by an energy or 'vital force' commonly found in CAM/TM systems such as Chinese medicine, Western herbalism, homeopathy, and naturopathy" (1998, p. 20). The concept of vitalism has also been observed to be closely associated with another CAM/TM-based concept, namely that the human body has the capacity for self-healing, and the task of the CAM/TM practitioner is to assist this process—a perspective that is fundamentally different from that of biomedicine (Vincent, Furnham & Richardson, 1998). Many CAM/TM therapies are also contained within a particular paradigm or worldview, with an accompanying holistic theory of disease in what is viewed as a "whole medical system" (whole-system CAM/TM research is now a new mode of research inquiry that has been taken up by leading CAM/TM researchers). Fulder (1984) found that CAM/TM systems use symptoms of disease as guides to the uncovering of a general "imbalance" within the whole body system. In the words of Vincent, Furnham & Richardson, "specific symptoms are seen as the most obvious manifestation of a general imbalance or dysfunction affecting the whole system" (1998, p. 21). One of the most common examples is found within the field of Chinese medicine, where *qi* energy becomes blocked within one's body system due to imbalance, and must then be "unblocked" or stimulated in order to restore the flow of energy in a direction that will be most healthy for the body system. Many CAM/TM systems and therapies also focus on prevention and positive states of health by striving to correct minor imbalances within the body's system before they manifest as an acute or chronic illness. Rather than medicalizing the body's normal functioning or positing perfect health as a normal state to be maintained at all costs with medical interventions, CAM/TM systems recognize the seemingly minor health imperfections that biomedicine tends not to manage effectively (e.g., persistent fatigue or low resistance to infection) but which, when addressed early, may play an important preventive role in maintaining health.

It should be noted that, as Kelner and Wellman (2000) and others (e.g., Vincent, Furnham & Richardson, 1998) point out, CAM/TM is not a homogenous phenomenon, although many CAM/TM systems do share philosophy and concepts. As Kelner and Wellman state: "individual [CAM/TM] therapies vary according to philosophy, terminology, practice, the degree of public acceptance, and the extent of efficacy" (2000, p. 6). The unique history of each modality is also diverse, since some types of CAM/TM are as much as 5000 years old, whereas other CAM types were founded little more than a century ago.

There have also been many attempts to classify and categorize the various types of CAM/TM, but no catch-all typology exists. Most recent attempts to classify CAM/TM into operational models and typologies draw on theoretical work done by CAM researchers in the late 1980s, throughout the 1990s and the early 2000s, when CAM/TM was increasingly being used by patients and CAM providers in western health care systems. Pietroni's early work on "holistic" medicine (1987; see also Pietroni, 1986) distinguishes between different "approaches" in CAM/TM, such as psychological (e.g., meditation), therapeutic (e.g., massage), diagnostic (e.g., blood analysis), and complete systems of healing (e.g., Chinese medicine). Vincent, Furnham & Richardson (1998) follow Pietroni's (1986) approach in their discussion of CAM/TM, as do Murray and Rubel (1992), who find four categories of CAM/TM based on specific treatments and techniques: (1) spiritual/psychological, such as faith healing; (2) nutritional, including dietary regimes and vitamin supplements; (3) biological/pharmacological, such as herbal remedies and drugs; and (4) physical interventions such as manipulative therapies, such as chiropractic. Murray and Rubel's model has become useful for CAM/TM advocates, who highlight the common ground that can be found when biomedicine is divided under the same headings, thus blurring the boundaries between CAM/TM and biomedicine. For instance, herbal CAM/TM therapies fall into the same category as biomedical drugs in Murray and Rubel's third, pharmacological, category.

Medical anthropologists, who have been key TM supporters since the early World Health Organization TM policies in the 1970s, have also developed theoretical typologies of CAM/TM relative to health care sectors. Helman (1990) in particular, following Kleinman (1980), finds three health care sectors, which may be applied to this discussion:

1. Folk: Practices deriving from Indigenous health knowledge that is not professionalized or taught in educational institutions.
2. Popular: Self-administered TM/CAM or biomedical therapies such as dietary supplements, over-the-counter remedies (e.g., aspirin), and general lay-knowledge about health.

3. Professional: "Professionalized" systems of medicine, long-dominated by biomedicine and other biomedical health professions, but now also including certain CAM/TM professions (such as chiropractic and naturopathy), all of which contain formalized knowledge systems taught in educational institutions, and which are often regulated. This health sector analysis is useful for showing how CAM/TM can legitimately exist in multiple contexts and settings.

Fulder (1996), drawing on Helman (1990), proposes a typology of five CAM/TM categories: (1) ethnic medical systems, such as acupuncture, Chinese medicine, and Ayurveda; (2) manual therapies such as chiropractic, reflexology, and massage therapy; (3) mind-body therapies such as hypnotherapy, psychic healing, and radionics; (4) nature-cure therapies such as naturopathy and hygienic methods; and (5) non-allopathic medical systems such as homeopathy and herbalism. Kelner and Wellman (2000, p. 6) modify Fulder's typology to organize CAM/TM therapies according to the specific context in which they are delivered: (1) clinical forms, such as chiropractic, homeopathy, acupuncture, and naturopathy; (2) psychological/behavioural forms including yoga, dance therapy, and biofeedback; and (3) social/community forms such as faith healing and folk medicine. Following the above early typologies, the American NCCIH developed its own CAM taxonomy, differentiating CAM by these categories: (1) whole medical systems; (2) mind-body medicine; (3) biologically based practices; (4) manipulative and body-based practices; and (5) energy medicine.

One of the more recent and arguably most in-depth health care taxonomies that includes both CAM and biomedical health practices was developed by Porcino and MacDougall (2009) after a lengthy five-year analysis. Their taxonomy, which they term the "integrated taxonomy of healthcare (ITHC)," contains four main areas in which health practices are differentiated: (1) systems; (2) domains; (3) modalities; and (4) techniques. The "domains" category is similar to the majority of categories summarized in earlier CAM typologies (i.e., most list the domain category of healing practice); however, Porcino and MacDougall's taxonomy goes substantially further and lists 11 domains.

Porcino and MacDougall's taxonomy differentiates between subtleties of "techniques" ("a specific action to achieve a particular outcome"), "modalities" ("a named scope of practice with defined standards of practice"), "domains" ("broad-based categories that encompass one or more modalities"), and "systems" ("a specified grouping of a number of distinct healthcare modalities" and domains) (2009, p. 21). Porcino and MacDougall's detailed taxonomy provides a theoretical orientation by sequentially including categories of increasing complexity, ultimately subsumed under health care "systems." The taxonomy also places biomedicine on an "equal footing" with any other medical or health care practice, as aspects of biomedicine can be placed in any of the four categories (i.e., biomedicine, as a health care system, equally has techniques, modalities, and domains, as does CAM/TM).

As Kelner and Wellman point out, such typologies "are not permanent" and will "continue to shift according to clinical, cultural, political and economic developments" (2000, p. 6). One of the most prominent and arguably fascinating reflections of shifting boundaries between CAM/TM and biomedicine is the recent development of integrative medicine (IM) or integrative health care (IHC), whereby certain types of CAM/TM are now taught at certain biomedical schools and are available in North American hospitals; CAM/TM practices are becoming part of the dominant health care system; and "new" IM practitioners and physicians are graduating, both prescribing and practicing multiple CAM/TM and biomedical modalities (Hollenberg, 2006, 2007).

Women and CAM

In this section, we discuss women's CAM use in western contexts, in comparison to TM use by women in other non-western areas of the world (as discussed in other chapters). Research findings from recent literature suggest that women are the most frequent users of CAM both for their health in general (Bishop & Lewith, 2010; Ohlen, Balneaves, Bottorffc & Brazierb, 2006; Thomas & Coleman, 2004) and their reproductive health in particular (De Boer & Lamxay, 2009; Smith & Cochrane, 2009).

Common modalities that women use include massage, vitamin and mineral supplements, herbal medicine, acupuncture/acupressure, aromatherapy, yoga, homeopathy, and chiropractic care (Mills, Dugoua, Perri & Koren, 2006; Ong, Chan, Yung & Leung, 2005). In addition, the literature shows that pregnant women generally use more than one type of CAM therapy (Gaffney & Smith, 2004; Nordeng & Havnen, 2004; Ong, Chan, Yung & Leung, 2005; Refuerzo et al., 2005; Wang, Dezinno & Fermo, 2005).

Studies also show how older women are the most likely to use CAM therapies (Furler et al., 2006; Lunny & Fraser, 2010) while menopause symptoms are among the top 15 medical conditions managed with CAM therapies in the United States (Ma, Drieling & Stafford, 2006). In their study conducted in Canada, Lunny and Fraser (2010) highlighted how out of the 423 menopausal women who were surveyed for their use of CAM therapies, 91 percent of them reported trying CAM therapies for their menopausal symptoms.

Reasons for women's use of CAM generally are varied and include the belief that these therapies provide a safer alternative to pharmaceuticals (Holst, Wringt, Nordeng & Haavik, 2009; Nordeng & Havnen, 2004) and a greater choice in regard to their health care choices (Ohlen, Balneaves, Bottorffc & Brazierb, 2006). Literature also suggests that CAM use reflects the holistic health beliefs of some women (Gaffney & Smith, 2004; Stratton & McGivern-Snofsky, 2008), which is consistent with other studies that show how the increasing popularity of CAM can be associated with changes in general attitudes to health (Coulter & Willis, 2007). Regarding reproductive health, studies show how pregnant women may choose CAM to have more control over their health and their childbearing experiences, and to use more natural (perceived as safer) treatment, especially during their pregnancy (Hollyer et al., 2002; Low Dog, 2009; Wiebelitz et al., 2009). As noted, women who use CAM are more likely to be older (Thomas & Coleman, 2004) but also have higher education and income (Bishop & Lewith, 2010); although other studies highlighted how women of young age (Boon et al., 2000; Buettner et al., 2006) are more often associated with CAM use.

Regarding pregnancy, literature shows how women who use CAM for their reproductive health had also used CAM therapies for other health reasons (e.g. Conover, 2003; Headley, Northstone, Simmons & Golding, 2004; Holst, Wringt, Nordeng & Haavik, 2009).

While considering the use of CAM for their reproductive health, women often rely on family, friends, and the media (Furlow et al., 2008; Maats & Crowther, 2002; Nordeng & Havnen, 2004). Health care practitioners also play an important role in influencing the decision of women to use CAM therapies (Holst, Wringt, Nordeng & Haavik, 2009).

CAM and Gender: Can CAM Practices Reproduce Traditional Gender Roles or Transform Them?

Existing health literature provides an overview of how **gender roles** can influence the use of and access to biomedical settings, yet not much is known about how gender affects the use of and access to CAM practices (Flesch, 2007). Only a few studies have noted the prevalence of women as both consumers and practitioners of CAM (Doel & Segrott, 2003; Ruggie, 2004).

Following Nissen (2011), the analysis of what literature exists about gender and CAM therapies suggests two hypotheses: (1) the use of CAM therapies by women is a means to reproduce traditional notions of femininity, according to which women are naturally nurturing and caregivers; or (2) CAM is a means to promote **empowerment** and self-agency in health for women.

Reproducing Traditional Femininity

According to studies conducted by Sointu and Woodhead (2008) and Sointu (2011), gender differences in the use of CAM may reflect gendered patterns of health behaviour in general. According to these authors, gendered identities play an important role in explaining the popularity of CAM practices among women, both as consumers and as practitioners. Women's inclination toward preventative health, well-being, and seeking CAM therapies may be interpreted in light of the discourse of "caring" femininity, which socially reproduces characteristics of femininity traditionally attributed to women (Sointu & Woodhead, 2008). According to O'Grady (2005), the discourse of caring femininity reinforces women's self-scrutiny toward what is considered to be an appropriate feminine behaviour, such as taking responsibility for the physical and emotional needs of others. Thus, one discourse of well-being achieved through CAM and holistic health practices reflects not only concern for physical health but also mirrors traditional ideas of femininity.

In turn, men's use of CAM practices has been seen as contrary to the ideal of **hegemonic masculinity**, in which concern for one's health is perceived as feminine and thus contrary to traditional ideals of manliness. Indeed, by focusing on emotional awareness, self-exploration, and intimacy, CAM practices have the potential to challenge the socially constructed ideals of hegemonic or dominant masculinity (Connell, 2002). As Sointu points out, "the turn to alternative and complementary medicines is thus entwined with ongoing negotiations of gendered subjectivity in today's late modern societies" (2011, p. 357). Similarly, the use of CAM practices by men and women may also reflect differing ideals of masculinity and femininity—the former being associated with strength, endurance, and performance. Zhang and colleagues (2015) examined the different motivations for and uses of CAM by patients, considering gender. Their data indicated that women were motivated to use CAM for reasons including general well-being and disease prevention. Conversely, men were more likely to use CAM to enhance their athletic performance—a motivation that may be interpreted as the enhancement of masculinity, based on physical performance and competition.

CAM as a Tool of Empowerment and Self-Agency for Women

Although some narratives of CAM use reflect traditional characteristics of femininity, other discourses embed CAM in the discourse of self-care, as a way to prioritize one's own needs rather than the needs of others, and a way to define the self independently from the wishes and expectations of others (Nissen, 2011). As Nissen

(2011) highlights, the theme of empowerment is a recurring one, both in biomedicine and CAM, inspired by the ideology of social action and the self-help movement that became increasingly popular in the 1960s and the 1970s. Being associated with an increased participation in the decision-making process of the patient (Hewitt-Taylor, 2004), the term "empowerment" points toward the capacity of women as patients to make informed decisions and to play a more active role in their health care decisions. It also pertains to increased self-knowledge and identity seeking (Nissen, 2011).

Feminist scholars emphasize how improvements in the ways that women manage their health can lead to more autonomy in health care and increase the control they have over their own lives (Ruzek, Clarke & Olesen, 1997).

Sointu (2011) stresses how CAM practices place the patient at the centre of the therapeutic act and promote values such as individual fulfillment, active agency, and participation. As such, CAM may provide an alternative framework to reconsider the ideal of femininity and create an alternative discourse of traditional femininity, which is oriented toward self-care rather than care for others. In this way, women can use CAM to affirm their own identity and find their own space, overcoming the ideology of "caring" femininity, which is centered on the idea of "being there for others." Gollschewski and colleagues (2008) argue that one of the main reasons for women's use of CAM is the feeling of personal control and responsibility for their own health, with the capacity to control the treatments and therapies used. The empowerment process may be considered as both a form of control and agency for women navigating the dominant biomedical model of health care, and a form of resistance against biomedical constructions of disease (Thompson, 2003) sustained by a sense of responsibility for one's body and health (Baarts & Pedersen, 2009). Consequently, it has been suggested that CAM can redirect feminine nurturing qualities toward the self rather than others, thus challenging the traditional gendered role of "caring" femininity (Sointu & Woodhead, 2008; Nissen, 2011).

Conclusion

Women's use of CAM as an act of agency and empowerment in health is consistent with both the long tradition of women as caregivers and efforts by women to (re-) establish themselves as legitimate healers. As feminist historians have noted, women have been attempting to reclaim their healing history for 500 years. It is a history of severe restriction, persecution, and, at times suppression (Pelicci, 2008). The "re-takeover" of midwifery by women over the past 100 years is a salient example of women reclaiming ownership of their own healing profession—as well as their own health and bodies. It is important to note here that although CAM/TM typologies do acknowledge Indigenous medical contributions, it is plausible that other forms of CAM/TM that originally derive from women's health knowledge have been either lost or subsumed by male-dominated systems.

The growing acceptance of CAM/TM and women's strong presence as consumers and practitioners of CAM/TM raise important questions about the relationship between gender and CAM/TM, and provide an opportunity to revisit interpretations of gender roles and discourses of femininity. As we have seen, the use of CAM/TM therapies by women may be viewed as conforming to the traditional model of femininity as naturally nurturing, or as challenging the biomedical model whereby CAM/TM becomes a tool to achieve self-awareness and self-care. These discourses of health and well-being in relation to gender roles shed light on the complexities of the uses and attitudes of women—and society in general—toward CAM/TM practices.

Critical Thinking Questions

1. How does CAM/TM differ from conventional biomedicine (western medicine)?
2. How does TM differ from CAM?
3. What are the obstacles to creating a comprehensive typology of CAM/TM systems?
4. What part does gender expectations and roles play in determining how a society perceives CAM/TM and which therapies gain acceptance in that society?
5. Why do women make up the majority of CAM/TM consumers and practitioners?

Glossary

Allopathic medicine: Also called biomedicine, or conventional medicine, it is a medicinal system that uses pharmacologically active agents to treat diseases.

Empowerment: The process of giving a person or group of people power and status in a particular situation.

Gender roles: The pattern of masculine or feminine behaviour of an individual that is determined by a particular culture and that is largely determined by a child's upbringing.

Hegemonic masculinity: The culturally idealized form of manhood that is socially and hierarchically dominant. The concept was popularized in gender studies by the sociologist R.W. Connell.

References

Baarts, C., & Pedersen, I. (2009). Derivative benefits: Exploring the body through complementary and alternative medicine. *Sociology of Health and Illness, 31*(5), 719–733.

Berliner, H.S., & Salmon, J.W. (1979). The holistic movement and scientific medicine: The naked and the dead. *Socialist Review, 43*, 31–52.

Bishop, F., & Lewith, G. (2010). Who uses CAM? A narrative review of demographic characteristics and health factors associated with CAM use. *Evidence Based Complementary and Alternative Medicine, 7*(1), 11–28.

Boon, H., Stewart, M., & Kennard, M. (2000). Use of complementary/alternative medicine by breast cancer survivors in Ontario: Prevalence and perceptions. *Journal of Clinical Oncology, 18*(13), 2515–2521.

Buettner, C., Kroenke, C., Phillips, R., Davis, R., Eisenberg, D., & Holmes, M. (2006). Correlates of use of different types of complementary and alternative medicine by breast cancer survivors in the nurses' health study. *Breast Cancer Research and Treatment, 100*(2), 219–227.

Clarke, J.N. (2004). *Health, illness, and medicine in Canada*. Don Mills, ON: Oxford University Press.

Connell, R.W. (2002). *Gender*. Cambridge: Polity.

Conover, E. (2003). Herbal agents and over-the-counter medications in pregnancy. Best practice & research. *Clinical Endocrinology & Metabolism, 17*(2), 237–251.

Coulter, I., & Willis, E. (2007). Explaining the growth of complementary and alternative medicine. *Health Sociology Review, 16*(3), 214–225.

De Boer, H., & Lamxay, V. (2009). Plants used during pregnancy, childbirth and postpartum healthcare in Lao PDR: A comparative study of the Brou, Saek and Kry ethnic groups. *Journal of Ethnobiology and Ethnomedicine, 5*(25). doi:10.1186/1746-4269-5-25

Doel, M.A., & Segrott, J. (2003). Self, health, and gender: Complementary and alternative medicine in the British mass media. *Gender, Places and Culture, 10*(2), 131–144.

Flesch, H. (2007). Silent voices: Women, complementary medicine, and the co-option of change. *Complementary Therapies in Clinical Practice, 1*(3), 166–173.

Fulder, S. (1984). *The handbook of complementary medicine*. London: Hodder and Stoughton.

Fulder, S. (1996). *The handbook of alternative and complementary medicine* (3rd ed.). Oxford: Oxford University Press.

Furler, M., Einarson, T., Walmsley, S., Millson, M., & Bendayan, R. (2006). Longitudinal trends in antiretroviral use in a cohort of men and women in Ontario, Canada. *AIDS Patient Care STDS, 20*, 245–257.

Furlow, M., Patel, D., Sen, A., & Liu, J. (2008). Physician and patient attitudes towards complementary and alternative medicine in obstetrics and gynecology. *BMC Complementary and Alternative Medicine, 8*(35). doi: 10.1186/1472-6882-8-35

Gaffney, L., & Smith, C. (2004). The views of pregnant women towards the use of complementary therapies and medicines. *Birth Issues, 13*, 43–50.

Goldstein, M.S. (1999). *Alternative health care: Medicine, miracle or mirage?* Philadelphia: Temple University Press.

Gollschewski, S., Kitto, S., Anderson, D., & Lyons-Wall, P. (2008). Women's perceptions and beliefs about the use of complementary and alternative medicines during the menopause. *Complementary Therapies in Medicine, 1*(6), 163–168.

Headley, J., Northstone, K., Simmons, H., & Golding, J. (2004). Medication use during pregnancy: Data from the Avon Longitudinal Study of Parents and Children. *European Journal of Clinical Pharmacology, 60*(5), 355–361.

Helman, C.G. (1990). *Culture, health and illness: An introduction for health professionals*. London: Wright.

Hewitt-Taylor, J. (2004). Challenging the balance of power: Patient empowerment. *Nursing Standard, 18*, 33–37.

Hollenberg, D. (1999). *Understanding "plural" medicine: Alternative and biomedical therapy use among chronic illness sufferers—A Canadian study* (unpublished Master's dissertation). University of Manitoba.

Hollenberg, D. (2006). Uncharted ground: Patterns of professional interaction among complementary/alternative and biomedical practitioners in integrative healthcare settings. *Social Science and Medicine, 62*, 731–744.

Hollenberg, D. (2007). How do private CAM therapies affect integrative healthcare settings in a publically funded healthcare system? *Journal of Complementary and Integrative Medicine, 4*(1), Article 5.

Hollenberg, D., Zakus, D., Cook, T., & Xu, X. (2008). Re-positioning the role of traditional, complementary and alternative medicine as essential health knowledge in global health: Do they still have a role to play? *World Health and Population, 10*(4), 62–75.

Hollyer, T., Boon, H., Georgousis, A., Smith, M., & Einarson, A. (2002). The use of CAM by women suffering from nausea and vomiting during pregnancy. *BMC Complementary and Alternative Medicine, 2*(5). doi: 0.1186/1472-6882-2-5

Holst, L., Wringt, D., Nordeng, H., & Haavik, S. (2009). Use of herbal preparations during pregnancy: Focus groups discussions among expectant mothers attending a hospital antenatal clinic in Norwick, UK. *Complementary Therapies in Clinical Practice, 15*(4), 225–229.

Kelner, M., & Wellman, B. (Eds). (2000). *Complementary and alternative medicine: Challenge and change*. Amsterdam: Harwood Academics Publishers.

Kleinman, A. (1980). *Patients and healers in the context of culture*. Berkeley, CA: University of California Press.

Low Dog, T. (2009). The use of botanicals during pregnancy and lactation. *Alternative Therapies in Health and Medicine, 15*(1), 54–58.

Lunny, C., & Fraser, S., (2010). The use of complementary and alternative medicines among a sample of Canadian menopausal-aged women. *Journal of Midwifery & Women's Health, 55*(4), 335–343.

Ma, J., Drieling, R., & Stafford, R. (2006). US women desire greater professional guidance on hormone and alternative therapies for menopause symptom management. *Menopause, 13*, 506–516.

Maats, F., & Crowther, C. (2002). Patterns of vitamin, mineral and herbal supplement use prior to and during pregnancy. *Australian and New Zealand Journal of Obstetrics and Gynaecology, 42*(5), 494–496.

Mills, E., Dugoua, J., Perri, D., & Koren, G. (2006). *Herbal medicines in pregnancy and lactation: An evidence based approach*. London, New York: Taylor & Francis.

Mitchinson, W. (1991). *The nature of their bodies: Women and their doctors in Victorian Canada*. Toronto: University of Toronto Press.

Murray, R.H., & Rubel, A.J. (1992). Physicians and healers—unwitting partners in health care. *New England Journal of Medicine, 326*(1), 61.

Nissen, N. (2011). Challenging perspectives: Women, complementary and alternative medicine, and social change. *Interface, 3*(2), 187–212.

Nordeng, H., & Havnen, G. (2004). Use of herbal drugs in pregnancy: A survey among 400 Norwegian women. *Pharmacoepidemiology and Drug Safety, 18*(6), 454–461.

O'Connor, B.B., Calabrese, C., Cardeña, E., Eisenberg, D., Fincher, J., ... Zhang, X. (Panel on Definition and Description, CAM Research Methodology Conference, April 1995). (1997). Defining and describing complementary and alternative medicine. *Alternative Therapies 3*(2), 49–57.

O'Grady, H. (2005). *Woman's relationship with herself: Gender, Foucault and therapy.* London & New York: Routledge.

Ohlen, J., Balneaves, L., Bottorffc, J., & Brazierb, A. (2006). The influence of significant others in complementary and alternative medicine decisions by cancer patients. *Social Science and Medicine, 63*(6), 1625–1636.

Ong, C., Chan, L., Yung, P., & Leung, T. (2005). Use of traditional Chinese herbal medicine during pregnancy: A prospective survey. *Acta Obstetricia et Gynecologica Scandinavica, 8*(4), 699–700.

Pelicci, G. (2008). Growth and transformation among women healers. *ReVision, 30*(1&2), 46–52.

Pietroni, P. (1986). Alternative medicine. *Practitioner, 230*(1422), 1053–1054.

Pietroni, P. (1987). Holistic medicine: New lessons to be learned. *Practitioner, 231*(1437), 1386–1390.

Procino, A., & MacDougall, C. (2009). The integrated taxonomy of healthcare: Classifying both complementary and biomedical practices using a uniform classification protocol. *International Journal of Therapeutic Massage & Bodywork: Research, Education, & Practice, 2*(3). Retrieved November 19, 2016 from www.ijtmb.org/index.php/ijtmb/article/view/40

Refuerzo, J., Blackwell, S., & Sokol, R. (2005). Use of over-the-counter medications and herbal remedies in pregnancy. *American Journal of Perinatology, 22*(6), 321–324.

Ruggie, M. (2004). *Marginal to mainstream: Alternative medicine in America.* Cambridge: Cambridge University Press.

Ruzek, S.B., Clarke, A., & Olesen, V.L. (1997). Social, biomedical and feminist models of women's health. In S.B. Ruzek, V.L. Olesen & A. Clarke (Eds), *Women's health: Complexities and differences* (pp. 11–28). Columbus, OH: Ohio State University Press.

Smith, C., & Cochrane, S. (2009). Does acupuncture have a place as an adjunct treatment during pregnancy? A review of randomized controlled trials and systematic reviews. *Birth, 36*(3), 246–253.

Sointu, E. (2011). Detraditionalisation, gender, and alternative and complementary medicines. *Sociology of Health and Illness, 33*, 356–371.

Sointu, E., & Woodhead, L. (2008). Spirituality, gender, and expressive selfhood. *Journal for the Scientific Study of Religion, 47*, 259–276.

Stratton, T., & McGivern-Snofsky, J. (2008). Toward a sociological understanding of complementary and alternative medicines by a sample of Australian women during pregnancy. *Australian and New Zealand Journal of Obstetrics and Gynaecology, 48*(6), 384–390.

Thomas, K., & Coleman, P. (2004). Use of complementary or alternative medicine in a general population in Great Britain. *Journal of Public Health, 26*(2), 152–157.

Thompson, C. (2003). Natural health discourses and the therapeutic production of consumer resistance. *The Sociological Quarterly, 4*(4), 81–107.

Vincent, C., Furnham, A., & Richardson, P. (1998). *Complementary medicine: A research perspective.* New York: John Wiley & Sons.

Wang, S., Dezinno, P., & Fermo, L. (2005). Complementary and alternative medicine for low-back pain in pregnancy: A cross-sectional survey. *Journal of Alternative and Complementary Medicine, 11*(3), 459–464.

Wiebelitz, R., Weyert, G., Brach, J., & Beer, A. (2009). Use of complementary and alternative medicine in obstetrics. *British Journal of Midwifery, 17*(3), 169–175.

World Health Organization (WHO). (2013). *WHO traditional medicine strategy 2014–2023.* Geneva: author.

Zhang, Y., Leach, M., Hall, H., Sundberg, T., Ward, L., Sibbritt, D., & Adams, J. (2015). Differences between male and female consumers of complementary and alternative medicine in a national US population: A secondary analysis of 2012 NIHS data. *Evidence-based Complementary and Alternative Medicine, 2015* (article ID 413173). doi: 10.1155/2015/413173

CHAPTER 2

Women as Healers in the Global Community: An Overview from Antiquity to the Present

Daniel Hollenberg, PhD
Ontario Health Human Resources Research Network, University of Ottawa, Canada

Learning Objectives

1. To analyze the role of women in the context of health and healing, from ancient times to the present day.
2. To explore examples of women as healers and explain how female healers have contributed to health care provision.

Introduction

Women have always played a prominent role in healing. As medical sociologist Juanne Nancarrow Clarke states, "there have always been women healers in society ... on stone tablets, carved in relief on ancient walls, and told in legends of ancient Egypt, Sumeria, Greece and Rome" (2004, p. 306). Other feminist scholars, such as Gabrielle Pelicci, concur. She states:

> There is evidence of communities of priestesses and women's councils that existed for millennia in Old Europe and other places. Almost all archeological sites in Italy, the Balkans and Central Europe, contain figurines etched with sacred symbols representing the sacred feminine. These objects can also be found in Asia

> Minor, the Near East, and to a lesser extent in Western and Northern Europe. (Pelicci, 2008, p. 46)

It is important not to generalize or stereotype women's roles in society. Keeping this in mind, there is evidence showing that women have uniquely and consistently been involved in health and healing throughout the history of humanity. Dichotomies of specific gender roles have been a disservice to both men and women at many times throughout history, but feminist scholars agree that women—both historically and currently—have played and continue to play a crucial role in preserving and maintaining the well-being of the human species. This historical observation does not negate the contributions by men to various aspects of health and healing throughout the ages. The point to be emphasized here is that, despite significant historical and socio-political limitations to and restrictions on women as healers in human society, both women and men historically have been and are currently involved in the practice of medicine, with women in particular taking on unique and important roles.

Women as Healers throughout History

Although certainly not exhaustive, the below examples demonstrate some of the roles of women as healers that were recorded in pre-modern times. Other examples of women as healers are documented elsewhere, and it is fair to state that numerous other examples were not recorded due to the historical and cultural oppression of female healers that later occurred.

It is thought that a small number of practising female physicians may have existed in the societies of ancient Greece and Rome, but no medical treatises written by or about these women have survived. The knowledge of female healers was viewed by the Greeks as "recruited wisdom which could be assimilated by a male as easily as by a female" (Dean-Jones, 1994, p. 35). Although there is information which suggests that "information from wise-women was taken into consideration in scientific accounts of the female body"—such as the testimony of wise-women and the acquired knowledge of midwives—the majority of expertise presented in the formal Greek historical medical literature was male-dominated (Dean-Jones, 1994, pp. 29, 34–35). Despite the lack of women healers noted in the Greek historical record, clear accounts of women as healers were noted in other, less formal historical references found in antiquity.

The earliest evidence for female healers in the western world comes from medieval Europe. As Pelicci (2008) notes, "women practiced midwifery and herbology during the eleventh, twelfth and thirteenth centuries ... the early part of the Middle Ages were times of excitement and diversity for women healers ..." (p. 46). Mumford (1983) also notes that women from powerful families in many European countries in this period often ran convents at which they were the main "infirmarian," functioning as physician, pharmacist, and health teacher. Medicinal herbs were grown and cared for in the convent gardens and the nuns provided nursing services.

Mumford (1983) describes a famous 11th-century medical school in Salerno, Italy, that accepted both men and women as medical students and teachers. During this time, one of the best-known medical teachers in the 11th century was a woman named Trotula, who not only taught medicine generally but also wrote an important gynecological-obstetrical treatise that became a major reference work for centuries to come. Shortly thereafter, between 1150 and 1160, the German abbess Hildegard of Bingen wrote the medical treatises *Physica* ("Medicine") and *Causae et Curae* ("Causes and Cures"), in which she discussed Galenic humoral theory, diagnosis, and treatment (Harper, 2011). Some centuries later in 1502, Ludwig V, the Count Palatine, compiled in Heidelberg a 12-volume book of medicine that included more than 1300 medicinal recipes attributed to female physicians (Harper, 2011). In 14th-century Italy, Roman women from important families were able to remain unmarried and work as doctors or professors. This social option was also available in other Italian medical schools, and also in the Muslim world such as in Cairo, Bagdad, Cordoba, Toledo, and Constantinople (Mumford, 1983). Female physicians from the Jewish faith were widely accepted in Italy and France, where, in the 1320s, one woman was recorded to have run a large medical school in Montpellier, France. Female physicians were also common in Germany and the Netherlands during the 14th century.

Throughout history, birthing assistance has almost everywhere been the responsibility of women, which can be viewed as an essential healing activity (Clarke, 2004). Women were involved with the process of birthing either as physicians or midwives, or both. The term **midwife** derives from old English and literally means "with the women;" the French equivalent is sage-femme, literally "wise-woman" (Clarke, 2004). Midwives in particular assisted women as they prepared for and gave birth, and as they learned to care for their new offspring. As Clarke notes, the practice of **midwifery** can be traced to antiquity (Clarke, 2004). Clarke observes that the Bible includes a number of references to midwives: for example, Exodus I:15–22 names two midwives, Shiprah and Puah, who refused to obey the order of the King of Egypt for all male infants to be put to death. Midwives, although formally excluded in ancient Greece, were also routinely mentioned in the medical texts of classical Greek and Roman physicians such as Hippocrates and Galen (Clarke, 2004). Until the Middle Ages, women who had given birth themselves were deemed acceptable attendants at other births, and this informal type of midwifery flourished in Europe until the 14th century (Clarke, 2004).

Yet, as Harper powerfully points out, studies such as that of Green (1989) clearly show that "the majority of female practitioners were not midwives. In fact, over two thirds of women medical practitioners were listed as barbers, surgeons, physicians, leeches, apothecaries …" (Harper, 2011, p. 109). Other scholars, such as Demos (2000), also concur. Describing Stoudt's 1997 study of female healers in medieval Germany, Harper states:

> The twelfth-century German legal records she examined reveal many women practicing medicine, most of whom practiced surgery, and specifically battlefield surgery. In her study are examples of a female practitioner in Frankfurt who healed mercenaries of their extensive battle wounds, and that of two other women who were locally famous for their surgical skills and wound draughts used in treating wounded soldiers. [...] One of the first literary references to female physicians in western Europe comes from Tacitus (c. 56–117 CE) who remarked that German women treated the wounds of men and "did not shrink away from counting and comparing the gashes." Whilst caring for illnesses and injury among family and friends was a customary duty of women in many cultures, Tacitus' special mention of this group of women who accompanied the soldiers and possessed specialized skills for healing battle-related wounds implies that some of those women may have been acting as professional healers. (Harper, 2001, p. 109)

Recognizing diversity within feminist scholarship, Clarke points out that some feminist scholars have re-examined women's historical contributions to health care and found that women have always been carers and healers (Clarke, 2004). Although men have clearly also been involved in healing activities throughout the ages, women have consistently been primarily carers for family members in times of sickness and have been an important source of information about health and healing remedies. Clarke (2004) argues that "the role of women as invisible healers, negotiators and mediators has long been overlooked" (p. 311). Although there is variation in women's specific activities, women are consistently involved in preparing food with adequate nutrients; sourcing seasonally appropriate garments for their families; providing soap, water, and other hygiene accessories; and teaching other family members about the ways and means of maintaining/promoting health and preventing illness (Clarke, 2004). As Clarke states, women "usually decide when medical intervention is required, make relevant appointments, and make sure family members are able to keep the appointments" (p. 312). Clarke (2004) argues that women's "health work" takes place when all family members are healthy as well as when they are not healthy. Moreover, in many industrialized countries, due to the combination of patients having shorter hospital stays and recent epidemiological trends favouring chronic rather than acute diseases, health care activities in the home environment are becoming more demanding for caregivers, of whom "the vast majority are women" (Clarke, 2004, p. 313).

With regard to health, healing, and caring activities related to labour, childbirth, and early infancy, it has now been widely documented that female midwives and **traditional birth attendants (TBAs)** deliver approximately 80 percent of babies worldwide (Helman, 1990). This wide-scale establishment of TBAs and midwives has occurred in spite of male domination of the reproductive health field since the 19th and 20th centuries, and recent professional struggles faced by professional midwives with regard to their professionalization and autonomy-seeking for self-regulation and professional control (Biggs, 1983; Bourgeault, Angus & Fynes, 1988; Clarke, 2004). Contemporary research has also demonstrated that births attended by female midwives/TBAs result in statistically significantly fewer episiotomies, less frequent use of anesthesia, lower health care and hospital costs, and more frequent breast feeding.

As the medical anthropologist Helman states, "most births world-wide—especially in rural areas of the developing world—are delivered in a very different way, usually by female [traditional] birth attendants, such as the *parteras* of Mexico, the *comadronas* of Puerto Rico, or the *nanas* of Jamaica" (1990, p. 151). TBAs have been documented assisting with labour, childbirth, and early infancy in almost every village and urban neighbourhood throughout Africa, Asia, and Latin America (Helman, 1990). The direct involvement of women in health care activities, in this case TBAs, has been so prevalent that when the World Health Organization (WHO) was first developing its traditional/Indigenous health policies in the late 1970s, WHO began to develop clear policy for the training of TBAs who at that time were noted to deliver approximately two thirds of the world's babies (WHO, 1978). As Helman notes, TBAs have also been recognized by governments in such countries as Ghana, Indonesia, Malaysia, Pakistan, the Philippines, Sudan, and Thailand where considerable numbers of TBAs have been trained and drawn upon for basic health services during the past 30 years (Helman, 1990).

Historical Challenges to Women as Healers

Despite the long association of women with caring and healing roles, deliberate socio-political efforts were made to restrict or forbid women practising any type of healing—including midwifery—starting in the Middle Ages. Theoretically, these efforts were generally rooted in a misogynistic worldview (see box 2.1).

Box 2.1 The Female Body in Ancient Greek Medical Theory

Foreshadowing 19th- and 20th-century medicine, the Greek philosopher Aristotle viewed reproduction as the sole purpose of a woman's womb; if a woman could not conceive, her body was considered "wasted" (Dean-Jones, 1994, p. 65) and it was believed that her uterus would rebel and attack other parts of her body (Findlay & Miller, 1994, p. 133). Furthermore, "empirical" observation of menstruation became the basis of "a biological construct which upheld the cultural characterization of a woman as inherently weaker, softer, and less stable than a man" (Dean-Jones, 1994, pp. 57–58).

Although a selection of medical treatises in the Hippocratic *corpus* (dating from the fifth to fourth centuries BCE) are relatively neutral in their descriptions of female patients and ailments, male writers such as Aristotle express clearly misogynistic views about the female body (Dean-Jones, 1994, p. 37). In terms of anatomy, the female body was viewed as a slightly modified—or defective—version of the male body. The ancient Greeks did not dissect human bodies and therefore only had a "vague understanding of the internal reproductive organs" (Dean-Jones, 1994, p. 43). Furthermore, to the extent that the male body was considered to be the prime specimen of human anatomy, a full analysis of the female body was not deemed necessary (Dean-Jones, 1994, p. 85). The ancient Greek understanding of female reproductive anatomy was more or less limited to the notion that "women have the same genitals of men, except that theirs are inside the body and not outside it" (Martin, 1987, p. 27).

Pelicci summarizes the situation in the Middle Ages in the following way:

> [T]he fourteenth through eighteenth centuries saw an orchestrated and thorough campaign to stamp out the woman healer. During this time of calamity, crime, crop failures and illness, women and witchcraft were blamed for the disasters of the earth. The newly established medical professionals and the Church tried to establish a monopoly on the healing professions, claiming that women healers were "idiots who gathered herbs and practiced religious nonsense." As a result of this unfortunate turn of events, women were forbidden to practice medicine. They were systematically tortured and burned by the hundreds and thousands for practicing healing arts. One medieval scholar estimates that more than one

> million women and healers were executed for the crime of helping other women. (2008, p. 46)

Harper (2011) also describes how, in medieval France, female healers were seen as a threat to "the universities and the growing professionalism of the male medical practitioners" as well as a reminder of the "long-standing connections between women, healing, and religion in pagan societies" (p. 11). In England, in the 15th century, Oxford and Cambridge Universities sent a petition to Parliament outlining the dangers of allowing "ignorant and unskilled persons" to practice medicine and surgery (Clarke, 2004, p. 306), in which women in particular were singled out to be excluded from the practice of medicine. In 1512, Henry VIII's Medical Act prohibited "undesirable and uneducated persons from doing medical work" (Clarke, 2004, p. 306); again, women were classified as one of the "categories of undesirables" and were accused of causing grievous harm in the name of "healing" (Clarke, 2004, p. 306). As Clarke and many feminist historians and social scientists have noted, these types of specific historical and socio-political movements directly excluded women from formal participation in health and healing as either physicians or midwives. In Harper's words:

> The rise of the universities and subsequent licensing of physicians excluded women, who were barred from study at the universities and thus from legally practicing within the field as medicine changed from a skill to a profession. [...] The terminology of these restrictions grouped all female healers together with "old wives, monks, rustics, herbalists and students not yet trained ... or coming from foreign parts ... ignorant of the science of medicine." [...] Although the emphasis seems to be on separating those practitioners who heal from those who could harm, the real effect of these regulations in excluding women is apparent in the trials of female physicians. (Harper, 2011, pp. 118–119)

Most notably, the Catholic Church of this time (15th century AD) drew on an official Catholic text written by the German monks Kramer and Sprenger, titled Malleus Maleficarem ("The Hammer of Witches"), to declare that women in particular were likely to be witches because they were especially vulnerable to consorting with the devil in a sexual way (Clarke, 2004) (see Ehrenreich & English, 1973b, for an early but classic in-depth historical discussion of this process, and also Demos, 2000). As Clarke (2004) states, "many of the people who were named witches, persecuted, and put to death were female healers and midwives, especially those from a peasant population" (p. 307). Additionally, caring and healing activities, which were often practised by women of this time, were thought to be evidence of witchcraft because they demonstrated a "lack of faith" (Clarke, 2004, p. 307). The subsequent European witch hunts, which lasted from 1479 to 1735, led to the deaths of approximately 300,000 people, most of whom were women (Clarke, 2004; Pelicci, 2008). Midwives were particularly targeted for prosecution as witches because they had access to purported "prized witchcraft material" such as placentas and the umbilical cords of newborn babies (Clarke, 2004, p. 307). Although it was during these centuries that British midwives gained formal recognition and legitimacy under the British Medical Act of 1512, they and their European counterparts were supervised by local churches that directly restricted any cultural practices that were believed to be associated with witchcraft. Meanwhile, the professionalization of midwifery in Britain was revoked in 1642, when the British College of Physicians gained authority to directly license midwives and, as Clarke states, "for the next 300 years the legitimacy, recognition, and power of the male midwives, now obstetricians, grew in England and Europe while those of female midwives declined" (Clarke, 2004, p. 341). In effect, male midwives took possession of the field of midwifery and established state legitimacy and recognition as a professional and autonomous group. As Ehrenreich and English (2010) argue, not only did thousands of women healers perish during this time, but an invaluable medical knowledge base was lost, leaving communities deprived of their healers—all at the same time as the purported Renaissance in Europe and the beginnings of the Scientific Revolution.

By the 1800s, the professionalization of male midwives in Britain and Canada, for example, had laid claim to a general practice that had largely replaced female midwives' management of health issues surrounding pregnancy, childbirth, and the treatment of diseases in women. This was partly achieved through attacking female midwives as "incompetent," blaming them for infant and maternal death, and labelling their child-rearing procedures as "outmoded" and "female rituals," even though the female midwife was often better trained (Moscucci, 1990, pp. 12, 66). The de-legitimization of female midwives was also linked to the notion of "female frailty" (Ehrenreich & English, 1973a, p. 23). Furthermore, male dominance in midwifery was achieved through the claim for "enlightened" procedures under the "watchful eye of the medical man," and the claim for the superiority of men and their abilities (Ehrenreich and English, 2010). Moreover, adding to this criticism were new political and economic agendas focused on establishing productive labour and a stable political order and population through women, while male medical practitioners were recognized as a means of control (Findlay & Miller, 1994, p. 116; Moscucci, 1990, p. 12). Yet some consistently argue that in the 19th century, "male physicians were both more dangerous and less effective than female lay healers" (Ehrenreich & English, 2010, p.16).

The development of male midwifery further combined the metaphor of machine with the use of actual mechanical devices such as forceps and the speculum. These devices replaced the female midwives' hands with male hands using tools, and became unique to the practice of male midwifery as a method of female domination where the medicalization of normal female health became commonplace (Martin, 1987, p. 54; Merchant, 1980; Moscucci, 1990, p. 112; Theriot, 1993, p. 6). An interesting irony was that while male midwives dominated midwifery and laid claim to their "obvious" expertise, they were largely ridiculed by male physicians for involving themselves in "unmanly women's work" of a "boring" and "degrading" nature (Moscucci, 1990, pp. 52, 56).

In the 19th and early 20th centuries, gynecology became the study of the "whole woman," fusing the physical, psychological, and moral aspects of femininity while collapsing the distinction between gender and sex (Moscucci, 1990, p. 103; Theriot, 1993, p. 6). The prevailing view, as stated by 19th-century gynecologist Robert Banes, was that "any disease occurring in a woman will almost certainly involve some modifications in the work of her sexual system ... on the other hand the ordinary or disturbed work of her sexual system will influence the course of any disease which may assail her" (Moscucci, 1990, p. 103, emphasis added). Thus, not only were women's reproductive organs inextricably connected to any and all disease, but disease itself—mental and physical—could be attributed to her body. This view was partly attributable to the claims by gynecologists that women's diseases were inseparable from the study of female physiology and pathology, and that sexual organs constantly interacted with the rest of the organism (Moscucci, 1990, pp. 103–104).

Notwithstanding the important role of women as healers throughout the ages, significant historical and socio-political movements such as those noted above have directly shaped and limited women's involvement in health and healing, up to the present day. Only in 1849 did Elizabeth Blackwell become the first female to graduate from an American medical school (Clarke, 2004). In Canada, women's medical colleges were affiliated with recognized universities such as Queen's University and the University of Toronto in 1883, in order to provide medical instruction to women; but women were not allowed to take examinations at a medical school of their choice until 1895 (Roland, 1988).

Although some historians attempt to downplay the deleterious effects of medical dominance as enacted by the profession of medicine on women healers and midwives (e.g., see Connor, 1994), others (see Dodd & Gorham, 1994) strongly disagree. Male physicians in the 19th century dominated female health, and in effect eliminated midwifery through various processes including professional closure tactics (e.g., scientific education) and dominance over obstetrical technologies (Dodd & Gorham,

1994). In Canada, although documents show that Montreal and Lunenburg, Nova Scotia, already had practising midwives in the first half of the 18th century (Oppenheiner, 1983), midwifery as a practice was still in the minority. From 1795–1895, in North America, the legal position of midwives was uncertain and changeable due to political restrictions from professionalizing male physicians who continued to dominate birthing and female reproductive health care generally (Barrington, 1985; Biggs, 1983; Connor, 1994; Ehrenreich & English, 1973b; Wertz & Wertz, 1977). In Britain, it took until 1893 for the British Nursing Association to garner enough political support for the creation of a new occupational category of "obstetric midwives or nurses" (Clarke, 2004, p. 342). Although British midwives were legitimized through regulation in the early part of the 20th century, they were not formally employed as a type of public health nurse until the National Health Service was formed in 1948 (Clarke, 2004). By the 1900s in Ontario, Canada, however, female midwives were virtually non-existent (Biggs, 1983). Even today in Canada and in many other countries, midwifery still struggles to maintain legitimacy, despite midwives having obtained formal legislation in most Canadian provinces and territories that assures their right to deliver services as qualified health care practitioners.

It is important to note today, both how and why midwifery is connected to historical developments and also CAM in particular. As noted earlier in this chapter, the practice of midwifery is identified as one of the earliest healing activities by women, alongside other healing activities practised by women such as herbology and wound care. In the 19th century, however, the surviving female-led midwifery was formally assumed by male physicians, and the female-led practice was appropriated and eliminated, similar to other non-**allopathic** (i.e., CAM) practices of the time (e.g., eclecticism; homeopathy). As midwifery today (e.g., in Canada) has re-professionalized and sought autonomy under state legislation and state-sanctioned self-regulation, midwifery has consistently had to "fight" the historical stigma of being a seemingly non-allopathic healing practice. This occurrence is ironic, considering that not only did midwifery shape such modern biomedical specialist fields as obstetrics and gynecology, but the field of midwifery itself is arguably one of the most biomedical CAM fields (as compared to acupuncture, for example). The above observation continues to affirm the pervasiveness of the patriarchal oppression of women healers.

Conclusion

Various historical, social, and political processes have dramatically restricted the capacities for women to act as healers in society, despite their centuries-long formal involvement in health and healing. Most notably, women's healing activities have been restricted due to the historical and contemporary effects of sexism, **patriarchy**, and state preference for the exclusive professionalization and power of biomedical forms of medicine, health, and healing as led by men in particular (see Clarke 2004; Coburn, 1998; Coburn, Rappolt & Bourgeault, 1997; Coburn, Torrance & Kaufert, 1983; Navarro, 1976). This is not to say, however, that women throughout the world have not resisted these obstacles and sought to (re-)establish themselves as important and significant healers within their respective communities. The recognition of women as healers also cannot ignore a historical record that clearly documents that women's health and bodies have been viewed negatively for more than two millennia (see box 2.1). These early misogynistic perceptions of women's health have directly influenced health care professionals' education and the clinical treatment of women up to the present day (for an extensive treatise on this topic, see Martin's 1987 book *The woman in the body*). It is clear that the establishment of women as healers has been a historical struggle that continues to this day.

Critical Thinking Questions

1. What roles have women historically played as healers?
2. What roles do women currently play as healers?
3. Why are female healers important?
4. What historical and socio-political factors caused the oppression of women as healers, and how have female healers resisted these forces?

Glossary

Allopathic: A historical term referring to what is now called "biomedicine" (western medicine), literally meaning "to treat with that which is different or opposite to the disease."

Midwife: A healing category that was historically the domain of women, focused on women's reproductive health, labour, birthing, delivery, and all aspects related to pre- and post-partum care of newborn and mother. The term "midwife" derives from old English and literally means "with the women."

Midwifery: The professional term referring to the practice of a midwife. The term likely originated in Europe in the 17th century.

Patriarchy: The dominance of men and/or male values.

Traditional birth attendant (TBA): A term used usually in non-western countries to refer to a healing category also historically practiced by women, focused on the same practices as those of a midwife. One distinction that has been noted between TBAs and midwives is that both may be in attendance at a birth, practising mutually related roles. Midwives sometimes have a greater scope of practice than TBAs depending on country and jurisdiction.

References

Barrington, E. (1985). *Midwifery is catching*. Toronto: NC Press.

Biggs, D.L. (1983). The case of the missing midwives: A history of midwifery in Ontario from 1795–1900. *Ontario History*, *75*, 21–35.

Bourgeault, I.L., Angus, J., & Fynes, M. (1998). *Gender, medicine, dominance and the state: Nurse practitioners and midwives in Ontario*. Paper presented at 14th World Congress of Sociology (July 1998), Montreal.

Clarke, J.N. (2004). *Health, illness, and medicine in Canada.* Oxford: Oxford University Press.

Coburn, D. (1998). State, authority, medical dominance, and trends in the regulation of the health professions: The Ontario case. In D. Coburn, C. D'Arcy & G. Torrance (Eds), *Health and Canadian society: Sociological perspectives* (pp. 332–346). Toronto: University of Toronto Press.

Coburn, D., Rappolt, S., & Bourgeault, I.L. (1997). Decline vs. retention of medical power through ratification: An examination of the Ontario case. *Sociology of Health and Illness, 19*(1), 1–22.

Coburn D., Torrance, G.M., & Kaufert, J.M. (1983). Medical dominance in Canada in historical perspective: The rise and fall of medicine. *International Journal of Health Services, 13*(3), 407–432.

Connor, J.T.H. (1994). Larger fish to catch here than midwives: Midwifery and the medical profession in nineteenth-century Ontario. In D. Dodd & D. Gorham (Eds), *Caring and curing: Historical perspectives on women and healing in Canada* (pp. 103–134). Ottawa: University of Ottawa Press.

Dean-Jones, L. (1994). *Women's bodies in classical Greek science.* Oxford: Clarendon Press.

Demos, J. (2000). *The enemy within: 2000 years of witch-hunting in the western world.* New York: Viking.

Dodd, D., & Gorham, D. (1994). Introduction. In D. Dodd & D. Gorham (Eds), *Caring and curing: Historical perspectives on women and healing in Canada* (pp. 1–15). Ottawa: University of Ottawa Press.

Ehrenreich, B., & English, D. (1973a). *Complaints and disorders: The sexual politics of sickness.* San Francisco: Harper & Row.

Ehrenreich, B., & English, D. (1973b). *Witches, midwives, and nurses: A history of women healers.* Old Westbury, New York: The Feminist Press.

Ehrenreich, B., & English, D. (2010). *Witches, midwives & nurses: A history of women healers* (2nd ed.). New York: The Feminist Press.

Findlay, D.A., & Miller, L.J. (1994). Medical power and women's bodies. In B. Singh & R. Bolaria (Eds), *Women, medicine, and health* (pp. 115–139). Halifax: Fernwood.

Green, M. (1989). Women's medical practices and health care in Medieval Europe. *Signs, 14*, 434–473.

Harper, A. (2011). The image of the female healer in western vernacular literature of the Middle Ages. *Social History of Medicine, 24*(1), 108–124.

Helman, C.G. (1990). *Culture, health and illness: An introduction for health professionals.* London: Wright.

Martin, E. (1987). *The woman in the body: A cultural analysis of reproduction.* Boston: Beacon Press.

Merchant, D. (1980). *The death of nature: Women, ecology, and the scientific revolution.* San Francisco: Harper & Row.

Moscucci, O. (1990). *The science of women: Gynaecology and gender in England, 1800–1929.* Cambridge: Cambridge University Press.

Mumford, E. (1983). *Medical sociology: Patients, providers, and policies.* New York: Random House.

Navarro, V. (1976). Social class, political power, and the state: Their implications in medicine. *Social Science & Medicine, 10*, 437–457.

Oppenheimer, J. (1983). Childbirth in Ontario: The transition from home to hospital in the early twentieth century. *Ontario History, 75* (March), 36–60.

Pelicci, G. (2008). Growth and transformation among women healers. *ReVision, 30*(1&2), 46–52.

Roland, C. (1988). Medicine, History of. In *The Canadian Encyclopedia* (2nd ed., p. 1330). Edmonton: Hurtig.

Stoudt, D. (1997). Medieval German women and the power of healing. In L. Furst (Ed), *Women healers and physicians* (pp. 13–42). Lexington, Kentucky: University Press of Kentucky.

Theriot, N.M. (1993). Women's voices in nineteenth-century medical discourse: A step toward deconstructing science. *Signs, 19*(1), 1–31.

Wertz, R.W., & Wertz, D.C. (1977). *Lying-in: A history of childbirth in America.* New York: The Free Press.

World Health Organization (WHO). (1978). *The promotion and development of traditional medicine.* Technical Report Series 622. Geneva: Author.

CHAPTER 3

Herbal Fertility Treatments in Colonial North America and Prospects for Modern Medicine

Cheryl Lans, PhD
Institute for Ethnobotany & Zoopharmacognosy, the Netherlands

Rachel Westfall, PhD
Yukon Bureau of Statistics, Canada

Learning Objectives

1. To learn about the botanical treatments used in colonial North America for all stages of reproduction, from pre-conception to birth, and their potential use for infertility treatments.
2. To learn about the historical relevance of these treatments.
3. To become more familiar with ethnomedicinal methodology through examining the ethnobotanical, phytochemical, and pharmacological data of selected plants.

Introduction

Herbal medicine historically has played a much greater role in supporting North American women's reproductive health than it does in contemporary times. With the rise of modern pharmacology and the consolidation of power and authority by the medical profession in the past century, herbalism has fallen out of favour.

Nonetheless, some traditional herbal medicines are still used as an alternative or complement to mainstream medicine.

In colonial North America (1492–1899), many plants were used to support fertility from pre-conception to birth. Early Americans merged Indigenous medicinal plants into a pharmacopoeia based on common European herbal remedies. This makes colonial North America a source of useful knowledge in terms of botanical uses of medicinal plants for reproductive health. This chapter reviews the botanical medicines used for fertility and sub-fertility from the early colonial period through to the 19th century. It provides an understanding of the therapeutic role and the potential uses of medicinal plants for reproductive health by analyzing the historical uses of these plants. This analysis shows the potential value of these plants, in a way that can facilitate their incorporation into an integrated approach of biomedicine and complementary and alternative medicine (CAM). Traditional uses of herbal medicine may have an important role for the treatments of infertility today, as medicinal plants can lower the cost and increase the success rate of **assisted reproductive technology (ART)** (Ried & Stuart, 2011). However, testing of plant therapies in controlled trials is rare and most fertility specialists do not know or ask what plants their patients are using (Shannon et al., 2010; Zeyneloglu & Onalan, 2014).

Allopathic drugs used in colonial North America were unregulated, and included dangerous substances like mercury, alcohol, cocaine, opium, and animal waste (Cox, 2004). Allopathic medicine was expensive and only used by colonialists when traditional medicine failed (Frader 1982; Ray 2009), and medicinal practices entailed harmful procedures (e.g., bleeding, purging, enemas, etc.). The problem of substandard medicines continued long after the colonial period as can be seen in the memoirs of author Dr. Oliver Wendell Holmes, dean (1847–1853) and later professor at the Harvard Medical School. As he observed, "I firmly believe that if the whole materia medica, as now used, could be sunk to the bottom of the sea, it would be all the better for mankind—and all the worse for the fishes" (as quoted in Neuhauser, 2006).

Methodology

In our research, we searched medical texts and papers from 1600–1899 using relevant keywords such as herb, healer, midwife, fertility, pregnancy, and miscarriage. Both physical and online texts in the libraries of the University of Victoria and the University of British Columbia, Canada, were selected. Online texts available from the libraries of major US universities and those in the public domain were also searched. An ethnomedicinal validation technique was used to identify traditional medicines with contemporary value. Validation included examination of the published phytochemical and pharmacological data to see whether the reported folk use of plants is safe and effective (Lans, Brown, Borde & Offiah, 2003).

Women's Gynecological Practices in Colonial Times

Women in colonial North America relied on midwives, neighbours, and homemade botanical remedies to enhance their fertility (England, 1922). The books consulted by these traditional practitioners to find appropriate treatments to treat women's reproductive problems included Buchan's *Domestic Medicine* (1769), Culpeper's *The English Physitian* (1652) and *The Complete Herbal* (1653), as well as Bartram's medicinal botanical guides, which included Indigenous remedies for women's reproductive health, published in Franklin's *Poor Richard's Almanack* and in Short's *Medicina Britannica* (Bartram, 1789/1909; Ray, 2009; Short & Bartram, 1751).

In colonial North America, curing people was open to anyone who could demonstrate a "gift for healing." Eclectic medical schools (see box 3.1) trained women and men, while Harvard and other established schools only trained men (Ehrenreich & English, 1973). Eclectic medicine incorporated plant-based remedies used by Indigenous Americans and other practices that were believed to benefit patients (Newton et al., 1856).

Box 3.1: Eclectic Medicine

Eclectic medicine was a branch of American medicine that made use of botanical remedies along with other substances and physical therapy practices. It was popular in the latter half of the 19th century. Eclectic medicine came under pressure from the American Medical Association for not following the standard curriculum, and ultimately lost students with the advent of penicillin and other new drugs.

When the number of European-trained doctors increased, conflicts arose between herbalists, midwives, doctors, and religious ministers in colonial North America due to their differing therapeutic knowledge and backgrounds. This culminated in the Massachusetts witchcraft trials of Boston midwife Anne Hutchinson and healers Ann Burt of Lynn, Elizabeth Morse of Newbury, Katherine Harrison of Wethersfield, and Margaret Jones of Charlestown (Augur, 1930; Meyer, 1973). The American Medical Association (AMA) was established in 1848, and county- and state-based associations of doctors re-established themselves and joined AMA. The few trained female doctors joined their male colleagues in limiting the ability of lay practitioners to practise medicine (Ehrenreich & English, 1973). In 1893, German-trained doctors established the Johns Hopkins medical school, which required too many years of expensive training to be accessible to poor students. New medical schools used the Johns Hopkins model and attracted funding from local philanthropists. The medical profession then established professional authority over midwifery and other branches of medicine by encouraging 13 states to pass medical licensing laws that outlawed "irregular" practice, restricted the entrance of women into medical schools, forbade midwifery, and established middle class and wealthy men as the only legal healers.

Colonial Botanical Remedies Used for Women's Fertility

Although herbal medicine came to be viewed as "unconventional" in North American medical practice, it has remained popular as an alternative and complement to modern pharmaceuticals. Many of the botanical medicines that were popular in the early colonial period remain in use today (Belew, 1999; van de Walle, 1997).

Some key botanical medicines used by colonial practitioners for women's fertility are discussed below. These plants are divided into the following categories:

1. Emmenagogues, contraceptives, and abortifacients
2. Maternity care, including miscarriage prevention and labour-induction herbs
3. Fertility enhancement

Emmenagogues, Contraceptives, and Abortifacients

Emmenagogues are used to stimulate menstruation; in some cases, they may be used to stimulate an abortion. The botanist Alfred Hall (c. 1843) recommended teas of tansy (*Tanacetum parthenium*), rue (*Ruta graveolens*), savin (*Juniperus sabina*), and pennyroyal (*Mentha pulegium*) for suppressed menses, and his contraceptive tincture was composed of crushed bloodroot (*Sanguinaria canadensis*) in a gin base (Brodie, 2001; Riddle, 1999).

New England physicians George Capron and David Slack recommended 14 different herbal teas for delayed menses (**amenorrhea** due to stress, poor nutrition, overwork, or early pregnancy) in their 1849 publication. An Ohio doctor wrote in *The American Druggists' Circular and Chemical Gazette* of 1859 that women should take a teaspoon of the tincture of bloodroot (*Sanguinaria canadensis*) thrice daily after ovulation to regulate menstruation (Klepp, 2001).

Dr. William Shippen, one of the first American doctors to supplant midwives (after women were restricted from medical school entrance and midwifery was forbidden), treated a case of obstructed menses with Razi's *trochisci e myrrha* (a formula containing rue [*Ruta graveolens*], dittany [*Cunila origanoides*] leaves, myrrh [*Commiphora abyssinica*], asafoetida [*Ferula assa-foetida*], sagapenum [*Ferula* spp.], castor [*Ricinus communis*], and opopanax [*Opopanax chironium*]) (Corner, 1951; Scholten, 1977). Razi (Abū Bakr Muhammad ibn Zakariyyā al-Rāzī) lived from 854–925 CE; Shippen did not use a "modern medicine" that midwives did not know about. Rue, dittany, myrrh, and asafoetida were all identified as emmenagogues in *Kings American Dispensatory* (Felter & Lloyd, 1898/1992).

The use of bloodroot (*Sanguinaria canadensis*) was also widespread among Indigenous Americans (Chippaways, Shawnees, and Osages), who used a strong decoction of bloodroot with ground ivy (probably *Glechoma hederacea*, introduced to North America before 1672) to abort before long journeys (Francis, 1822). Francis (1822) did not give the Latin name of the plant he refers to as ground ivy that was being used by Indigenous Americans.

Juniper berries (*Juniperus communis*) were used by eclectic physicians to treat gonorrhea and **leucorrhea**, while oil of savin (*Juniperus sabina*) was used to treat suppressed menses (Felter & Lloyd, 1898/1992). New York-born doctor Joel Shew warned against the use of oil of savin for amenorrhea in his 1853 midwifery book, since savin and pennyroyal (*Mentha pulegium*) were commonly used abortifacients (Brodie, 2001). Many herb usages transferred from Indigenous Americans were given the common name "squaw." These included squaw bush (*Viburnum opulus*) and squaw mint (*Hedeoma pulegioides),* also called American pennyroyal (Klepp, 2001). Both were used to regulate the menstrual cycle and procure abortions.

Viburnum opulus and *Viburnum prunifolium* were also used to prevent miscarriages that reoccurred at the same stage of development of the fetus (Marsden, 1879). A Dr. E. Nelson reported to his colleagues at a meeting that *Viburnum opulus* had prevented miscarriage in several of his patients and was tolerated better than *Viburnum prunifolium* (Anonymous, 1888). A Dr. Hulbert reported that *Viburnum opulus* was used for **dysmenorrhea** and he also used *Viburnum prunifolium* and *Discorea villosa* to treat dysmenorrhea (Anonymous, 1888). He also reported that in 1886 (two years before his talk) there had been an extensive discussion that promoted the use of *Viburnum prunifolium* for threatened abortion (Anonymous, 1888).

Cook's *Physiomedical Dispensatory* (1869) lists American pennyroyal (*Hedeoma pulegioides*) in combination with blue cohosh (*Caulophyllum thalictroides*) for painful menstruation, diminished **lochia**, and prolonged labour. Squaw root was the common name of both *Cimicifuga racemosa* (also called black cohosh, used by colonial women and eclectic physicians to relieve sickness and heartburn in pregnancy, various menstrual disorders, and tendency to miscarriage) and *Caulophyllum thalictroides* (which was used to provoke menstruation, to relieve period pain, and to speed delivery) (Felter & Lloyd, 1898/1992). Dr. Lawrence Bohun, a 17th-century Virginia physician, and Philadelphia pharmacist Elias Durand experimented with local plants like *Cimicifuga racemosa* as a treatment for amenorrhea (England, 1922; Gill, 1972). *Cimicifuga* was listed in *King's American Dispensatory* for toning the reproductive tract, restoring suppressed menses, and treating dysmenorrhea (Felter & Lloyd, 1898/1992). *Caulophyllum thalictroides* was used as an emmenagogue; a treatment for uterine leucorrhea, amenorrhea, and dysmenorrhea; and an aid to induce labour in combination with *Mitchella repens* (partridge berry or squaw vine) (Felter & Lloyd, 1898/1992).

Squaw vine (*Mitchella repens*) and squaw weed (*Erigeron philadelphicus*) were used for menstrual pain by the Navajo (Meyer, 1973) and early settlers (Klepp, 2001). A commercial tablet called ponca contained *Mitchella repens*, caulophyllin, and viburnin. Ponca was prescribed for uterine disorders, threatened abortion, and miscarriage. Another uterine tonic called Helonias elixir contained *Mitchella repens*, *Viburnum opulus*, *Caulophyllum thalictroides*, and *Helonias dioica*. This was also used to prevent successive miscarriages (Bates & Tilden, 1874).

Philadelphia-fleabane (*Erigeron philadelphicus*) was used to suppress menstruation by the Cherokee and to treat menstrual problems by the Houma (Fenton, 1942; Moerman, 1998). A Dr. Currey of Knox, Tennessee, prescribed oil of erigeron for hemorrhage after four miscarriages experienced by his patients and found it effective in three cases. He learned of the remedy from a report in the *Transactions of the College of Physicians of Philadelphia* (Currey, 1857).

Plants used by the Indigenous Americans such as the Oklahoma Delaware included black haw (*Viburnum prunifolium*) root, used to strengthen the reproductive tract, relax the uterus and thus reduce menstrual pain, and bring the fetus to full term, and *Acorus calamus* root, used for suppressed menses. The Delaware, Mi'kmaq, Modheman, and Shinnecock peoples treated gynecological disorders with motherwort (*Leonurus cardiaca*) (Moerman, 1998). The use of this plant among Indigenous Americans was also consistent with its use among eclectic physicians who used it to treat amenorrhea and dysmenorrhea.

Women were also experts in using medicinal plants for reproductive health, and some established businesses that sold herbal remedies. One famous example is Deborah Read Franklin who operated a store out of her husband's Benjamin Franklin's print shop. She sold gentian root (*Gentiana* species) and seneca root (*Polygala senega*) as emmenagogues from the Philadelphia post office in 1740. As proof of its popularity, seneca root was still being sold (as snakeroot cordial) by pharmacies a century later

(Klepp, 1994). It was listed by Tully as an abortifacient if accidentally taken during pregnancy (1857).

Apothecary shops and doctors in 1850 used powdered *Sanguinaria canadensis* for many ailments and conducted pharmaceutical studies. Senecionin—a tincture made from the leaves and roots of liferoot (*Senecio aureus*)—was sold as an emmenagogue, and it was reported to tone the uterus and restore menstruation ("Descriptions of new remedies," 1863; Klepp, 1994). J.M. Nickell's (1880) botanical reference for druggists and physicians called *Senecio aureus* a female regulator. It was used in homeopathic formulations. One recipe for "female weakness" contained wild sarsaparilla (*Aralia nudicaulis*), white water-lily (*Nymphaea odorata/Castalia odorata*), and life root (*Senecio aureus*) (Meyer, 1973).

A uterine tonic sold by Dios Chemical Co from St. Louis, Missouri, was called Dioviburnia and contained *Viburnum prunifolium*, *Viburnum opulus*, *Dioscorea villosa*, *Aletris farinosa*, *Helonias dioica*, *Mitchella repens*, *Caulophyllum thalictroides*, and *Scutellaria lateriflora* (Shrady, 1891).

Maternity Care: Miscarriage Prevention and Labour-Induction Herbs

False unicorn (*Chamaelirium luteum*) was used by eclectic physicians to treat leucorrhea, amenorrhea, and dysmenorrhea; it was also used to treat repeated miscarriage and to alleviate morning sickness (Felter & Lloyd, 1898/1992). The Cherokee used dittany (*Cunila origanoides*) to support labour and delivery. Bethroot (*Trillium pendulum*) was used by Indigenous American women to induce labour (Felter & Lloyd, 1898/1992).

Caulophyllum thalictroides (blue cohosh) was listed in the *United States Pharmacopoeia* in 1882 as a labour inducer, copying Indigenous Americans who used it to relieve menstrual cramps and ease childbirth pains (Dugoua et al., 2008). *King's American Dispensatory* noted its use amongst Indigenous Americans to stimulate labour, while also noting its usefulness in treating amenorrhoea, dysmenorrhea, and a variety of other uterine problems (Felter & Lloyd, 1898/1992).

King's American Dispensatory provided specific indications and doses for the use of *Cimicifuga racemosa* (black cohosh) to induce labour, for effective uterine contractions, and for after-pains (Felter & Lloyd, 1898/1992).

Fertility Enhancement

Black haw (*Viburnum prunifolium*) was listed in *King's American Dispensatory* as a uterine tonic to treat menstrual pain and was used in small doses over a period of time to remedy habitual miscarriage (Felter & Lloyd, 1898/1992). False unicorn (*Chamaelirium luteum*) was listed by numerous scientists in the *Dispensatory* as a remedy for repeated miscarriage (Felter & Lloyd, 1898/1992). Motherwort was listed to treat amenorrhea and suppressed lochia (Felter & Lloyd, 1898/1992) (see table 3.1).

Table 3.1 Colonial Botanical Remedies Used for Women's Fertility

Latin name/ botanical name	Common name	Uses
Tanacetum parthenium	Tansy	Emmenagogue
Ruta graveolens	Rue	Emmenagogue
Juniperus sabina	Savin	Emmenagogue; abortifacient
Mentha pulegium	Pennyroyal	Emmenagogue; abortifacient
Sanguinaria canadensis	Bloodroot	Contraceptive; emmenagogue; abortifacient
Cunila origanoides	Dittany	Emmenagogue
Commiphora abyssinica	Myrrh	Emmenagogue
Ferula assa-foetida	Asafoetida	Emmenagogue
Ferula spp.	Sagapenum	Emmenagogue
Ricinus communis	Castor	Emmenagogue
Opopanax chironium	Opopanax	Emmenagogue
Glechoma hederacea	Ground ivy	Abortifacient
Juniperus communis	Juniper	Treatment for gonorrhea and leucorrhea
Viburnum opulus	Cramp bark (Squaw bush)	Menstrual regulator; abortifacient; miscarriage prevention; dysmenorrhea
Hedeoma pulegioides	American pennyroyal (Squaw mint)	Menstrual regulator; abortifacient; dysmenorrhea, diminished lochia, and prolonged labour
Viburnum prunifolium	Black haw	Miscarriage prevention; remedy for habitual miscarriage; dysmenorrhea; strengthen the reproductive tract; prevent early labour
Discorea villosa	Wild yam	Dysmenorrhea
Caulophyllum thalictroides	Blue cohosh (squaw root)	Dysmenorrhea, diminished lochia, and prolonged labour; emmenagogue; leucorrhea; amenorrhea; labour induction; prevent successive miscarriages
Cimicifuga racemosa	Black cohosh (squaw root)	Relieve sickness and heartburn in pregnancy; tendency to miscarriage; toning the reproductive tract; amenorrhea; dysmenorrhea; induce labour; promote effective uterine contractions; relieve after-pains
Mitchella repens	partridge berry (squaw vine)	Labour induction; dysmenorrhea; uterine disorders, threatened abortion, and miscarriage; prevent successive miscarriages

continued

Latin name/ botanical name	Common name	Uses
Erigeron philadelphicus	Philadelphia fleabane (squaw weed)	Dysmenorrhea; used to suppress menstruation; treat menstrual problems; treat hemorrhage after miscarriage
Helonias dioica	Unicorn root	Prevent successive miscarriages
Acorus calamus	Sweet flag	Emmenagogue
Leonurus cardiaca	Motherwort	Amenorrhea; dysmenorrhea; suppressed lochia
Gentiana species	Gentian	Emmenagogue
Polygala senega	Seneca	Emmenagogue; abortifacient
Senecio aureus	Liferoot	Emmenagogue; "female weakness"
Aralia nudicaulis	Wild sarsaparilla	"Female weakness"
Nymphaea odorata/ Castalia odorata	White water-lily	"Female weakness"
Chamaelirium luteum	False unicorn	Leucorrhea; amenorrhea; dysmenorrhea; treat repeated miscarriage; alleviate morning sickness
Cunila origanoides	Dittany	Support labour and delivery
Trillium pendulum	Bethroot	Induce labour

Ethnomedicinal Validation of Plants Used for Fertility Enhancement

This section examines the efficacy of some of the herbal remedies used for fertility enhancement described above. The methodology used entails examining the phytochemical and pharmacological data from published studies to see if there is a scientific basis for the reported folk use of these plants (Lans, Brown, Borde & Offiah, 2003).

Antioxidants

High antioxidant levels are associated with greater pregnancy success (Comhaire & Mahmoud, 2003). For example, Dutch sub-fertile couples on the "Mediterranean" diet (high intakes of vegetable oils, vegetables, fruits, nuts, fish, and legumes; low intake of dairy and moderate intake of alcohol) had a 40 percent increased probability of achieving pregnancy after **in vitro fertilization (IVF)** or intra-cytoplasmic sperm injection (ICSI) treatment. Women had high concentrations of folate and vitamin B6 in blood and **follicular fluid** (Vujkovic et al., 2010). The plants discussed in this chapter that have a documented antioxidant activity include *Juniperus virginiana* leaves and twigs, *Senecio aureus*, and *Aralia racemosa* roots (McCune & Johns, 2002; Nachman, 1983). Some plants with antioxidant activity can be used to treat infertility since oxidative stress has a negative effect on oocyte maturation, fertilization, embryo development, and pregnancy (Comhaire & Mahmoud, 2003).

Vitex Agnus-castus and *Viburnum Prunifolium*

Three studies have shown that vitex increases luteal phases and luteal progesterone synthesis (Bergmann et al., 2000; Milewicz et al., 1993; Westphal, Polan, Trant & Mooney, 2004). Vitex has therefore improved conception rates and live birth rates, validating its traditional use. Black haw (*Viburnum prunifolium*) is a fast-acting, safe, and effective herb that is used in contemporary herbal medicine to prevent miscarriage and relieve labour pains (Green, 1886; Hoffmann, 2003; Westfall, 2001). Black haw contains salicin and scopoletin, both of which relax and sedate uterine muscle and other smooth muscles (Cometa et al., 2009; Duke, 1992). The most appropriate clinical trials for the testing of black haw are those in which the patients are suffering from infertility linked to frequent miscarriages.

Chamaelirium Luteum and *Leonurus Cardiaca*

False unicorn (*Chamaelirium luteum*) contains steroidal compounds (Challinor et al., 2012). Steroidal saponins may influence human hormones. Though it is considered effective in preventing miscarriage, due to its rarity, the use of false unicorn is discouraged in modern herbalism (Westfall, 2001).

Motherwort (*Leonurus cardiaca*) is used to support childbirth in modern herbalism. The alkaloid leonurine contained in motherwort has shown uterine stimulant effects *in vitro*. The alkaloid stachydrine—also found in motherwort—may stimulate oxytocin release (Blumenthal, Goldberg & Brinckmann, 2000).

Cimicifuga Racemosa and *Caulophyllum Thalictroides*

Many plant-derived compounds (such as **flavonoids**) can act like endogenous hormones. Black cohosh (*Cimicifuga racemosa*) has been identified as a source of phytoestrogen, and the question of whether black cohosh binds to estrogen receptors is still being settled (Bolle, Mastrangelo, Perrone & Evandri, 2007). A study found that a dry extract of black cohosh improved clinical pregnancy rates, endometrial thickness, and serum progesterone when used with clomiphene citrate in ART (Shahin, Ismail, Zahran & Makhlouf, 2008).

Blue cohosh (*Caulophyllum thalictroides*) enhances estradiol binding to estrogen receptors and has demonstrated estrogenic activity. It contains an active oxytocic compound that is responsible for increasing uterine tone, and also contains alkaloids, steroidal glycosides, and several triterpene glycosides (Matsuo, Watanabe & Mimaki, 2009).

Though blue and black cohosh have both been used in contemporary herbalism to induce labour (Westfall, 2001), midwives have reported adverse effects from their use such as nausea, increased meconium-stained fluid, and transient fetal tachycardia (accelerated heart rate). Case reports of health problems in newborns associated with maternal use of blue cohosh are possibly due to caulosaponin and caulophyllosaponin, constituents of blue cohosh that cause coronary blood vessel constriction and myocardial toxicity (Gunn & Wright, 1996; Jones & Lawson, 1998).

Angelica Archangelica

Wild celery (*Angelica archangelica*) contains isoquercitrin, a flavonoid that inhibits the activity of leukotriene LTD4 (Bili et al., 1998). Leukotrienes are compounds that cause contractions by stimulating receptors in arteries and increasing vascular permeability. LTD4 was found in follicular fluids of stimulated women undergoing IVF. This compound may act on follicular maturation (Bili et al., 1998). Further studies are needed to determine whether isoquercitrin is the relevant compound and if it supports pregnancy.

Conclusion

Colonial North Americans used a range of botanical medicines to regulate and promote fertility as well as for other gynecological problems. With the rise of modern pharmacology and the consolidation of power and authority by the North American medical profession, herbalism fell out of favour over the past century. However, herbal remedies have remained popular as an alternative or complement to conventional medicine. Herbal medicines are cost effective and appeal to people who want to use natural or organic methods of healing. The European Union scientifically reviewed all of the herbal medicines sold between 1978 and 1990. A German expert committee called Commission E subsequently published 380 monographs on the safety and efficacy of herbs that are legally prescribed in Germany. These monographs were translated and republished by the American Botanical Council in the 1990s, became well known, and provided information that individuals and small companies involved in herbal medicine could use. The monographs, combined with the increasing cost and greater public knowledge of the side effects of allopathic medicine, have increased the use of herbal medicine.

Ethnobotanical texts, herbals, and key resource documents such as *King's American Dispensatory* (Felter & Lloyd, 1898/1992) include a wealth of information about how botanical medicines have been used to support women's reproductive health. Some of these uses have carried over into modern herbalism, and in a few cases, there is clinical (Vitex) or pharmacological evidence (Black haw) of their efficacy. In other cases, such as that of blue cohosh, modern evidence indicates that the harmful side effects of the remedy outweigh its usefulness.

Several of these plants are presently used unofficially with assisted reproductive technology and could be incorporated into an integrated approach with biomedicine. However, there are only a limited number of studies that prove the scientific efficacy and safety of these plants. Many of the plants used in colonial North America merit further study in a clinical setting.

Critical Thinking Questions

1. Why do you think the cultural environment of colonial North America facilitated the use of herbs for fertility, infertility, and sub-fertility?
2. How can women's historical knowledge be recovered for contemporary assisted reproductive technology?
3. The few qualified female doctors of colonial North America sided with their male professional colleagues in preventing lay practitioners from helping patients. Why do you think that they did this? Would you do the same in similar circumstances?

Glossary

Amenorrhea: The absence of a menstrual period in a woman of reproductive age.

Assisted reproductive technology (ART): Methods used to achieve pregnancy by artificial or partially artificial means. It is reproductive technology used primarily for infertility treatments, and is also known as fertility treatments.

Dysmenorrhea: A medical condition of pain during menstruation.

Emmenagogues: Herbs that stimulate blood flow in the pelvic area and uterus; some stimulate menstruation.

Flavonoids: A class of plant secondary metabolites, which are organic compounds not directly involved in the normal growth, development, or reproduction of an organism.

Follicular fluid: A liquid that surrounds the ovum in an ovarian follicle, a spherical cellular aggregations found in the ovaries.

In vitro fertilization (IVF): A process by which an egg is fertilized by sperm outside the body: *in vitro* means "in glass" (i.e., a test tube). The process involves monitoring and stimulating a woman's ovulatory process, removing ovum or ova (egg or eggs) from the woman's ovaries, and letting sperm fertilize them in a fluid medium in a laboratory. The fertilized egg (zygote) is cultured for a few days and is then implanted in the woman's uterus.

Leucorrhea: A medical term that denotes a thick whitish or yellowish vaginal discharge.

Lochia: The vaginal discharge after giving birth containing blood, mucus, and uterian tissue.

References

Anonymous. (1888). *The archives of gynecology, obstetrics and pediatrics.* New York: Leonard & Company.

Augur, H. (1930). *An American Jezebel: The life of Anne Hutchinson.* New York: Brentano's.

Bartram, W. (1909). *Observations on the Creek and Cherokee Indians.* New York: American Ethnological Society. (Original work published 1789.)

Bates, J., & Tilden, H.A. (Eds). (1874). *Journal of Materia Medica*, 15. New Lebanon, NY: Tilden & Company.

Belew, C. (1999). Herbs and the childbearing woman. Guidelines for midwives. *Journal of Nurse Midwifery, 44*(3), 231–252.

Bergmann, J., Luft, B., Boehmann, S., Runnebaum, B., & Gerhard, I. (2000). [The efficacy of the complex medication Phyto-Hypophyson L in female, hormone-related sterility. A randomized, placebo-controlled clinical double-blind study]. *Forsch Komplementarmed Klass Naturheilkd, 7*(4), 190–199. German.

Bili, H., Tarlatzis, B.C., Daniilidis, M., Fleva, A., Bontis, J., Tourkantonis, A., & Mantalenakis, S. (1998). Cytokines in the human ovary: Presence in follicular fluid and correlation with leukotriene B4. *Journal of Assisted Reproduction and Genetics, 15*(2), 93–98.

Blumenthal, M., Goldberg, A., & Brinckmann, J. (2000). *Herbal medicine: Expanded Commission E monographs.* Newton, MA: Integrative Medicine Communications.

Bolle, P., Mastrangelo, S., Perrone, F., & Evandri, M.G. (2007). Estrogen-like effect of a *Cimicifuga racemosa* extract sub-fraction as assessed by *in vivo, ex vivo* and *in vitro* assays. *Journal of Steroid Biochemistry and Molecular Biology, 107*(3–5), 262–269.

Brodie, J.F. (2001). Menstruation interventions in the nineteenth-century United States. In E. van de Walle & E. Renne (Eds), *Regulating menstruation: Beliefs, practices, interpretations* (pp. 39–63). Chicago: University of Chicago Press.

Buchan, W. (1769). *Domestic medicine/The family physician.* Edinburgh: Balfour, Auld, and Smellie.

Capron, G., & Slack, D. (1849). *Popular medicine/The American family physician.* New York: Ray & Bro.

Challinor, V.L., Stuthe, J.M.U., Parsons, P.G., Lambert, L.K., Lehmann, R.P., Kitching, W., & De Voss, J.J. (2012). Structure and bioactivity of steroidal saponins isolated from the roots of *Chamaelirium luteum* (false unicorn). *Journal of Natural Products, 75*(8), 1469–1479.

Cometa, M.F., Parisi, L., Palmery, M., Meneguz, A., & Tomassini, L. (2009). *In vitro* relaxant and spasmolytic effects of constituents from *Viburnum prunifolium* and HPLC quantification of the bioactive isolated iridoids. *Journal of Ethnopharmacology, 123*(2), 201–207.

Comhaire, F.H., & Mahmoud, A. (2003). The role of food supplements in the treatment of the infertile man. *Reproductive Biomedicine Online, 7*(4), 385–391.

Cook, W. (1869). *The physiomedical dispensatory.* Cincinnati, OH: Wm .H. Cook. (Digitized by *Medical Herbalism: A Journal for the Clinical Practitioner,* Boulder, CO.)

Corner, B.C. (1951). *William Shippen, Jr., pioneer in American medical education: A biographical essay with notes, and the original text of Shippen's student diary, London, 1759–1760, together with a translation of his Edinburgh Dissertation, 1761.* Philadelphia: American Philosophical Society.

Cox, J. (2004). That quacking sound in colonial America. *Colonial Williamsburg,* Spring 2004. Retrieved from www.history.org/Foundation/journal/Spring04/quackery.cfm

Culpeper, N. (1995). *Culpeper's complete herbal: A book of natural remedies of ancient ills.* Lincolnwood, IL: NTC/Contemporary Publishing Company. (Original work published 1652.)

Currey, R.O. (Ed.). (1857). *The southern journal of the medical and physical sciences, 5.* Knoxville, TN: Kinsloe & Rice.

Descriptions of new remedies introduced into the practice of medicine, with their therapeutic effects. (1863). *The Lancet, 81*(2059), 190.

Dugoua, J.J., Perri, D., Seely, D., Mills, E., & Koren, G. (2008). Safety and efficacy of blue cohosh (*Caulophyllum thalictroides*) during pregnancy and lactation. *Canadian Journal of Clinical Pharmacology, 15*(1), 66–73.

Duke, J.A. (1992). *Handbook of phytochemical constituents of GRAS herbs and other economic plants.* Boca Raton, FL: CRC Press.

Ehrenreich, B., & English, D. (1973). *Witches, midwives and nurses: A history of women healers.* New York: The Feminist Press at the City University of New York. Retrieved from www.marxists.orf/subject/women/authors/ehrenreich-barbara/witches-htm

England, J.W. (Ed.) (1922). *The first century of the Philadelphia College of Pharmacy 1821–1921.* Philadelphia: Philadelphia College of Pharmacy and Science.

Felter, H.W., & Lloyd, J.U. (1992). *King's American dispensatory.* Oregon: Eclectic Medical Publications. (Original work published 1898.)

Fenton, W.N. (1942). *Contacts between Iroquois herbalism and colonial medicine.* Washington, DC: Smithsonian Institution.

Frader, L.L. (1982). Review of the book *Female complaints: Lydia Pinkham and the business of women's medicine,* by S. Stage. *The New England Quarterly 55*(1), 137–140.

Francis, J.W. (1822). Observations on the medicinal properties of the *Sanguinaria canadensis* in a letter to Mr. Fitzgerald Bird. *The New York Medical and Physical Journal 1,* 170–173.

Gill, H.B. (1972). *The apothecary in colonial Virginia.* Charlottesville, VA: The Colonial Williamsburg Foundation.

Green, W.E. (1886). The uses of *Viburnum prunifolium. British Medical Journal, 1*(1316), 542.

Gunn, T.A., & Wright, I.M.R. (1996). The use of black and blue cohosh in labour. *New Zealand Medical Journal, 109*, 410–411.

Hoffmann, D. (2003). *Medical herbalism: The science and practice of herbal medicine*. Rochester, VT: Healing Arts Press.

Holmes, O.W. (n.d.). *Medical essays, 1842–1882*. Retrieved from www.gutenberg.org/files/2700/2700.txt

Jones, T.K., & Lawson, B.M. (1998). Profound neonatal congestive heart failure caused by maternal consumption of blue cohosh herbal medication. *Journal of Pediatrics, 132*, 550–552.

Klepp, S.E. (1994). Lost, hidden, obstructed, and repressed: Contraceptive and abortive technology in the early Delaware Valley. In J.A. McGaw (Ed.), *Early American technology. Making and doing things from the Colonial Era to 1850* (pp. 68–113). Chapel Hill, NC: University of North Carolina Press.

Klepp, S.E. (2001). Colds, worms, and hysteria: Menstrual regulation in eighteenth-century America. In E. van de Walle & E. Renne (Eds), *Regulating menstruation: Beliefs, practices, interpretations* (pp. 22–38). Chicago: University of Chicago Press.

Lans, C., Brown, G., Borde, G., & Offiah, V.N. (2003). Knowledge of traditional medicines and veterinary practices used for reproductive health problems. *Journal of Ethnobiology, 23*, 187–208.

Marsden, J. (1879). *Handbook of practical midwifery*. New York: Boericke and Tafel.

Matsuo, Y., Watanabe, K., & Mimaki, Y. (2009). Triterpene glycosides from the underground parts of *Caulophyllum thalictroides. Journal of Natural Products, 72*(6), 1155–1160.

McCune, L.M., & Johns, T. (2002). Antioxidant activity in medicinal plants associated with the symptoms of diabetes mellitus used by the Indigenous peoples of the North American boreal forest. *Journal of Ethnopharmacology, 82*(2–3), 197–205.

Meyer, C. (1973). *American folk medicine*. New York: Thomas Y. Crowell Company.

Milewicz, A., Gejdel, E., Sworen, H., Sienkiewicz, K., Jedrzejak, J., Teucher, T., & Schmitz, H. (1993). [*Vitex agnus castus* extract in the treatment of luteal phase defects due to latent hyperprolactinemia. Results of a randomized placebo-controlled double-blind study]. *Arzneim-Forsch, 43*(7), 752–756. German.

Moerman, D.E. (1998). *Native American ethonobotany*. Portland, OR: Timber Press.

Nachman, R.J. (1983). Tetrahydroligularenolide and related eremophilanes from *Senecio aureus. Phytochemistry, 22*(3), 780–782.

Newton, R.S., Powell, W.B., Freeman, Z., Sanders, J.M., & Coe, G. (Eds). (1856). *The eclectic medical journal*. Cincinnati: Wm. Phillips and Co.

Neuhauser D. (2006). Oliver Wendell Holmes MD 1809–94 and the logic of medicine. *Quality and Safety in Health Care, 15*(4), 302–304.

Nickell, J.M. (1880). *J.M. Nickell's botanical ready reference*. Chicago: Ottaway & Company.

Ray, L. (2009). *Podophyllum peltatum* and observations on the Creek and Cherokee Indians: William Bartram's preservation of Native American pharmacology. *Yale Journal of Biology and Medicine, 82*(1), 25–36.

Ried, K., & Stuart, K. (2011). Efficacy of traditional Chinese herbal medicine in the management of female infertility: A systematic review. *Complement Therapies in Medicine, 19*(6), 319–331.

Riddle, J.M. (1999). *Contraception and abortion from the ancient world to the Renaissance.* Cambridge, MA: Harvard University Press.

Scholten, C. (1977). On the importance of the obstetrick art: Changing customs of childbirth in America, 1760–1825. *William and Mary Quarterly, 34*, 426–445.

Shahin, A.Y., Ismail, A.M., Zahran, K.M., & Makhlouf, A.M. (2008). Adding phytoestrogens to clomiphene induction in unexplained infertility patients—a randomized trial. *Reproductive Biomedicine Online, 16*(4), 580–588.

Shannon, J., El Saigh, I., Tadrous, R., Mocanu, E., & Loughrey, J. (2010). Usage of herbal medications in patients undergoing IVF treatment in an Irish infertility treatment unit. *Irish Journal of Medical Science, 179*(1), 63–65.

Short, T., & Bartram, J. (1751). *Medicina Britannica: Or a treatise on such physical plants* [...]. Philadelphia: B. Franklin & D. Hall. Retrieved from opac.newsbank.com/select/evans/6783

Shrady, G.F. (Ed.). (1891). *Medical Record: A Weekly Journal of Medicine and Surgery, 40*(15). New York: W. Wood.

Tully, W. (1857). *Materia medica, or, Pharmacology and therapeutics.* Springfield, MA: Jefferson Church, MD.

van de Walle, E. (1997). Flowers and fruits: Two thousand years of menstrual regulation. *Journal of Interdisciplinary History, 28*(2), 183–203.

Vujkovic, M., de Vries, J.H., Lindemans, J., Macklon, N.S., van der Spek, P.J., Steegers, E.A., & Steegers-Theunissen, R.P. (2010). The preconception Mediterranean dietary pattern in couples undergoing *in vitro* fertilization/intracytoplasmic sperm injection treatment increases the chance of pregnancy. *Fertility and Sterility, 94*(6), 2096–2101.

Westphal, L.M., Polan, M.L., Trant, A.S., & Mooney, S.B. (2004). A nutritional supplement for improving fertility in women: a pilot study. *Journal of Reproductive Medicine, 49*(4), 289–293.

Westfall, R.E. (2001). Herbal medicine in pregnancy and childbirth. *Advances in Therapy, 18*(1), 47–55.

Zeyneloglu, H.B., & Onalan, G. (2014). Remedies for recurrent implantation failure. *Seminars in Reproductive Medicine, 32*(4), 297–305.

CHAPTER 4

Being "There" for Pregnant Women: Canadian Midwives in Indigenous and Settler Communities

Cecilia Benoit, PhD
Department of Sociology, University of Victoria, Canada

Dena Carroll, BA, MBA
Aboriginal Health Consultant, Victoria, Canada

Rachel Westfall, PhD
Yukon Bureau of Statistics, Canada

Learning Objectives

1. To develop an understanding of hidden historical narratives that are worthy of telling and relevant to the health and well-being of pregnant women and their families living in pre-industrial times in Canada.
2. To create a space in your thinking for midwives to be acknowledged as historical actors in their own right and midwifery as a profession that has much more diverse history than is commonly portrayed.
3. To appreciate the similarities but also crucial differences in the history of midwifery and maternity care in early Indigenous and settler communities in Canada.

Introduction

Pregnancy and childbirth are core female events fundamental to the survival of the human species, yet the social organization of these events shows amazing variation across time and place (Benoit et al., 2015; Wrede, Benoit & Sandall, 2001). One obvious dimension of this variation concerns the care that women have available to them to help make a successful transition to motherhood. While specialized care provided by medical doctors falls within this domain, an additional form of maternity care that is often overlooked in our technologically focussed society is women's desire for **social support** or "social care" in their local communities.

Few would dispute that access to medical specialists and advanced technology have been of positive benefit for women experiencing difficult pregnancies, achievements associated with the urbanization and scientization of modern life. Yet social support from family members, extended kin, neighbours, and primary health care providers such as lay midwives and doulas has been in the past and remains today fundamental to the health of all childbearing women, regardless of biological condition. This is the case not only in high-income countries such as Canada but around the world, and is promoted by the World Health Organization as well as other key international organizations working to improve the health and well-being of women and girls in their home countries (Benoit et al., 2015).

Below we give evidence that social support is a key **social determinant of health** (Raphael, 2004) for childbearing women and is central to what women say they want in regard to **maternity care** services (Bourgeault, Benoit & Davis-Floyd, 2004; De Vries, Benoit, van Teijlingen & Wrede, 2001). However, not all Canadian women have access to social support at the community level; rather, the evidence shows that social support, much like other social determinants, is stratified along lines of social class, ethnicity and race, and geographical location, among other factors. While much of the feminist literature on pregnancy and childbirth has highlighted the gendered "patriarchal" underpinning of medicine and depicted the female midwife as women's "natural" ally during pregnancy and childbirth (e.g., Oakley, 1984; Witz, 1992), in this chapter we use an intersectional approach to analyze important differences among women in the historical record of access to midwifery care (Benoit, 1994; Bourgeault, Benoit & Hirschkorn, 2009; Hankivsky et al, 2010).

Because of the rich and distinct historical records relating to maternity care systems in Indigenous and non-Indigenous communities across Canada, as well as the fact that there are clear differences among Canadian women of non-Indigenous and Indigenous statuses in regard to access to high quality maternity care, including midwives "being there," we discuss each separately while highlighting overarching themes common to all women.

The chapter makes three contributions to learning: (1) it provides an understanding of hidden historical narratives that are worthy of telling and relevant to the health and well-being of pregnant women and their families living in pre-industrial times in Canada; (2) it encourages understanding of midwives as historical actors in their own right and midwifery as a profession that has much more diverse history than commonly portrayed; and (3) it appreciates the similarities but also crucial differences in the history of midwifery and maternity care in early Indigenous and settler communities in Canada.

Maternity Care in Early Indigenous Communities

Prior to contact with European settlers, there existed an informal system of maternity care across Canada's diverse Indigenous communities. Pregnant women had access to an extensive local network of family members, neighbours, and healers who embraced a worldview where birthing was considered a cultural and spiritual process rather than an individual act or medical event. One such healer was the traditional birth attendant or midwife, who was typically trained through a lengthy apprenticeship that included technical as well as extensive socio-cultural training. The midwife's role was typically reserved for female elders who had personal childbearing experience, and who held positions of respect and honour in their communities. As anthropologist Jo-Anne Fiske (1992) states when writing about the pre-contact Carrier peoples of British Columbia, "reproductive roles were central to women's claims to social prominence. Carrier women who successfully raised their families and provided care and nurturance to the needy became influential as family spokespersons. The wisdom of older women was proclaimed in legend and song and institutionalized in the valued role of the grandmothers of the tribe" (p. 201).

Although seldom occupying the role of midwife until their own children were grown, candidates tended to be chosen much earlier on for apprenticeship. Young girls, for example, often attended the births of their female relatives in order to build a solid basis of both technical skills and local knowledge of rituals, language, customs, herbal medicines, and spiritual norms related to reproduction. According to one elder, the young apprentice was sometimes taught to recognize the **birth energy**, described as a special communication between the labouring woman and her baby (Benoit & Carroll, 1995).

Anthropologist Franz Boas (1966, p. 61), in his Kwakiutl ethnography, described the complex social organization of pregnancy and childbirth in Indigenous societies on the Pacific Northwest coast, including the traditional stories and dances such as the Atlak'im masks and Legends of the G*exsem of the Kwakiutl people, used to illustrate the spiritual and cultural connection between midwife, mother, and newborn. Boas relates that a pregnant woman was also required to follow specific regulations, rituals, and obligations, pay careful attention to her activities, and avoid certain social networks and foods, in order to ward off danger to her baby (Boas, 1966). Other related cultural practices included naming the baby and the baby's relationship to the environment, and refraining from intervening in the natural process of growth by not cutting the baby's hair (Boas, 1966). Among the Cree, the midwife's tasks included gathering wood, making and beading the tikinagan, preparing the "birthing hands," honouring the placenta, using traditional medicines to aid birth, preparing the rabbit skins, gathering moss, and preparing special foods (Kioke, 1999).

The midwife was also closely involved with the newborn's family circle during the four-week post-partum "healing period," and midwifery care was often extended throughout the child and mother's life cycles. The small size of the communities and the close proximity of the people were important factors facilitating this type of care. In addition, the midwife oversaw a variety of preparations for labour and delivery and the welcoming of the new baby into the community.

When colonial governments began taking an interest in Indigenous health care provision, this community-based and culturally appropriate care was undermined, and the organization of maternity care became isolated from other aspects of community life. Beginning in the late 19th century, Indigenous family structures were negatively impacted by the imposition of colonial laws and policies aimed at assimilation of Canada's Indigenous peoples (Waldram, Herring & Young, 1995). Indigenous peoples became defined as federal responsibility under the 1876 Indian Act, and the federal government assumed an increasingly large role in the lives of Indigenous people on reserves. Indian agents, employed by the federal government, were appointed to oversee the affairs of Indigenous communities; they often worked hand-in-hand with medical doctors brought in from the outside. Christian missionaries were an additional powerful force in Indigenous people's lives. Many Indigenous midwives and other healers increasingly found themselves threatened, punished, or brushed aside by one or other of these foreigners (Wells, 1994). Of course, there were exceptions. Such was the case of one Tsimshian midwife from Vancouver Island, Mary Wiha, who died in 1917 at the age of 87. Her obituary made note of the fact that she "practiced for years the profession of mid-wife, and was most successful, treating upwards of 200 cases without a single mishap. Her services were greatly appreciated by the medical men on the coast at that time" (*Prince Rupert Evening Empire*, Dec. 27, 1917—see Atkinson, 2003). The obituary suggests that midwife Mary Wiha continued to hold a vital place in her Indigenous community even with the presence of colonial agents.

However, in many other parts of British Columbia, midwives were frequently treated as charlatans and their original birthing practices dismissed as outdated and even harmful to pregnant women in their community. Elders were discouraged from passing traditional knowledge to the young. Eventually, the government established residential schools, where Indigenous children, often against their own and their parents' wills, were sent to be educated in non-Indigenous traditions, languages, and customs (Hiebert, 2003).

As part of a general federal strategy to provide primary care to Indigenous peoples, by the late 1950s Health and Welfare Canada had established nursing stations in rural and northern Indigenous communities. Pre- and post-natal care was provided by station nurses, many of whom were immigrant nurse-midwives. The research literature is mixed regarding their effectiveness in meeting the social care as well as more technical needs of local women. Some report that the nurse-midwives remained "outsiders," failing to work with traditional midwives and gain the confidence and trust of the pregnant women they had come to serve (Waldram, Herring & Young, 1995). Yet other researchers note that some nurse-midwives, especially those who remained for long periods, became accepted into the community and were respected by local healers and childbearing women (Hiebert, 2003).

New federal government policies in the early 1970s led to the closing down of most nursing stations. The combination of factors mentioned above meant that Indigenous women no longer had viable alternatives at the community level to deliver their babies close to their homes. Instead, they were placed under increasing pressure to leave their communities and deliver their babies in large hospitals located in distant urban settings. Some resisted and continued to give birth in their own communities, attended by elder midwives and members of their family and community (O'Neil & Kaufert, 1996). For those women who left their communities to give birth, loneliness and disruption of their family's life were commonplace (Daviss, 1997). They travelled, usually by plane and without their families, to urban centres where they were attended by English-speaking professional nurses and physicians who knew little about the language and traditions of Indigenous peoples. This remains the situation in most remote communities to this day.

Maternity Care in Settler Communities

Immigrant groups began settling in present-day Canada in the 1700s. Over time, settlers began to develop systems of maternity care that were a combination of customs and traditions learned in their country of origin and the practices found in their new homeland. In some cases, Indigenous midwives provided much needed services to colonial settlers (Biggs, 2004).

As in Indigenous communities, the traditional lay midwives who emerged to care for childbearing women in settler communities were mostly older women who had little or no formal education but who nevertheless demonstrated strong skills, were well integrated into their ethnically diverse local communities, and sometimes were informally "elected" by the women they served (Biggs, 2004; Mitchinson, 2002). One of the first references to lay midwifery in this part of the world appears in a deed published by a Mr. Massicotte, "which reveals that the women of Ville-Marie [Montreal], in solemn concave assembled, on February 12th, 1713, elected a midwife Catherine Guertin for the community" (Abbott, 1931, p. 28).

Physicians' capacity to influence government legislation over health matters, including the organization of care for pregnant women, began as early as 1795 in Upper Canada (present-day Ontario), with the introduction of the first Medical Act to regulate the practices of "physic" and "surgery." This act essentially made it illegal to practise midwifery without an official licence to do so. Due to the impracticality of such a ruling, the small degree-holding urban-based segment of the medical profession was left vulnerable to public criticism and the act was eventually repealed in 1806 (Canniff, 1894, p. 22). From 1806–1866, traditional lay midwifery remained immune from the licensing laws of the Ontario Medical Board. However, by 1866, permission awarded by the provincial government to unlicensed female midwives had been withdrawn and midwifery practice was henceforth restricted exclusively to academically trained physicians. Medical schools were closed to women until the later part of the 19th century; no female physicians were licensed in Ontario until the 1880s, and few women worked in this capacity for many decades to come. Thus, licensed male physicians enjoyed an official monopoly over childbirth and other medically designated health events (Biggs, 1983). Nonetheless, even in the larger urban areas of Ontario, competition between physicians and midwives as to who had authority for home-births continued for several decades after Confederation. Although physician-attended births were eventually to become the norm, for some time midwives continued to attend women in rural and remote areas of the province, as well as the urban poor who could not afford physician attendance fees.

Outside Ontario, midwives in other settler communities remained active much longer. In Quebec, for example, traditional lay midwives (***sage-femmes***) continued to remain unregulated in legislative terms, and were controlled by local clergy and by birthing women themselves. In 1879, the Quebec College of Physicians and Surgeons, following events in Ontario, placed midwifery practice in the hands of physicians (Laforce, 1990). Nevertheless, for the next half century, Quebec midwives in rural areas were permitted to practise, provided that their competence was physician-certified. Such was the case as well in New Brunswick and Saskatchewan, where as late as 1924 at least 50 percent of births were not attended by medical doctors (Biggs, 1983).

In central Canada in the 1930s, prominent Canadian health reformers started advocating for "health teams," comprised of midwives, physicians, and public health nurses working out of community clinics. However, medical and nursing associations, worried that competition from midwives might reduce work for their own memberships, lobbied against these recommendations. Ultimately, the hospital-based physician-obstetrical nurse team replaced the community midwife as primary attendant during childbirth, initially among the urban middle classes and eventually reaching other sectors of society. The obstetrical nurse became known as the "doctor's handmaiden" and was expected to show "wifely obedience to the doctor, motherly self-devotion to the patient and a form of mistress/servant discipline to those below" (Buckley, 1979, p. 134). The commonly adopted perspective promoted by the medical and nursing professions was that "the art of midwifery belongs to prehistoric times" (Biggs, 1983, p. 32). Nonetheless, women continued to aid one another during pregnancy and in childbirth. Though obstetrical nurses were officially subordinate to doctors and were denied the technical training required to be effective autonomous birthing care providers, in practice many continued to serve as women's primary attendant at birth, sometimes with the attending physician's acquiescence. While physicians were able to lay claim to the territory of childbirth, they were, in practice, unable to service the entire population. In reality, physician services were available to those who could afford them, and those who did not reside in areas that were geographically remote or too sparsely populated to support a successful physician's practice. One such case was in Essex County, Ontario, where Agnes Deslippe Dupuis (1869–1954), a wife and mother of nine, worked as a midwife throughout her adult life. Agnes, who was trained to administer anaesthesia, worked both on her own and with a Dr. MacDonald when he was in the region and a case warranted his attention (M. Everest, personal communication, June 2004). Accordingly, in the mid-20th century, as was the case in Indigenous communities, the federal government made special provision for nurse-midwives to practice in remote non-Indigenous communities where physician services were unavailable (Bourgeault & Fynes, 1997).

The historical record is even more complex when we look at settler communities in the western and eastern provinces. Access to formal health care and trained health care professionals (including midwives as well as physicians) was limited in relation to how far women lived from towns and villages. Often stories arose about male relatives who were forced to travel large distances to "fetch" the midwife, if time and weather permitted, while the woman laboured alone or perhaps with a neighbour standing by. In many cases, the birth attendant simply did not arrive on time, and those at hand did what they could to facilitate the delivery. Social historian Nancy

Langford (1995), who researched childbirth on the Canadian prairies from 1880–1930, noted that although homestead birthing women hoped to find experienced midwives, some were successful and others not. Some women were forced to rely on inexperienced neighbours who did not always want to be midwives but took on the role out of necessity. Mrs. Elizabeth Akitt of Edmonton, Alberta, who was attended by a doctor and a nurse with midwifery training, indicated that, "I know what lots of women have gone through by not having a doctor. Sometimes, there was just a neighbour; no midwife" (as quoted in Rasmussen, Savage & Wheeler, 1976, p. 78). In recalling the beginning of labour, a first-generation settler in Alberta indicated to Eliane Leslau Silverman (1984) that "some good friends were with us; one of them wasn't exactly a midwife, but people used to call her that" (p. 66). Similarly, Eileen Lillian Cleary of Beaver Harbour, Halifax County, Nova Scotia, helped deliver seven of her nieces and nephews in the late 1940s and early 1950s out of both necessity and generosity, and also helped seven other local women birth their babies (K. Robb, personal communication, July 2003).

Traditional maternity care practices also survived well into the 20th century in Newfoundland and Labrador, which arguably has better records of this form of health care for childbearing women compared with anywhere else in the country (McNaughton, 1989). Midwives from Canada's most easterly province were often given the epithet of "granny" or "auntie," signalling the wisdom and practical skill that comes with age and experience, as well as denoting the respect that these women often held within their outport and rural communities. Like their Indigenous counterparts, many Newfoundland and Labrador traditional midwives learned their craft from female relatives or senior midwives as well as through personal experience (most had given birth themselves, often many times over); they thus learned by observation and by simply doing the work. According to one granny midwife from the west coast of Newfoundland, "I first learned to doctor the women and others in the village from my dear mother. I learned to give a newborn a steeped brew from weeds—caraway seeds perhaps [and to be] always present during birth, consoling and guiding the mother" (Benoit, 1990, p. 185). Newfoundland and Labrador midwives were often called upon to provide an array of nursing services to local families, most of whom had no access to professional forms of health care: "I had to do the other things besides bringing along babies 'cause there was no nurse there for a long time. So I had to do that work too. When anybody got sick, they'd call" (as quoted in Benoit, 1991, p. 57). Similarly, accordingly to midwife Aunt Gertie Legge from Heart's Delight in eastern Newfoundland, "we understood sickness and set bones and everything, and even did animals" (as quoted in Benoit, 1983, p. 23). Clara Tarrant, a granny midwife from St. Lawrence, Newfoundland, described her experience this way: "I got into a situation when I just had to [do midwifery] and there was nobody but myself. I had been at a birth and had seen deliveries and I had children. Seeing is believing but feeling is the naked truth" (as quoted in Benoit, 1983, p. 24).

As on the island of Newfoundland, until well into the 20th century, most Labrador families resided in small fishing villages or rural farming communities separated from each other by considerable distances. Access to the services of local midwives was crucial to survival. Bertha Anderson or "Aunt Bertha," as she was affectionately known in her home community of Makkovik, Labrador, was one such local midwife; she travelled by dog team, boat, or overland "to answer a call of mercy" (Chard, 1978). Susan Andersen (1914–2000), another local Labrador lay midwife, is recorded as having delivered 50 babies in her lifetime, many of them at the "White Elephant," a multipurpose building located in Makkovik where women from nearby fishing villages came to deliver their babies.

While variation existed in skill level and dedication to task, what stands out about these examples of social care from the prairies and eastern coastal communities is the willingness of female elders to provide technical care and social support to birthing women in need. Often there was little or no remuneration for these culturally relevant services that emerged from within local communities themselves. In regions where physicians were unable or unwilling to set up lucrative practices and nursing stations did not exist, women rarely went entirely without care, and traditional systems of midwifery were perpetuated. As shown next, this went on largely unnoticed by health policy makers, whose ultimate aim was to extend physician and hospital services to Canadian women and their families.

Medicare and the Solidification of Medical Dominance

Federal and provincial governments eventually responded to inequities in access to physician and hospital services through the establishment of a system of universal health coverage. First, in 1957, the federal government of Canada introduced the Hospital Insurance and Diagnostic Act. This act provided for a number of medical services associated with hospitalization and medical testing. The payment structure determined by the federal government was a cost-matching scheme whereby provincial governments were reimbursed 50 percent for some fixed portion of the expenditures. Of crucial importance, however, physicians' fees were not covered under the act of 1957. Universal health insurance finally arrived in Canada with the passage of the federal Medical Care Act of 1968 (implemented in 1972). The act teamed national principles with provincial administration through an innovative program, eventually known as Medicare. Importantly, under this second act, physicians' fees were insured. Pregnant women in Canada thus, for the first time, had free access to physician and hospital services. The "conditions" or five fundamental principles of the Medicare plan included universality (everyone would be covered), portability (from province to province), comprehensiveness, accessibility, and public administration.

It is crucial to note that though initially resistant to the implementation of a "socialized" health care system for Canada (there was even an infamous doctors' strike to protest the government Medicare plan), physicians across the country eventually gained much by this new welfare state policy. First of all, their services were reimbursed through the public purse, thereby virtually guaranteeing them economic security. Secondly, Medicare solidified physicians' dominance over maternity care services, granting them a virtual monopoly over the provision of the country's care of pregnant women. This monopoly was reinforced by the first point: the reimbursement of physicians but not midwives for services rendered limited women's choices regarding style of care. Thirdly, physicians retained their right to remain private entrepreneurs, establishing their practices wherever they deemed appropriate, where they would provide a range of medical services to women that the physicians themselves—not the women—decided upon as necessary. This point is notable as it did nothing to alleviate the pre-existing disparity in the availability of physician services between rural and urban areas. Finally, hospitalization of childbirth had long been a goal of the Canadian medical profession. Medicare solidified the medically dominated hospital as the linchpin to the entire maternity care system (Benoit et al., 2005). One important reason for doctors to promote hospital birth rather than domiciliary care was a consequence of the need for the physicians to be able to use substitute health care providers to assist them in the care of birthing women and their newborns. Canadian physicians thus gave their support to the training of obstetrical nurses (rather than community midwives), a strategy that was supported by the nursing lobby itself (Benoit, 1991; Bourgeault & Fynes, 1997; Bourgeault et al., 2004).

It should be noted here that it is a common misconception that the rise in physician attendance at births led to lower rates of maternal mortality. This belief has been critically examined by a number of authors. In the Canadian context, Suzann Buckley's (1988) examination of Ottawa birth records from the 1930s illustrated how socio-economic factors played a large role in determining the likelihood that a woman (and by inference, her baby) would survive childbirth. Similarly, Strong-Boag and McPherson (1986) considered the trend toward hospital deliveries in Vancouver between 1919 and 1939. Their statistics demonstrate that maternal mortality rates dropped at a rate that exceeded the increase in hospital births over this period of time. British Columbia had the highest rates of hospital birth in the country over that timespan, at 84.4 percent of live births by 1940, yet the province had one of the highest maternal mortality rates, with Vancouver's rates of hospitalization and maternal mortality exceeding those of rural areas. These studies indicate that in Canada, like elsewhere, the trend toward hospitalization and physician attendance was not a "cure" for the problem of childbirth related mortality; rather, it served the professional interests of the medical profession.

Recent developments in the last two decades have resulted in changes in traditional medical dominance over maternity care services (Benoit et al., 2010). Studies in both Indigenous and non-Indigenous communities indicate that childbearing women are keen to take advantage of viable alternatives to physician attendance and hospital birth if they are available to them in their own communities. Nationally, the occupation of midwifery has gained cultural legitimacy and in most Canadian provinces and territories, midwives currently have an opportunity to attain professional education and regulation, and their services have been publicly funded (see table 4.1). Yet the occupation still remains unregulated and unfunded in some areas, and less than 5 percent of births in Canada are currently attended by a midwife. A substantial proportion of women in all parts of the country who want access to a trained publicly funded midwife are currently unable to find one. Indigenous women, women with lower education, younger mothers, women without a partner,

Table 4.1 Midwifery across Canada, 2014

Province/Territory	Regulated	Public funded
Newfoundland and Labrador	No	No
Prince Edward Island	No	No
Nova Scotia	Yes	Yes, limited
New Brunswick	No	No
Quebec	Yes	Yes
Ontario	Yes	Yes
Saskatchewan	Yes	Yes
Manitoba	Yes	Yes
Alberta	Yes	Yes
British Columbia	Yes	Yes
Yukon	No	No
Northwest Territories	Yes	Yes
Nunavut	In process	Yes

Source: Canadian Association of Midwives: www.canadianmidwives.org/province/

Table 4.2: Caesarean Section Rates in Canada, 2012

Geography	Rate-female percent (95% confidence interval)
Canada	27.2 (27.1–27.4)
Newfoundland and Labrador	30.4 (29.0–31.7)
Prince Edward Island	30.3 (27.8–32.8)
Nova Scotia	27.0 (26.1–28.0)
New Brunswick	28.0 (26.9–29.0)
Quebec	23.9 (23.6–24.2)
Ontario	28.2 (28.0–28.5)
Manitoba	21.9 (21.3–22.6)
Saskatchewan	23.9 (23.2–24.6)
Alberta	28.3 (28.0–28.7)
British Columbia	32.5 (32.0–32.9)
Yukon Territory	19.6 (15.7–23.6)
Northwest Territories	21.7 (18.5–24.8)
Nunavut	9.9 (7.8–11.9)

Source: Canadian Institute for Health Information. (1996–2014). Health Indicators Interactive Tool. Available from http://yourhealthsystem.cihi.ca/epub/.

Notes

1. Due to recent changes in boundaries, data for Manitoba regions (4601-4605) is not available for years prior to 2012 for this indicator.
2. For PEI, the Yukon, the Northwest Territories, and Nunavut, the entire province or territory is included as a region.

and women living in rural and remote areas or socio-economically disadvantaged communities have the least access to public midwifery services (Benoit, 2015; Benoit et al., 2015). Moreover, efforts to address the lack of socially oriented care through the integration of midwifery care into the health care system have thus far been insufficient, as midwives are too few in number, and few midwives are trained in Indigenous knowledge ways.

At the same time, the number of family doctors involved in **maternity care** delivery has significantly declined across Canada, as have the number of hospitals offering maternity care services, while the percentage of deliveries attended by obstetricians has increased substantially. For example, obstetricians currently attend 80 percent of hospital births in Ontario. Caesarean section rates have also steadily increased, with total national rate increasing from 17.6 percent in 1995, to 21.1 percent in 2000 and 27.1 percent in 2011–2012 (see table 4.2). The current rate of caesarean section births ranges from a high of 32 percent in British Columbia and 31 percent in Newfoundland and Labrador, to a low of 23.1 percent in Saskatchewan and 21.41 percent in Manitoba (Benoit, 2015). According to the World Health Organization, caesarean section rates below 10 percent indicate underuse of this life-saving procedure, while rates above 15 percent are deemed to show overuse (Benoit et al., 2015).

Conclusion

As is clear from the above historical overview, midwives were the main maternity care provider in what is now Canada before the arrival of European settlers and up to the modern period, providing crucial technical care but also **social support** to enhance the health and well-being of women and babies in homes and local communities. **Modernization** was accompanied by the demise of midwives and childbirth as a socio-cultural event and the **medicalization of human reproduction**. In recent decades, this turn of events has shifted, with obstetricians replacing family doctors as the maternity providers, and labour and delivery restricted to fewer and fewer hospitals. One outcome is troublesome: high caesarean rates which are linked to unnecessary morbidity for mothers. Efforts to alleviate these problems through the integration of midwifery care into the health care system have thus far been insufficient, as midwives are too few in number, they are concentrated in urban centres, and their services are not equally available in all provinces/territories. As we have noted elsewhere (Benoit et al., 2010; Benoit et al., 2012; Benoit et al., 2015), many difficulties remain before the kind of social care available to Canadian women in earlier times again becomes a reality for all. Future health planning will need to undertake this formidable task.

Acknowledgements

We wish to thank our community partners who helped us design and carry out the research for this chapter. We are also grateful to those who participated in the background interviews. Without their stories, this work would not have been possible. Finally, we acknowledge the observant feedback from the editors.

Critical Thinking Questions

1. How have historical socio-political factors shaped our understanding of the organization of maternity care in pre-colonial Indigenous and settler communities?
2. Why is it important to take a social determinants and intersectionality perspective on the organization of maternity care in Canada's past?
3. Explain why childbearing is as much a social and cultural process as a biological one.
4. What are the enduring themes about family and community that cut across the history of maternity care in Indigenous and non-Indigenous communities?

Glossary

Birth energy: A special communication between the labouring woman and her baby in pre-colonial Indigenous communities.

Maternity care: Informal and formal care during pregnancy, labour, and delivery and into the post-partum period.

Modernization: A vision of progress that involves the transition from a "pre-modern" or "traditional" to a "modern" society.

Medicalization of human reproduction: Pregnancy and childbirth defined as an illness event that required frequent medical supervision and technological intervention.

Sage-femmes: Traditional lay midwives in early settler communities.

Social determinants of health: Economic and social conditions and their distribution among the population that influence individual and group differences in health status.

Social support: Support that involves a four-part typology of supportive functions of social relationships: (1) emotional support; (2) instrumental support; (3) companionship support; and, (4) informational support.

References

Abbott, M. (1931). *The history of medicine in the province of Quebec*. Montreal: McGill University.

Atkinson, M. (2003). *"The mother of this place": (Paykw) Mary Wiha, professional midwife and Tsimshian role model*. Prince George, BC: University of Northern British Columbia.

Benoit, C. (1983). Midwives and healers: The Newfoundland experience. *Healthsharing, 5*(1), 22–26.

Benoit, C. (1990). Mothering in a Newfoundland community: 1900–1940. In K. Arnup, A. Levesque & R. Roach Pierson (Eds), *Delivering motherhood: Maternal ideologies and practices in the 19th and 20th centuries* (pp. 173–189). London and New York: Routledge.

Benoit, C. (1991). *Midwives in passage: The modernisation of maternity Care*. St John's, NL: Memorial University, Institute of Social and Economic Research.

Benoit, C. (1994). Paradigm conflict in the sociology of service professions: Midwifery as a case study. *Canadian Journal of Sociology, 19*(3), 303–329.

Benoit, C. (2015). Modern maternity care in Canada. *Transition, 45*(4), 3–6.

Benoit, C., & Carroll, D. (1995). Aboriginal midwifery in British Columbia: A narrative still untold. *Western Geographic Series, 30*, 221–246.

Benoit, C., Wrede, S., Bourgeault, I., Sandall, J., van Teijlingen, E. & De Vries, R. (2005). Understanding the social organisation of maternity care systems: Midwifery as a touchstone. *Sociology of Health & Illness, 27*(6), 722–737.

Benoit, C., Declercq, E., De Vries, R., Sandall, J., van Teijlingen, E., & Wrede, S. (2015). Maternity care as global health policy issue. In E. Kuhlmann, R. Blank, I. Bourgeault & C. Wendt (Eds), *The Palgrave international handbook of health policy and governance* (pp. 85–100). Basingstoke: Palgrave.

Benoit, C., Stengel, C., Phillips, R., Zadoroznyj, M., & Berry, S. (2012). Privatization & marketization of post-birth care: The hidden cost for new mothers. *International Journal for Equity in Health, 11*(1), 61. doi:10.1186/1475-9276-11-61

Benoit, C., Zadoroznyj, M., Hallgrimsdottir, H., Treloar, A., & Taylor, K. (2010). Medical dominance and neoliberalisation in maternal care provision: The evidence from Canada and Australia. *Social Science & Medicine. 71*, 475–481.

Biggs, C.L. (1983). The case of the missing midwives: A history of midwifery in Ontario from 1795–1900. *Ontario History, 65*(2), 21–35.

Biggs, C.L. (2004). Rethinking the history of midwifery in Canada. In I. Bourgeault, C. Benoit & R. Davis-Floyd (Eds), *Reconceiving midwifery: Emerging models of care* (pp. 17–45). Kingston and Montreal: McGill-Queen's University Press.

Boas, F. (1966). *Kwakiutl ethnography*. H. Codere (Ed.). Chicago: University of Chicago Press.

Bourgeault, I., & Fynes, M. (1997). The integration of nurse- and lay midwives in the US and Canada. *Social Science and Medicine, 44*(70), 1051–1063.

Bourgeault, I., Benoit, C., & Davis-Floyd, R. (Eds). (2004). *Reconceiving midwifery: The new Canadian model of care*. Kingston and Montreal: McGill-Queen's University Press.

Bourgeault, I., Benoit, C., & Hirschkorn, K. (2009). Comparative perspectives on professional groups: Current issues and critical debates. *Current Sociology, 57*, 475–485.

Buckley, S. (1979). Ladies or midwives? Efforts to reduce infant and maternal mortality. In L. Kealey (Ed.), *A not unreasonable claim: Women and reform in Canada, 1880s–1920s* (pp. 131–149). Toronto: The Women's Press.

Buckley, S. (1988). The search for the decline of maternal mortality: The place of hospital records. In W. Mitchinson & J.D. McGinnis (Eds), *Essays in the history of Canadian medicine* (pp. 148–197). Toronto: McClelland and Stewart.

Canniff, W. (1894). *History of the medical profession in Upper Canada, 1783–1850.* Toronto: W. Biggs.

Chard, S. (1978). Tribute to Aunt Bertha: Bertha Anderson, Makkovik, 1872–1950. *Them Days Magazine, 4*(1), 56–58.

Daviss, B. (1997). Heeding warnings from the canary, the whale, and the Inuit: A framework for analyzing competing types of knowledge about childbirth. In R. Davis-Floyd & C. Sargent (Eds), *Childbirth and authoritative knowledge: Cross-cultural perspectives* (pp. 441–473). Berkeley: University of California Press.

De Vries, R., Benoit, C., Van Teijlingen, E., & Wrede, S. (Eds). (2001). *Birth by design: Pregnancy, maternity care and midwifery in North America and Europe.* London: Routledge.

Fiske, J. (1992). Carrier women and the politics of mothering. In G. Creese & V. Strong-Boag (Eds), *British Columbia reconsidered: Essays on women* (pp. 198–216). Vancouver: Press Gang Publishers.

Hankivsky, O., Reid, C., Cormier, R., Varcoe, C., Clark, N., Benoit, C., & Brotman, S. (2010). Exploring the promises of intersectionality for advancing women's health research. *International Journal for Equity in Health, 9*(5), 1–15.

Hiebert, S. (2003). Ncn Otinawsuwuk (receivers of children): Taking control of birth in Nisichawayasihk Cree Nation (doctoral dissertation). University of Manitoba, Winnipeg, MB. Retrieved from http://mspace.lib.umanitoba.ca/handle/1993/29574?mode=full

Kioke, S.J. (1999). Revisiting the past: Discovering traditional care and the cultural meaning of pregnancy and birth in a Cree Community (Master's dissertation). Queen's University, London, ON.

Laforce, H. (1990). The Different stages of the elimination of midwives in Québec. In K. Arnup, A. Levesque & R. Roach Pierson (Eds), *Delivering motherhood: Maternal ideologies and practices in the 19th and 20th centuries* (pp. 36–50). London and New York: Routledge.

Langford, N. (1995). Childbirth on the Canadian prairies, 1880–1930. *Journal of Historical Sociology, 3*, 278–302.

McNaughton, J. (1989). The role of the Newfoundland midwife in traditional care, 1900–1970 (doctoral dissertation). Memorial University of Newfoundland, St. John's, NL. Retrieved from http://research.library.mun.ca/799/

Mitchinson, W. (2002). *Giving birth in Canada, 1900–1950.* Toronto: University of Toronto Press.

Oakley, A. (1984). *Captured womb.* London: Blackwell.

O'Neil, J., & Kaufert, P. (1996). The politics of obstetric care: The Inuit experience. In W. Mitchinson, P. Bourne, A. Prentice, G. Cuthbert Brandt, B. Light & N. Black (Eds), *Canadian women: A reader* (pp. 416–429). Toronto: Harcourt Brace.

Raphael, D. (Ed.). (2004). *Social determinants of health. Canadian perspectives.* Toronto: Canadian Scholars Press Inc.

Rasmussen, L., Savage, C., & Wheeler, A. (Eds). (1976). *A harvest yet to reap: A history of prairie women.* Toronto: The Women's Press.

Silverman, E. (1984). *The last best west: Women on the Alberta frontier, 1880–1930.* Montreal and London: Eden Press.

Strong-Boag, V., & McPherson, K. (1986). The confinement of women: Childbirth and hospitalization in Vancouver, 1919–1939. *BC Studies, 69–70*, 142–174.

Waldram, J., Herring, D., & Young, T.K. (1995). *Aboriginal health in Canada: Historical, cultural and epidemiological perspectives.* Toronto: University of Toronto Press.

Wells, R. (1994). *Native American resurgence and renewal.* Metuchen, NJ: The Scarecrow Press, Inc.

Witz, A. (1992). *Professions and patriarchy.* London: Routledge.

Wrede, W., Benoit, C., & Sandall, J. (2001). The state and birth/the state of birth: Maternal health policy in three countries. In R. De Vries, C. Benoit, E. van Teijlingen & S. Wrede (Eds), *Birth by design: Pregnancy, maternity care, and midwifery in North America and Europe* (pp. 28–50). London: Routledge.

PART II

GLOBAL SOUTH

The second part of this book presents case studies representing current practices in women's reproductive health care in the Global South. It investigates the relationship between various socio-cultural settings and the philosophical and theoretical principles and therapeutic practices followed by women and CAM/TM practitioners in this region, as well as the extent to which women's access to and uses of CAM/TM are cross-culturally similar or different. In particular, these case studies underscore how therapeutic practices and health care choices are deeply intertwined with social relationships and cultural meanings.

The chapters that follow explore the experiences of local women, traditional midwives, spiritual healers, herbalists, and other practitioners of CAM/TM with an emphasis on the areas of fertility, pregnancy, birth, and post-natal care. These different settings for the use of TM are the backdrop for distinctive care practices that are embedded in a dynamic set of relationships among the many social actors involved (including the women themselves, their health care providers, families, and the communities in which they live). The chapters highlight the diversity of knowledge and models of care that are considered to be appropriate for women's health, and that vary from one context to the other.

In the chapters of this section, the pluralistic dimensions of health care for women's reproductive health are analyzed in terms of the heterogeneous therapeutic behaviour of both patients and practitioners, emphasizing how aspects of the various traditions (e.g., herbal medicine, traditional midwifery, spiritual healing) are incorporated in the healing process and used by women. Therapeutic practices operate at different levels and co-exist. In rural Turkey[1] (chapter 9), spiritual healing co-exists with folk medicine in the treatment of women with fertility issues, whereas in Indonesia (chapter 8) herbal medicine (jamu) is a well-established form of TM used alongside biomedicine by women for pre-natal and post-natal care. Biomedical clinics and hospitals are also interlinked with traditional midwifery practices in Brazil (chapter 5), Ecuador (chapter 6), Bolivia (chapter 7), and Ghana (chapter 10).

This section also observes the interaction between therapeutic itineraries and gender power relations, especially how ideas of female reproductive health are influenced by the authority of male healers and the patriarchal society in which they live. Chapter 9 highlights the social and moral pressures for Turkish women to be mothers. These pressures drive many women to seek faith-based healing for infertility, including—in extreme cases—the exorcism of an evil spirit (**jinn**) by a religious healer (**hodja**). The topic of infertility is also discussed by inscribing it within patriarchal gender roles existing in traditional Turkish communities.

The emergence of complementary, alternative, and integrative medicine within biomedical institutions and practices has had significant theoretical and practical implications, and presents important challenges for attending to the complexities of women's reproductive health, especially within indigenous populations.

Managing maternity care outside of a hospital setting is one challenge that is currently being addressed in the Global South. Improving the quality of pre-natal and post-natal care, and understanding the indicators of maternal and peri-natal health are central issues for reproductive health. Although giving birth in a biomedical hospital might be more appropriate for certain diagnosed risks in pregnancy, in other cases a hospital setting itself is a cultural and social obstacle for the mother-to-be, and can make the process of childbirth an alienating experience. Chapter 5 presents the case study of Casa Angela, a birth centre in Brazil, guided by the philosophy of anthroposophy, which employs birth attendants. The practices of pre-natal and post-natal care at Casa Angela, the relationship between the women and the health care professionals, and the values assigned to this place by local women are discussed through approaches in sensorial anthropology. On a similar theme, chapters 7 and 10 investigate the multi-level factors that motivate local women living in urban areas in Bolivia and Ghana, respectively, to use the services of traditional birth attendants instead of prioritizing giving birth in a hospital.

The scope for and challenges to integrating traditional midwifery practices and biomedicine is explored in chapter 6, which investigates efforts that have been made in Ecuador to reduce the cultural marginalization of traditional midwifery and promote forms of co-operation between indigenous medicinal systems and biomedicine. Chapter 10 also explores Ghanaian traditional birth attendants' experiences of the current interactions between the two systems of care, providing valuable insight into how collaborations might be improved for the provision of women's reproductive health services.

Note

1. There is still some ongoing debate as to whether Turkey is part of the Global North or Global South. This dichotomy in itself is problematic especially in the case of some countries, Turkey being one of them. As part of Europe, with a highly industrialized and developed sector, Turkey is considered as belonging to the Global North. However, there also is a significant rural area in Turkey where many people still hold to traditional practices and beliefs. As well, factors such as income inequality, literacy rates, and curtailing of press freedom would place Turkey more in the Global South category. Turkey ranks 72nd in a list of countries on the Human Development Index (just above Sri Lanka).

CHAPTER 5

Childbirth in Brazil: Voices of Brazilian Women

Natália Rejane Salim, PhD
Nursing Faculty, Federal University of São Carlos, São Paulo, Brazil

Julie Laplante, PhD
Department of Sociology and Anthropology, University of Ottawa, Canada

Learning Objectives

1. To increase knowledge about childbirth care and places of birth, and make it possible to reflect more deeply on midwifery in a Brazilian context.
2. To understand the place of the social sciences in midwifery studies, focusing on different contexts of childbirth.
3. To understand that childbirth is a complex biosocial event.

Introduction

The Portuguese expression for giving birth, *dar a luz*, literally means "bringing into the light," and encompasses the entire process of childbirth from the beginning of the first contraction until the baby is born. It is a process that is marked by interactions between people and places. The act of giving birth itself is characterized by an exchange of knowledge between social actors—that is, mother and child—and the health professionals who interact with each other in the events leading to the delivery of the child.

By listening to the voices of women—who are the most important people in these stories—we can gain a better understanding of the experiences of childbirth and the exchanges between the different social actors involved in the process. Recent years have seen increasing awareness of how the process of childbirth has become part of the domain of biomedicine. The ideology embedded in the Cartesian revolution has led to the perception of the human body as a machine, and therefore has created a fragmented understanding of the human being (Capra, 2006, p. 116). Thus, life events such as childbirth have become subject to the dominion of medical power and are under its scrutiny.

In this chapter, we will describe briefly the three different avenues of obstetric care in São Paulo, where the research took place, namely hospital births, a birth centre within a hospital setting, and an independent birth centre called Casa Angela.[1] The approach to birthing at Casa Angela will be the focus of this chapter, with the two other settings providing contrast and perspective. Casa Angela follows the principles of anthroposophy to provide care for its patients. Anthroposophy is a philosophy founded by Rudolf Steiner that postulates the existence of an intellectually comprehensible spiritual world that can be accessed through inner development. The main fields to which anthroposophy is applied are pedagogy and health.

Secondly, we will consider a sensorial anthropological approach, which focuses on the experience of giving birth. Thirdly, we will explain the methodological approach we used in this study and analyze women's stories and experiences of giving birth in a hospital versus giving birth at Casa Angela. Finally, we will discuss the views of local women about different ways of giving birth in city of São Paulo.

Childbirth in Brazil

A look at history shows us that the ways of thinking about pregnancy and childbirth are constantly changing. Although the act of giving birth has always been part of human female life, practices and customs surrounding childbirth have varied throughout history and cross-culturally (Mott, 2002). Generally speaking, until the 1800s, childbirth in Brazil (as well as in numerous western countries) predominantly took place in the home. Social and health care changes such as the emergence of medicine as a profession led to the hospital being viewed as a safer location for childbirth. In Brazil, the creation of hospitals started at the end of the 18th century and took place in complex ways. A hospital was constituted as a spatial structure, as a "therapeutic tool" of intervention over the patient and the disease, and as a curing machine (Foucault, 1979, p. 79–98). The first maternity hospitals (known as "lying-in hospitals") were inaugurated in London, England, in 1749. Thanks largely to this association with hospitals, childbirth gained the status of illness, a risky medical event that should be controlled through routines, procedures, and interventions (Salim, 2014).

In Brazil, childbirth predominantly occurred at home until the late 19th century. It was assisted by women known as *aparadeiras, comadres*, or ***parteras*** (midwives). The merger between midwifery and medicine that occurred during the 17th and 18th centuries in Europe was made official in Brazil in 19th century (Brennes, 1991).

The arrival of the Portuguese court in the country was soon followed by the creation of schools of medical surgery in Bahia and Rio de Janeiro, from which the first "male midwife physicians" graduated (Brennes, 1991). In 1832, the teaching of obstetrics to women was officially endorsed by those two medical schools, which began to train professional midwives (***obstetrizes***). The first midwife educated in Brazil was the illustrious Madame Durocher. She was born in France and known to dress in men's clothing. She was the first woman to be received at the Imperial Academy of Medicine in 1871 (Brennes, 1991; Mott 1999).

Hospital birthing became an ideal to be achieved and considered a synonym for civilization and medical progress (Mott, 2002). As a result, the biomedical model became widespread and foundational to the teachings and practices of care in obstetrics. The role of midwives became restricted because they were considered unreliable.[2]

Current data on childbirth in Brazil show a large number of unnecessary caesarean section procedures (C-sections) and other questionable medical interventions such as **episiotomies** and the use of the **Kristeller manoeuvre**.

Researchers are trying to understand why the number of C-sections in Brazil is much higher than in other countries (do Carmo, et al., 2012; Domingues, et al., 2014). In Brazil, C-sections account for almost 80 percent all of deliveries in the private sector and 35 percent in the public sector (Victora, et al., 2011, p. 1864). Studies show that Brazilian women express a preference for a vaginal birth (Diniz & Chacham, 2006; Zorzam, 2013). However, the perception of childbirth and labour pain as unnecessary suffering and childbirth as a risk event, as well as the convenience for physicians of scheduling C-section procedures to suit their timetables, seem to result in C-sections being performed despite the women's preference for a natural birth.

Adding to this picture, recent research has shown that one in four Brazilian women suffers violence during delivery, typically in the form of verbal abuse from health care providers (Perseus Abramo Foundation, 2010). For example, many women reported that a health care professional responded to their crying out in labour by saying, "you screamed when you conceived the baby, now shut up and stop screaming to deliver your baby" (Perseus Abramo Foundation, 2010).

In response to the hegemony of biomedicine, important changes and initiatives have occurred in the political, social, and educational realms in Brazil in recent decades.

The 1990s were marked by an awakening of political and civil society toward the promotion of health policies focused on the reduction of **medicalization of childbirth** in Brazil[3] For example, in 1997 the campaign "Normal is a normal childbirth" was inaugurated by the Ministry of Health[4] Two years later, in 1999, the campaign launched a petition for the establishment of birth centres in the country, with the focus on "humanized practices" and the right of women to be accompanied by a companion during their labour. The year 2000 saw two important milestones: a "national pact" to reduce the number of medically unnecessary C-section births, and the first conference about humanization in childbirth (Rattner, 2009). All of these events set the stage for the emergence of a humanization movement of midwifery in Brazil. The Brazilian objective of "returning to the roots" is about rediscovering the human component of giving birth; it is about awakening the senses, memories, and stories; it is about prioritizing human beings and natural processes over medical technology. Women's movements and the formation of networks comprising professionals and educators to promote the right of choice for women during childbirth have revealed that obstetric care in Brazil is undergoing a new process of transformation, this time returning to traditional models. In 2005, the University of São Paulo reopened the midwifery training program, which had been closed for three decades.[5]

An Anthropological Approach

In order to understand the ways and experiences of giving birth and the health care practices involved in this process, we examine a combination of different anthropological approaches, such as sensorial anthropology, the anthropology of childbirth intermeshing with principles of phenomenology, the theories of place, as well as ontology of care.

In the late 1960s, an increased scientific interest around childbirth emerged in anthropology and investigations started to appear in the social sciences. Anthropological studies help in understanding local cultures and how culture is reflected in childbirth practices and health care models. These studies helped delineate a new sub-field of study, the anthropology of childbirth. We refer here in particular to the work of two important anthropologists in this field, namely Brigitte Jordan and Robbie Davis-Floyd. Jordan (1993) conducted her research in different countries (Mexico, the United States of America, and Sweden) and elaborated the concept of "authoritative knowledge" in childbirth (see box 5.1). She discusses how a biomedical model and technology came to dominate the childbirth process while discrediting and devaluing other ways of giving birth and providing health care. In this context, one kind of knowledge (i.e., biomedical knowledge) was viewed as superior and

Box 5.1: Authoritative Knowledge

In different situations different forms of knowledge can be created. Authoritative knowledge is when a unique sort of knowledge becomes accepted by the elite in society and thus socially dominant. This implies that other forms of knowledge are devalued and depreciated. In the context of birth, authoritative knowledge indicates who possesses the power to decide how and what technology and biomedical devices, such as drugs, to use during the delivery process.

dominated other forms of knowledge (i.e., traditional and experiential knowledge).

The anthropologist Robbie Davis-Floyd (1992) explored technocratic childbirth in American society through the biomedical paradigm which views the body as a machine. In her words, "the hospital has become the factory, the mother's body has become the machine, and the baby has become the product of an industrial manufacturing process" (p. 6).

Following both Jordan's and Davis-Floyd's insights into potential power/knowledge relations applicable to childbirth practices, we understand that places are continuously re-shaped through the relationships of human beings within their environment. According to Ingold (1992), the relationship between people and their environment happens through an interaction with other human beings and objects (pp. 39–40). This means that the human experience of being in the world occurs in a multisensorial and dynamic way which, in turn, means that knowledge is not acquired but is produced by the relationship of human beings with the environment that surrounds them and which they experience through their senses. From this perspective, sensory relations occupy an important place, so what becomes an important issue in the field of anthropology is the place of the ethnographer as an active agent.

The anthropologist Sarah Pink brings attention to issues of place and space in anthropology. In *Doing sensorial ethnography*, Pink (2009) discusses the notion that the site cannot be defined because it is constituted by flows that interrelate, among things, people, and what is inside and outside. Given the dynamics of how sites are being built, the author brings up the question of the role of the ethnographer, who would not only have the role of participant but also that of author in the location of the study (Pink, 2009, pp. 29–30). Contextualizing this reflection to the research in the field of health becomes essential. Childbirth is a sensorial experience that happens in the body as a whole and evokes different sensorial responses and reactions. The encounters among the different social actors that happen during childbirth in

Box 5.2: The Sensorial Anthropological Approach

The sensorial anthropological approach proposes that knowledge is achieved through practice by being involved with outside environment. The body as a whole and its ongoing relationship with the environment is what makes each human being feel one's self in the world. This means that knowledge is not acquired: it happens while the individuals interact with the environment to inhabit the world. Thus knowledge consists of the process of living in the world (Ingold, 2010).

different spaces are sensorial encounters that highlight the importance of multiple senses in defining the interactions and the practices of health care (see box 5.2).

Annemarie Mol's proposal for an ontology of a multiple object follows a similar line of thought. It refers to ways that ontologies (categories of existence such as "body" or "disease") are brought into being in different contexts of childbirth. In *The Body Multiple*, Mol (2002) proposes the idea of following ontologies of practice as they are made to appear in certain places and times. This study follows how childbirth is made to appear in multiple ways as it varies with regard to the actors involved and with relation to multiple settings (Mol, 2002). In different contexts, social actors interact; these relationships and interactions translate into care practices and influence the way that each human being relates to the world and lives in the world. In line with this approach and the ones explained beforehand, we analyze the experiences of giving birth in three different settings in a neighbourhood of the city of São Paulo, paying particular attention to Casa Angela.

Methodology

Fieldwork for this research was conducted as part of a doctoral study by the lead author from March 2011 to March 2012. Three different sites were selected to observe the different ways of giving birth:

1. Birth centre: Casa Angela is located in a community area and is not part of a hospital. It offers women a relaxed, home-like environment that has the flexibility to adapt care to each woman's needs. The care team consists of certified midwives and nurses. The contact between the team and the pregnant women is very close and warm throughout the entire process of pre-natal care, childbirth, and post-partum care.

2. Obstetric centre: This is a hospital unit that was built based on biomedical concepts, as is shown in its material components, standards of practice, and forms of organization of services. The medical team has the power of decision in this context. This means that decisions about care and interventions during childbirth are decided solely by the medical team.
3. Humanized birth centre: This is a hospital unit that encourages natural childbirth with minimal intervention, but is equipped with technological support and medical staff for emergency situations. The care team consists of certified midwives and physicians.

All three centres are located in the southern part of the city of São Paulo, where the population comes from varied socio-economic backgrounds. Data were collected by means of participant observation and structured interviews. Eighteen women participated in this study. Most were between 20 and 30 years of age and were residents in neighbourhoods in proximity to where they chose to give birth. Participants were selected randomly using the following criteria: the woman had given birth in one of the three settings, she had an uncomplicated pregnancy and did not deliver a stillborn child, and she was aged 18 years or older and agreed to participate in the study. Three of the interviewees lived in slums, one lived in northern São Paulo, six were immigrants from states in the northeast region of Brazil, and one had travelled from the north region. Eight of the women interviewed were housewives. The occupations of the other women were as follows: one was a cook, one was a hairdresser, one was a caregiver for the elderly, one was a manufacturing worker, one was a nutritionist, and two were students. Three of the employed women who were interviewed from Casa Angela worked at the Monte Azul Community Association—one in the library and two in the daycare.

As a researcher, the lead author's experience of Casa Angela differed from that in the hospital-based centres. At Casa Angela she felt as if she was in her own home. She was invited to join the meetings, attend meals, help in the care of women, and join the celebrations. At the hospital she found herself excluded: she had to show identification at the entrance and wait for authorization to access the building. On one occasion, she was expelled from the obstetric centre by health care providers, yet on a different day another staff member invited her in and even provided her with a white coat so that she could stay on the premises without arousing suspicion.

Giving Birth at Casa Angela: Historical Background

In June 1983, a young German midwife, Angela Gehrke, arrived in Brazil. Born premature in Kassel, Germany, in February 1956, she moved to France after completing high school. There she met French obstetrician Frederick Leboyer, who inspired and motivated her to follow training in midwifery. In 1982, the young midwife made a trip to a small island in the Caribbean. She had brought in her travel bag a book titled Favela-Kinder (shanty town children), which changed her career path. The author of this book was Professor Ute Craemer, who also founded the Monte Azul Community Association located in the southern district of the city of São Paulo. Angela sent a letter to Monte Azul asking to become a volunteer. Her request was rejected, with the explanation that all the local women gave birth in hospitals. Not satisfied with this response, she decided to investigate matters for herself. As she later wrote, "when there is no place for someone, then we have to make a place" (da Silva & Galvão, 2010, p. 32).

Over time, Angela helped more than 1,500 women to give birth in the Monte Azul community. Her dedication and hard work resulted in her obtaining a small room at the out-patient health facility in Monte Azul as an alternative birthing facility. In 1997, with much effort, donations, and help from community residents, she built the first official birth centre of the state of São Paulo.

The Monte Azul Community Association now offers four different programs: education, culture, arts, and the environment. All actions in the community are guided by the philosophy of anthroposophy.[6]

European immigrants implemented anthroposophy (see box 5.3) in Brazil. Gradually, the Anthroposophical Society became established in the cities of São Paulo, Rio de Janeiro, and Porto Alegre. The development of anthroposophy was mainly in São Paulo where most of the initiatives and study groups were located and the city continues to have the majority of anthroposophists in the country.[7]

Box 5.3: Anthroposophy

The Greek word *anthroposophy* means "knowledge of man." Anthroposophy was developed by the philosopher Rudolf Steiner, who was born in Croatia and raised in Austria. Anthroposophy covers the spiritual and physical realities of human beings based on the assumption that every person is able to be an agent of change in the world. For Steiner, the concept of culture involves the areas of philosophy, medicine, social sciences, agriculture, teaching, and arts and comprises both the spiritual and the physical.

In anthroposophy, childbirth is considered the beginning and the first phase of development of a child, which extends until the age of seven. The birth process is understood to begin when a being "in the spiritual level" (fetus stage) wants to come into the world. Angela's view of labour as an intensive and transforming event that involves and reflects on society as a whole corresponded with the anthroposophical perspective (Hotmisky, 2001).

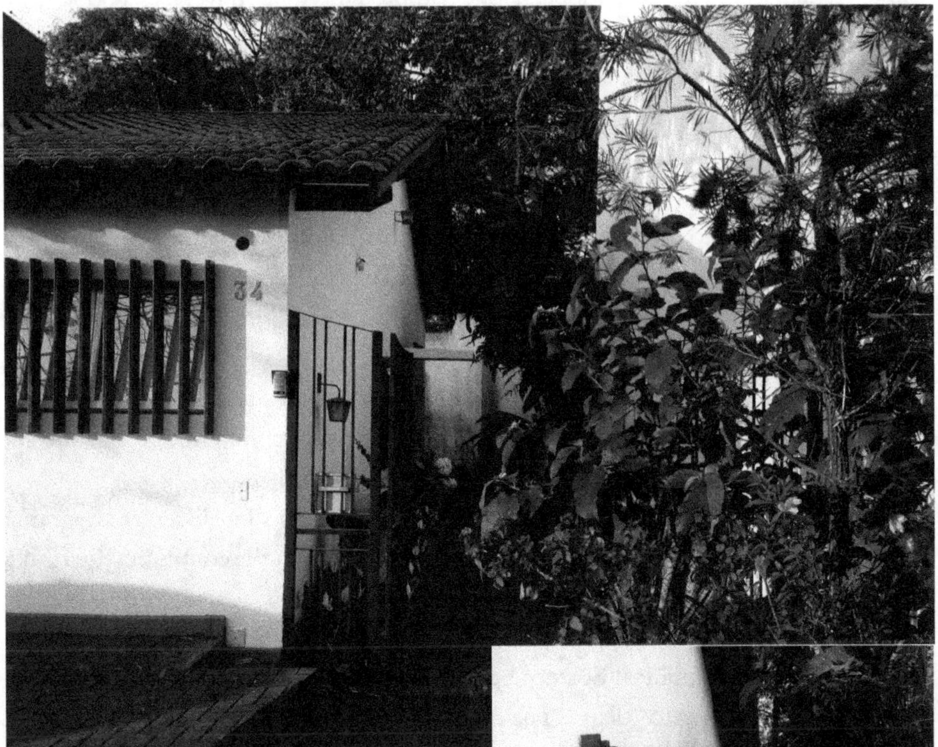

Photo 5.1: Exterior of Casa Angela.

Source: Photo by Natália Salim.

(All photos were taken by the researcher and are used with permission of the local co-ordination unit.)

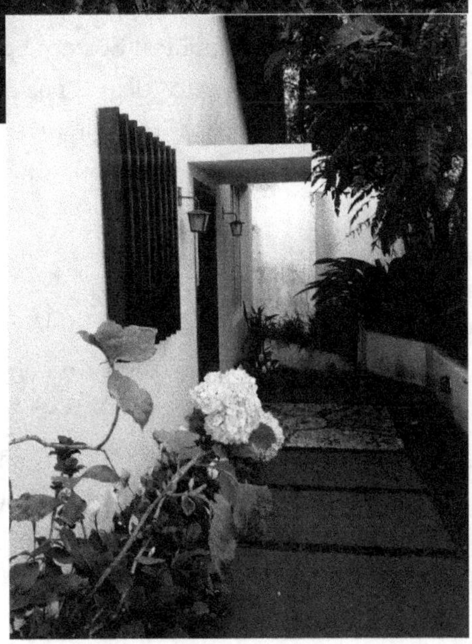

Photo 5.2: Exterior of Casa Angela.

Source: Photo by Natália Salim.

The Senses Involved in Childbirth

The data showed different values, meanings, and practices of childbirth care in obstetric care in each of the contexts studied. The women's stories emphasized the importance of their relationships with the professionals caring for them and with the environment in which they gave birth. For Juliana, giving birth at Casa Angela was an awakening experience. She stated:

> The way that they cared of me was inexplicable. During the whole time they explained to me what they were doing and what was happening. This made you fully aware at the time of the delivery. (Juliana, Casa Angela)

Rachel, who gave birth in a hospital birth centre, particularly noted the therapeutic measures which the nurses oversaw. She stated:

> They were two nurses watching me, making me doing exercises and putting me in the shower. What I liked and what helped a lot was the shower, I let the hot water fall on my back and that helped dilation a lot. (Rachel, obstetric centre)

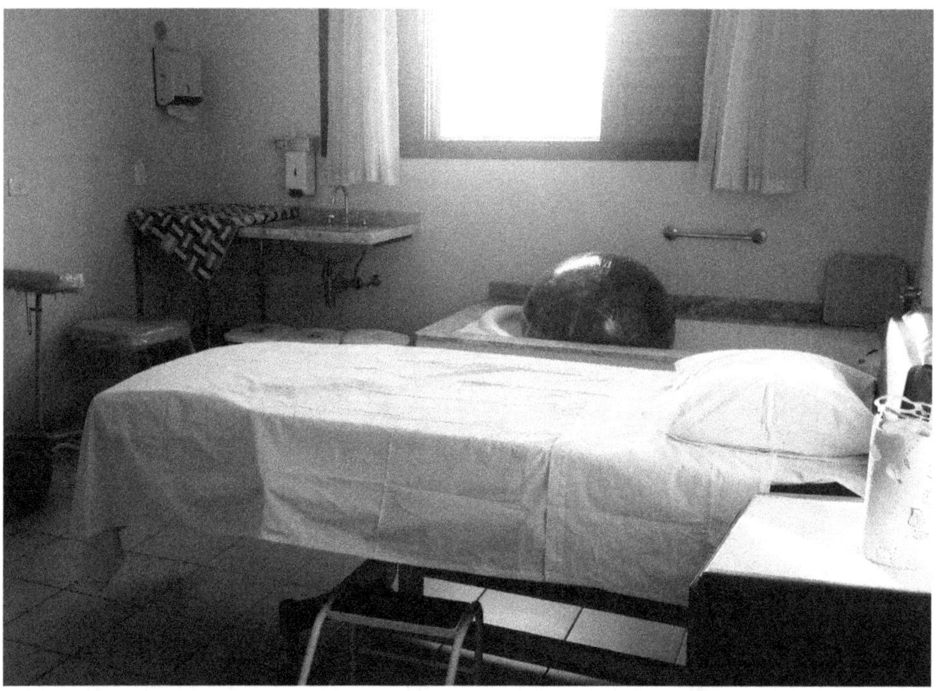

Photo 5.3: Delivery Room at Casa Angela.

Source: Photo by Natália Salim.

Luana talked about the reassurance she felt as a result of dialogue with her nurse. This highlights the importance of such individualized attention, as she explained:

> The nurse always talked to me and explained what was happening. The nurse would see me, put me in the bath, and this is what was important for me. If I had been alone I would have felt much more pain. (Luana, humanized birth centre)

By contrast, Bruna reported that she felt alone during labour:

> I was in pain and I called the nurse and she did not come. No one was with me, the doctor saw that I was in pain and did not come to help me. (Bruna, humanized birth centre)

There were different care practices and concepts about childbirth in the three different places. The views of the women were similar to attitudes and practices observed by the researcher. For example, the hospital settings were more bureaucratic, impersonal, and centred on biomedicine. Marina, giving birth at the obstetric centre, had this to say:

> The doctor stuck his arm in to pull out my baby; it was a lot of pain, and a lot of doctors pushed me. A doctor arrived and said, "the baby will be born soon." He pushed my stomach with his arm … she was born. (Marina, obstetric centre)

Vania, another patient at the same centre, said:

> The doctor told me not to disturb the other patients and make them feel uncomfortable. I could not scream as it was not allowed. (Vania, obstetric centre)

The women's narratives clearly show how relationships between patients and health care providers include a dynamic network of different actors and artifacts.[8] This reveals the multiplicity of practices of care in the birth scene in different settings. Often strict protocols appear as deterrents for choice and negotiations during the birthing process.

The conversations between the lead author of the chapter with women interviewed revolved around the importance of the senses during the event of giving birth. They shared their memories about the sensations attached to their experiences of giving birth.

> I remember that what struck me the most was how when the contraction came it was like a wave, coming very strong. The pain was so intense. By the time the contraction ended I do not remember anything. It was like waking up from a sleep and I woke up again. My delivery was my own birth, I think now I have become more aware of myself. (Bianca, Casa Angela)

Going through childbirth shows how different senses come into play, including improvisational skills and self-resilience as coping mechanisms for labour pains:

> I think that after childbirth I can face all challenges, I think there is no greater pain than childbirth. (Giulia, obstetric centre)

> The pain during delivery comes back and then disappears. The birth was a life lesson for me that you have to be yourself and not worry about what others say. (Luana, humanized birth centre)

The women's descriptions of their birthing experiences often emphasize how their sensations and feelings—as well as their own knowledge and control over their own bodies—were ignored. The narratives mirror the existence of hierarchical and power relationships between doctor and patient, where the patient is not conceived in her whole but only as a body deprived of feelings. This experience of the dichotomous relationship between the physical and the emotional spheres was more common in the hospital setting.

> I do not know what the strength of normal birth is; it's the baby who has the strength. I found it absurd that they ordered me to push before the baby got into the position. I did not want to lie; I wanted to stand up and they said "stay where you are!", "You cannot cry!", "You cannot scream!" "You can't do this or that." "Make the effort, push!" (Vanda, obstetric centre)

The women's experiences during giving birth seemed closely influenced by the different settings and contexts of childbirth.

> I liked the physical space of the hospital because it is not dirty. What ruins it is the behaviour of some people who work there. You must be aware that the service is different depending on the location. Not in every place they listen to you or ask how you're feeling or if you need something. In my case, I needed to go to the bathroom and the nurse refused to help me. (Giulia, obstetric centre)

Women spoke of the different comments they heard about the different places and how the experiences of relatives and acquaintances influenced their perceptions about these places.

> I heard about the horrible things about that hospital before. Even the nurse joked with me about that and said: "This is not a slaughterhouse." People said: "Are you going there? You're crazy." (Luana, humanized birth centre)

The biomedical discourse describing childbirth as a risky physiological event is evident in the interviews, where women were often discouraged from having a home birth. The technology available at the hospital, along with the expertise of a doctor, sometimes overrides the desire of women to have a "normal" birth at home, or at least it creates conflicts or discussions within families.

> My husband was worried and thought that it was dangerous [to give birth at home]. He was afraid, but I made up my mind and I was not scared. (Sara, Casa Angela)

> My mother was upset, she said: "How can you go to prenatal care where there is only a midwife?" I was afraid that a complication could arise but I knew they are trained to provide prompt care and have an incubator. (Carla, Casa Angela)

Casa Angela evoked, in the mind of the women interviewed, a familiar place in which the care providers were seen as familiar and friendly individuals. This relationship of intimacy between women and health care providers played an important role in the birth experience of these women:

> Here at Casa Angela they know my story, they know me and it's like a family; it's just that we do not have the same blood. (Ana, Casa Angela)

The women found Casa Angela to be alive and coherent with everyday life, comparing it with and differentiating it from the hospital environment. Women reported that they had their identities and their belongings respected, and contrasted it with the traditional hospital model. In this context, childbirth is seen as a natural event that is part of the life course.

> I think in Brazil there isn't a place where we are as well treated as there. I think it's an idea that has to be implemented in all places. I think birth centres need to be separated from the hospitals, they are a place of life. (Giulia, Casa Angela)

> I had my first child at the hospital and it was very different. At the hospital your husband leaves[9] you there, you need to leave your clothes and you can't take your personal belongings with you. You're alone for many hours during the contractions. (Sara, Casa Angela)

Conclusion

The women's narratives allow us to understand the different relationships that were established between women and health care providers, and to reflect on how different environments generate different feelings and experiences lived by women during the delivery process.

The settings available for childbirth provide different care practices which are embedded in a dynamic set of relationships among different social actors involved (e.g., women, health care providers, administrative staff, families) and available material objects (e.g., showers, bathtubs, balls, medicines, sonar) and other artifacts that make up the contexts of birth. It also became evident that there is a diversity of knowledge and models that are considered to be appropriate for the birth process.

In conclusion, each centre is characterized by a variety of health practices that shape the birth experiences. The "return to roots" movement, which advocates for a more natural birth practices, here epitomized by Casa Angela, shows how yet a new way of giving birth such as humanized birth centres co-exists side by side with a high-tech hospital birth setting in which midwives work together with medical doctors. As such, our research has shown how sensorial experiences of places and social relations represent an important aspect of giving birth as much as the physiological processes. Thus, both need to be considered equally, as the women's voices in this study tell us.

Notes

1. The voices and stories shared in this chapter are part of the lead author's PhD thesis entitled: *Childbirth contexts: Experiences, senses and practices of care*. The research was developed in three different contexts of care delivery in an economically disadvantaged region of the city of São Paulo.
2. The gap left by the phasing out midwifery courses was somewhat filled by the emergence of a midwifery specialization for nurses. Nurse-midwives continue to be trained in Brazil today, on a one-year course. However, it is important to note that the traditional midwives have always been present and active, especially in indigenous communities.
3. The term *humanization* has many senses. When it is used in the obstetrics field, it refers to a main objective of promoting childbirth as a dignified and respectful experience.

4. This was a campaign to encourage and incentivize women to have natural births (i.e., vaginally) and thus to reduce the number of medically unnecessary C-sections.
5. The midwifery training program in São Paulo city, which remained open until 1970, belonged to the School of the Faculty of Medicine. The profession is facing many struggles to establish in women's health field again in Brazil. For more information, see Gualda, D.M.R., Narchi, N.Z., & de Campos, E.A. (2013). Strengthening midwifery in Brazil: Education, regulation and professional association of midwives. *Midwifery, 29*(10), 1077–1081.
6. See www.sab.org.br/portal/index.php
7. See www.monteazul.org.br/home.php
8. Artifacts typically present in a childbirth scenario include doppler, birth chair, and birth bed.
9. Women are often not permitted to keep their personal belongings with them on hospital wards, and are generally required to wear a hospital gown instead of their own clothes, thus adding to the institutionalized feeling of the experience.

Critical Thinking Questions

1. Why is listening to women's voices about their own experiences of giving birth important in studies adopting an anthropological perspective?
2. How can anthropological approaches help us understand a childbirth context?

Glossary

Episiotomy: A cut in a woman's perineum (the area between the vagina and anus). The cut makes the opening of the vagina a bit wider. In many places episiotomy is routine; however, there is no evidence showing the benefits of its liberal use.

Kristeller manoeuvre: A uterine fundal pressure. It is a practice used without evidence and can be associated with harm to the woman and her baby.

Medicalization of childbirth: The medicalization of childbirth can be explained as a way to consider childbirth as a risky and pathological event. Thus, health practices are based only on the biological sphere, medical knowledge and technology become dominant, and the professional health care providers such as doctors and nurses are the central figures in the childbirth context. This can lead to the devaluation of the knowledge of women.

Partera* and *obstetriz: Brazilian words for midwife. Generally partera refers to a traditional midwife and obstetriz to a professional midwife.

References

Brennes, A.C. (1991). História da Parturição no Brasil, Século XIX. *Cadernos de Saúde Pública, 7*(2), 135–149. Portuguese.

Capra, F. (2006). O modelo biomédico. In F. Capra (Ed.), *O Ponto de Mutação* (26th ed.) (pp.116–155). São Paulo: Cultrix. Portuguese. (Original work published 1982.)

da Silva, A.G., & Galvão, M.L. (2010). *A parteira do Monte Azul*. D. Rattner & M.L. Galvão (Eds). Salvador, Brazil: JM Gráfica e Editora.

Davis-Floyd, R. (1992) *Birth as an American rite of passage*. Oakland, CA: University of California Press.

Diniz, S.G., & Chacham, A.S. (2006). O corte por cima e o corte por baixo: O abuso de cesáreas e episiotomias em São Paulo. *Questões de Saúde Reprodutiva, 1*(1), 80–91. Portuguese. Retrieved from www.mulheres.org.br/revistarhm/revista_rhm1/revista1/80-91.pdf

do Carmo Leal, M., da Silva, A.A., Dias, M.A., da Gama, S.G., Rattner, D., ... Szwarcwald, C.L. (2012). Birth in Brazil: National survey into labour and birth. *Reproductive Health*, *9*(15). doi: 10.1186/1742-4755-9-15

Domingues, R.M.S.M., Dias, M.A.B., Nakamura-Pereira, M., Torres, J.A., d'Orsi, E., ... Leal, M. (2014). Processo de decisão pelo tipo de parto no Brasil: Da preferência inicial das mulheres à via de parto final. *Cadernos de Saúde Pública*, *30*(Suppl. 1), S101–S116. Portuguese. Retrieved from https://dx.doi.org/10.1590/0102-311X00105113

Foucault, M. (1979). O nascimento do hospital. In R. Machado (Ed. & Trans.) *Microfísica do poder* (pp. 79–98). Rio de Janeiro, Brazil: Edições Graal.

Hotmisky, S.N. (2001). *Parto e Nascimento no ambulatório e na casa de parto da associação comunitária Monte Azul: Uma abordagem antropológica* (Master's dissertation). Universidade de São Paulo: São Paulo, Brazil. Portuguese.

Ingold, T. (1992). Culture and the perception of the environment. In E. Croll & D. Parkin (Eds), *Bush base, forest farm: Culture, environment, and development* (pp. 39–57). New York: Routledge.

Ingold, T. (2010). Da transmissão de representações à educação da atenção. *Educação Porto Alegre*, *33*(1), 6–25. Portuguese.

Jordan, B. (1993). *Birth in four cultures*. Prospect Heights, IL: Waveland Press.

Mol, A. (2002). *The body multiple: Ontology in medical practice*. Durham & London: Duke University Press.

Mott, M.L. (1999). O curso de partos: deve ou não haver parteiras. *Cadernos de pesquisa*, *108*, 133–160. Portuguese.

Mott, M.L. (2002). As parteiras e a assistência ao parto em São Paulo nas primeiras décadas do século XX. *Revista do Instituto Histórico Geográfico Brasileiro*, *163*(415), 67–84. Portuguese.

Persus Abramo Foundation/Núcleo de Opinião Pública da Fundação Perseu Abramo. (2010). *Pesquisa mulheres brasileiras nos espaços públicos e privados*. São Paulo, Brazil. Portuguese. Retrieved from www.fpabramo.org.br/o-que-fazemos/ pesquisas-de-opiniao-publica/pesquisas-realizadas/pesquisa-mulheres-brasileiras-nos-es

Pink, S. (2009). Principles for sensory ethnography: Perception, place, knowing, memory and imagination. In S. Pink, *Doing sensory ethnography* (pp. 23–43). London: Sage Publications.

Rattner, D. (2009). Humanizing childbirth care: Brief theoretical framework. *Interface—Comunicação, Saúde, Educação*, *13*(1), 595–602.

Salim, N.R. (2014). *Contextos de nascimento: experiências, sentidos e práticas de cuidado* (doctoral dissertation). Universidade de São Paulo, São Paulo, Brazil. Portuguese.

Victora, C.G., Aquino, E.M.L., Leal, M. do C., Monteiro, C.A., Barros, F.C., & Szwarcwald, C.L. (2011, 28 May). Maternal and child health in Brazil: Progress and challenges. *Lancet*, *377*(9780), 1863–1876. http://dx.doi.org/10.1016/S0140-6736(11)60138-4

Zorzam, B.A. de O. (2013). *Informações e escolha no parto: perspectivas das mulheres usuárias do SUS e da Saúde Suplementar.* (Master's dissertation). Universidade de São Paulo: São Paulo, Brazil. Portuguese.

CHAPTER 6

Intercultural Birth Practices and Reproductive Health in Ecuador

Costanza Torri, PhD
Department of Sociology, University of New Brunswick, Canada

Learning Objectives

1. To analyze how **traditional birth attendants** (***parteras***) have been incorporated into biomedical health services in Ecuador, and the power relationships between traditional medicine and biomedicine existing there.
2. To examine the processes of knowledge exchange between indigenous medicine and biomedicine within this intercultural health initiative and the possible transformations produced by these intercultural practices.
3. To analyze the conditions necessary to reduce the cultural marginalization of traditional midwifery and develop effective forms of co-operation between indigenous medicine and biomedicine.

Introduction

In the past few years in Ecuador, efforts have been made to reduce the cultural marginalization of traditional midwifery and to enhance more effective forms of co-operation between indigenous medicinal systems and biomedicine in order to promote "intercultural health." This concept of health emerged in Latin America in the 1990s and has recently achieved wide popularity, especially after the decentralization of health services (Turner, 2004). Within this context, intercultural health is understood as practices in health care that bridge or integrate aspects of traditional medicine and biomedicine, where both are considered as complementary and legitimate (see Hollenberg, Zakus, Cook & Xu, 2008/09).

It is worth asking to what extent these initiatives have been effective in promoting integration between indigenous/traditional health practitioners and biomedical staff, and what sorts of challenges the implementation of intercultural programs has faced. In order to answer these questions, this chapter presents a case study of San Luis Hospital in Otavalo, Ecuador, which operates an intercultural reproductive health initiative. This initiative was created with the objective of reducing local maternal morbidity and mortality by increasing the number of hospital births among indigenous women, while also ensuring that the cultural concerns of indigenous women giving birth in a biomedical setting were met.

The Public Health Ministry of Ecuador foresees implementing this practice in other hospitals nationwide. So far, intercultural maternity centres have spread from Otavalo to the provinces of Chimborazo, Amazonia, and Esmeraldas.

Intercultural Health Practices in Reproductive Health

Approximately 40 million people in Latin America and the Caribbean belong to the nearly 600 indigenous peoples of the continent, many of whom are located in Mexico, Peru, Guatemala, Bolivia, and Ecuador (Economic Commission on Latin America and the Caribbean [ECLAC], 2005) (see box 6.1). Traditional medicine is still practised in many indigenous communities in Latin America, despite the presence of biomedicine (Athais, 2004). Indigenous health care systems are characterized by a holistic conception of health, which does not view the body, mind, and spirit as separate entities but as integrated parts of the health ecosystem and the spiritual realm (Montenegro & Stephens, 2006).

According to the Pan American Health Organization (PAHO), "the concept of intercultural health involves equitable relationships which are respectful of the political, economic, social, and cultural differences between different cultures or ethnic groups in order to build a more just society" (PAHO, 2003, p. 30). "Intercultural" practices emphasize the importance of "cultural rights" and point to the government's responsibility to provide adequate health care through access to institutional medicine (Cujilema & Ochoa Dávila, 2003; Cunningham, 2002; PAHO, 2001). In Ecuador, the right to health care that considers the worldview and cultural factors of its users is guaranteed by the National Constitution (2008).[1]

The issue posed by intercultural health is not only political and economic but also epistemological, as it challenges the differential value assigned to knowledge that comes from groups within different socio-economic and cultural positions.

Central to Foucault's (1991) notion of discourse is the critique of an official or dominant knowledge system, and the investigation of forms of knowledge that are considered as subjugated or marginal. Salinas Mulder and colleagues (2000) emphasize the danger of an unequal relationship that usually accompanies the co-existence of diverse therapeutic traditions. According to these authors, intercultural health practices can be characterized by a form of domination by biomedicine vis-à-vis the indigenous medical system, thus creating a form of "hierarchical medical pluralism" (Brown, 2008; Cheung-Blunden & Juang, 2008; Conrad, 2007).

The history of the indigenous population in Ecuador has been marked by discrimination (Marschke, Szablowski & Vandergeest, 2008). Socio-cultural segregation as well as forced assimilation became the twin tools of domination by the European-origin population (Jeffrey, 2007; Rector, 2003). This social inequality is also reflected in the way that indigenous traditional practitioners are negatively perceived by biomedical health care providers, who are often non-indigenous.

In Ecuador, as in other developing countries, midwifery continues to play an important role in providing health care to women (Bailey, de Bocaletti, Barrios & de Cross, 2005; Cavender & Albán, 2009; Nigenda, Ruiz, Rosales & Bejerano, 2005). Worldwide, 53 percent of births are attended by biomedical health care providers, but only 40 percent of births occur in hospitals or health centres (Calvet-Mir, Reyes-García & Tanner, 2008). In Ecuador, only 30.1 percent of indigenous births occur in hospitals or health centres. In 2006, over 40 percent of women in the provinces of Bolivar, Chimborazo, Cotopaxi, and Esmeraldas, and about 30 percent of women across the Amazon region gave birth at home (Ministerio de Salud Pública, 2008a). The reasons for choosing to give birth at home are related to cultural, economic, and geographic factors (Foster, Anderson, Houston & Doe-Simkins, 2004; Rodríguez, 2009; Torres & De Vries, 2009; Walsh & Downe, 2004).

Box 6.1: Demographics

Ecuador is multicultural and multiethnic. According to the Seventh Population Census carried out by Ecuador's Instituto Nacional de Estadística y Censos (INEC) in 2009, 6.1 percent of the population over 15 years of age is considered to be indigenous, 5 percent Afro-Ecuadorian and mulatto, 77.7 percent ***mestizo***, and 10.8 percent white.

Otavalo is a largely indigenous town in the Imbabura province of Ecuador with a population of roughly 40,000 inhabitants. It is located in northern Ecuador, 90 kilometres from Quito, the capital. In Imbabura province, the indigenous population in 2009 amounted to 45 percent of the total population (Ministerio de Salud Pública, 2011).

In South America, reproductive health policies and programs that are more inclusive vis-à-vis the culture of the indigenous population are starting to be practised and enforced in health systems, especially at the local level (Davis-Floyd, 2003; Ministerio de Salud Pública, 2008b). Efforts have been made to expand and adapt the health services with the inclusion of symbolic and cultural elements and indigenous practices (Bailey, Szaszdi & Glover, 2002; Cosminsky, 2001).

Criticisms about the actual degree of implementation of intercultural health practices in Latin America have been emphasized in the literature (Doel & Segrott, 2003; Green, Bradby, Chan & Lee, 2006). Green (1989) stresses that even if medical pluralism is acknowledged, development plans often continue to embrace an old and misguided set of conceptions about traditional medicine and indigenous cultures (Alegria, Canino & Shrout, 2008; Belliard & Ramírez-Johnson, 2005; Hahn & Inhorn, 2010).

Against this background, this chapter aims to contribute to the debate of intercultural health practices by analyzing this case study in Ecuador. The following questions will be examined:

1. How have traditional birth attendants (*parteras*) been incorporated into biomedical health services? Are *parteras* still fulfilling the same functions they historically performed in their communities, or has their role changed as a result of collaboration with biomedical health care providers at the hospital? How have power relationships between traditional medicine and biomedicine been negotiated in this intercultural health initiative?
2. To what degree has a process of knowledge sharing between *parteras* and the biomedical staff taken place and what have been the consequences in terms of therapeutic practices for both indigenous medicinal systems and biomedicine?
3. Under what conditions is it possible to reduce the cultural marginalization of traditional midwifery in order to enhance more effective forms of co-operation between indigenous medicinal systems and biomedicine?

Case Study Presentation

The city of Otavalo is located 90 kilometres from Quito. According to the latest census data for 2008, it has 39,354 inhabitants, of which 52 percent are indigenous and 48 percent are non-indigenous. The area of Otavalo has one hospital and ten health centres. The hospital of San Luis, built in 1953, is located in the northern part of the city. According to the Ministry of Public Health (Ministerio de Salud Pública, 2011), the hospital offers "basic" health services, having 120 beds and offering four specialties: internal medicine, obstetrics, pediatrics, and general surgery.

In order to provide better care for indigenous women who are, in some cases, reluctant to access biomedical health care due to cultural barriers (among other reasons), an intercultural health unit was established in the maternity ward of San Luis Hospital in 2008. This initiative was funded by the United Nations Population Fund (UNFPA) and led by the hospital's biomedical team, in coordination with the provincial Department of Health of Imbabura (office of Intercultural Health) and the municipal government of Otavalo at the local level, as well as the Ministry of Public Health at the national level. The main features of this intercultural reproductive health model include (1) the participation of traditional *parteras* at delivery in the hospital; (2) the possibility for patients to decide on which position (i.e., vertical or horizontal) to give birth in; (3) the possibility for husbands and family members to be present during labour; and (4) the option to give birth in a separate room, decorated like a traditional bedroom in the indigenous culture, while assisted by biomedical health care providers and *parteras*.

The official statistics at San Luis Hospital show that of the 128 vertical births (see box 6.2) that took place in 2011, 42 patients (32.8 percent) were non-indigenous women and 86 patients (67.1 percent) were indigenous—in other words, a large majority of the vertical births occur among indigenous women. Official hospital data show that the percentage of indigenous women coming from rural areas to give birth at the hospital has increased since the beginning of this program, rising from 32.8 percent in 2008 to 45.4 percent in 2009, and to 47.2 percent in 2010, according to the statistics available at the San Luis Hospital.

Methods

The fieldwork for this study was carried out at San Luis Hospital between May and July of 2011. Fifty-seven interviews were conducted: 10 with *parteras*, 16 with pregnant women, 24 with women who had recently given birth, and 7 with biomedical

Box 6.2: Vertical Birth

Giving birth in a vertical position is commonly practised among indigenous people in Latin America. Vertical birth positions include squatting, resting on hands and knees, and standing. It is believed that a vertical position uses gravity to encourage labour to progress and ensure that the baby's head stays evenly pressed against the cervix. This pressure leads to a more consistent dilation and speedier labour.

health care providers (two doctors and five nurses) who worked in the delivery ward at San Luis Hospital.

Data were collected through semi-structured and structured interviews, and through observation at San Luis Hospital. Half of the patients interviewed were non-indigenous women, and the other half were women from an indigenous background. These women were waiting for their pre- or post-natal check-ups, and so were either pregnant at the time of interview or had given birth no more than approximately two months prior to being interviewed. The participants in this study were selected on the basis of age, education, and socio-economic background—this last factor being assessed on the basis of their current occupation and the average income of the household in which they lived. The age of the interviewees ranged from 21 to 43 years old.

Most of the *parteras* interviewed were in their early 60s (two thirds of the interviewees); the majority of the remaining *parteras* were in their early 70s. Their level of education was generally primary education (almost half of the interviewees; the other half were illiterate). Most interviewees had been practising traditional medicine for more than 40 years. The *parteras* were selected based on the geographic area where they lived (rural versus urban areas), the number of years of experience they had as traditional birth attendants, and their reputation within the community in Otavalo.

With prior consent, the interviews were recorded, transcribed, and subsequently translated into English. In order to ensure the anonymity of the participants in the study, their names have been omitted. Data have been summarized thematically, with illustrative quotations to capture the perspectives represented in the interviews.

Results and Discussion

Perceptions of *Parteras* Regarding Their Experience at the Hospital

All of the *parteras* emphasized that their motivation for being at the hospital was not based on economic considerations but on their willingness to provide a service for local women. Indeed, the *parteras* did not receive any remuneration for their work and were only reimbursed for their travel fees. However, the lack of monetary recognition might undermine the acceptance and sustainability of this intercultural health experience in the long term. One *partera* in her mid-40s affirmed: "I come here at the hospital totally on a volunteer basis. I have to come here three times a week and stay at the hospital overnight.... My husband is not happy at all and he says that I should stay at home or attend in the village instead of wasting my time and energy at the hospital without being paid."

Contrary to what happens in the community, where the *parteras* are completely in charge of every stage of the delivery, the *parteras* working in the hospital sometimes felt a lack of independence and were restricted in their role. Two thirds of the *parteras* interviewed drew attention to how their tasks at the hospital were generally limited to the care prior to delivery. They stated that they were rarely involved in the delivery itself, which was mainly carried out under the close supervision of biomedical health care providers. Some *parteras* found this limiting, but others described their role as complementary to that of the biomedical health care providers: the *parteras* were primarily concerned with the labour (e.g., alleviating pain with massage and herbal decoctions) whereas the biomedical staff attended to the delivery itself. It should be noted that the extent of *partera* participation in the delivery was left to the discretion of the biomedical staff, and so could vary considerably according to the decision of doctors on duty at the time of the delivery. For their part, the biomedical health care providers who were interviewed stated that the preferences of the patients played an important role in determining the degree of participation of the *parteras* during the delivery.

Although the relationship between the *parteras* and the biomedical staff at the hospital was perceived as far from equal by the *parteras*, the very presence of *parteras* in an institutional space previously denied to them nevertheless represents real progress in the process of social recognition of their role outside the indigenous community.

Exchange of Knowledge between *Parteras* and Biomedical Health Care Providers

The interviews with the biomedical health care providers and *parteras* drew attention to the limited exchange of knowledge between the *parteras* and biomedical staff. Although the *parteras* were offered some initial training on topics such as risk factors during pregnancy, HIV/AIDS, and violence against women, this was considered by them to be very limited. Two thirds of the *parteras*, especially the younger women in their 40s, expressed interest in enhancing their skills and being trained in other gynecological domains. This desire was not shared by the older *parteras*.

The interviews also highlighted how some *parteras*, again the younger ones in particular, had become more interested in learning about allopathic drugs, such as those used by biomedical health providers to expedite delivery (e.g., oxytocin) and reduce pain and bleeding. These *parteras* also wanted to be able to use these drugs in the community, believing that this would help women during their delivery. The administration of drugs without a biomedical practitioner's supervision is a particularly sensitive issue because of the risk of harmful interactions between these drugs and specific health conditions such as high blood pressure and diabetes.

Part of the *parteras*' attraction to being able to provide drugs may also derive from a desire to appear "modern" and "competent" in a society that looks with approval on biomedicine. This interpretation is consistent with the findings of a study carried out by Cosminsky (2001) in Guatemala. She writes, "[healers] are using certain aspects of the physician's role as their model, and thus acknowledging and reinforcing his prestige. However, it is primarily the technology and pharmaceuticals that they have adopted, reflecting both their own and their clients' faith in those aspects of Western medicine" (Cosminsky, 2001, p. 185).

Vertical Delivery and Other Traditional Practices

The doctors interviewed affirmed that the *parteras* taught them how to carry out vertical births. The practice of vertical delivery was praised by some doctors as being easier for the patients because it facilitated a faster delivery. The chief gynecologist at the ward stated that "vertical delivery, adopted by the Kichwa tradition, is a natural and instinctive process that makes physiological sense because it uses the force of gravity."

This positive perception of vertical delivery was also shared by some nurses (three), who expressed their interest in learning more about this traditional practice. These nurses explained that when they assisted in vertical deliveries at the hospital they noticed that the birthing process was easier and it involved less bleeding. Another advantage observed by the nurses was that the perineal tissues stretched more effectively, often reducing discomfort for the patients and/or the need for post-partum surgical repairs.

Despite this, two biomedical health care providers admitted that they did not feel comfortable with assisting women in vertical deliveries. They had not received training about vertical delivery at university because it was an indigenous practice and thus not considered relevant to biomedical practice. This finding is consistent with some ethnographies of pregnancy and delivery, which point out the divergence between the biomedical model that dominates the provision of formal health care and the traditional beliefs and practices surrounding birth (Bailey, de Bocaletti, Barrios & de Cross, 2005; Lorentzen, 2008). These differences in birth practices and beliefs are often a matter of concern for public health care professionals who fear that "traditional culture" may represent an "obstacle" to health, and for those who advocate for interventions to replace existing indigenous beliefs with more accurate information derived from biomedicine.

Intercultural Reproductive Health: Perceptions of Patients

Data show that a large number of non-indigenous patients found the presence of *parteras* psychologically reassuring. Patients felt that *parteras* were culturally and socially closer to them than the nurses or doctors, and said that they felt more secure and at ease with the *parteras* as a result. The non-indigenous women drew attention to the fact that *parteras* were able to administer a massage to reduce pain before the delivery. Patients also appreciated having the *parteras* available at the hospital because of their knowledge about medicinal plants and their uses during pregnancy and delivery.

Despite the general appreciation of *parteras* both by indigenous and non-indigenous patients, only a limited number of non-indigenous women delivered their babies in a vertical position or were willing to experiment with different delivery positions. This attitude could be explained by the fact that vertical delivery is still widely associated with indigenous culture and viewed as an indigenous practice. As Ginsburg and Rapp have noted (1995), reproduction beliefs represent an important site of defence and affirmation of cultural identity. My interviews indicated that few non-indigenous women wanted to be associated with indigenous culture. As one non-indigenous woman in her mid-30s from Otavalo stated: "I wanted to be attended by a *partera* as I like the *parteras* and they have a very good reputation but my mother-in-law said that mainly indigenous people are attended by *parteras* and give birth in a vertical position, not the mestizo and those who live in the city … so finally I gave birth with a doctor." Her words show how the process of choosing a medical system (i.e., indigenous medicine versus biomedicine) depends not only on cultural factors and beliefs but is also influenced by aspects such as identity perception and definition of indigeneity within a given society.

Non-indigenous women perceived the role of *parteras* more as "helpers" for biomedical health care providers, and preferred to rely more on biomedical staff at the moment of delivery. A preference for being exclusively assisted by a biomedical health care provider was shared by a quarter of the indigenous patients interviewed, especially those who were younger (aged 19–25 years old), living in the urban area, and had a higher education (secondary school or above). These patients felt that biomedical health care providers were more competent and knowledgeable, and that "modern" medicine was more "effective." They emphasized that although *parteras* had an important role to play at the hospital, it should be more as a back-up role for the biomedical staff instead of a prominent role, especially during the delivery.

By contrast, indigenous women from rural communities, with a lower level of education, and aged around 35 or older generally preferred to be assisted by the *parteras*. These women also preferred to give birth in a vertical position. This choice was justified by the firm belief, as one indigenous woman put it, that "*parteras* don't possess a formal knowledge as doctors do but they have a lot of experience in deliveries and dealing with pregnant women that sometimes doctors don't have." Here we can see how the notion of "legitimate knowledge" in regards to traditional midwifery practices and biomedicine is problematic and highly subjective; this notion is socially constructed and therefore socially contestable.

The interviews show that there are a variety of perceptions regarding the kind of knowledge that is valued and accepted. On the one hand, for some women, "legitimate" knowledge meant scientific knowledge, produced by and sanctioned through professional research (i.e., the knowledge of biomedical staff). For these patients, knowledge from non-scientifically validated origins is dismissed because it has not been validated through methods deemed acceptable by "experts." On the other hand, there are other women who regard the "experiential" knowledge of *parteras*, based on experience and constant practice, as more valuable.

Lessons Learned and Recommendations

A more integrative and culturally aware approach for reproductive health could be beneficial to improving the reproductive health of indigenous women. In order to achieve this change in the existing biomedical system, a number of barriers need to be overcome. Some recommendations would include the following considerations.

Intercultural Health Can Lead to Resistance and the Health System May Reflect Prejudices Present in Society

Beyond the existence of Ministry of Health guidelines and protocols to tailor health services to indigenous needs, the attitude of biomedical health care providers and society toward indigenous culture is central for the creation of health services that can truly be defined as "intercultural." This paradigm shift does not occur automatically but needs time to be fully understood and accepted by society.

Critics of intercultural health care practices assert that knowledge transfer may disregard the fact that social actors—including traditional birth attendants—make sense of their world as they interact with others (Davis-Floyd, 2003). Because meanings are rooted in people's perception of reality, and are in turn shaped by socio-cultural contexts, knowledge transfer needs to take into account people's meanings and visions of reality. When this is ignored, knowledge transfer may reinforce a vision of intercultural health based on a hierarchy of knowledge and practices, and competing knowledge systems (see box 6.3).

Box 6.3: Knowledge Transfer

Knowledge transfer (KT) is a term used to encompass a very broad range of activities as the means by which expertise, knowledge, skills, and capabilities are transferred from the "knowledge base" (experts in general, a university, a research centre, or a research technology organization, etc.) to those in need of that knowledge (an individual, group of people, company, or not-for-profit organization, etc.). (Mohan and Kumar, 2015).

Critics of KT caution that knowledge should not be confused with information and contend that it is not possible to "transfer" experiential knowledge to other people (Stake, 2005). Information consists of facts or understood data, whereas knowledge involves flexible and adaptable skills and is shaped by a person's ability to apply information.

It is important to keep in mind that for indigenous peoples, health is a complex phenomenon; it comprises not only an individual's physical and mental well-being, but also one's balance with nature, with the community of which one is a part, and with the rich and complex spiritual realm to which one is connected. The worldview or "cosmovision" of indigenous people is intrinsic to their well-being, and their concept of health must be understood within a social and cultural context (Janni & Bastien, 2004).

The emphasis on intercultural health should not focus solely on providing translation services in the indigenous language or in creating a space, such as a delivery area, which resembles an indigenous dwelling. On the contrary, efforts need to be aimed at enhancing the level of understanding and acceptance of traditional midwifery practices and indigenous birth beliefs among biomedical health care providers. It is also important to question the conviction that legitimate knowledge can only arise through methods accepted as valid by scientific researchers. A dynamic pluralism of knowledge in society would require a degree of openness around what constitutes knowledge, what is worth knowing, and how claims to knowledge are validated. Academic disciplines and professional bodies could no longer maintain their status as epistemologically closed systems with a monopoly on authority.

The Importance of Ensuring Links between *Parteras*/Communities and Health Centres

The services offered at San Luis Hospital and other intercultural reproductive health centres cannot be known by indigenous women if community-level birth attendants do not disseminate the information. Mainstreaming knowledge about the existence of these services within indigenous communities is important if an effective and sustainable intercultural health initiative involving traditional birth attendants and the local hospital is to be built. *Parteras* play an important intermediary role between health centres and indigenous women, and their presence both at the community level and hospital level can be very important in strengthening trust between indigenous communities and the biomedical staff.

Social networks composed of community leaders, local women, and *parteras* can also play a key role in sustaining this new approach of intercultural reproductive health, as well as in monitoring the functioning of this health model. Further studies should be undertaken with the objective of gaining more insight into the institutional contribution of this social network approach in promoting an intercultural health initiative, and to identify potential opportunities and challenges involved.

In order to achieve an intercultural health system, medical schools need to incorporate indigenous views into their curriculum. One of the reasons given by medical staff for resisting vertical childbirth was that this type of delivery technique is not taught in medical schools. There is a lack of knowledge and understanding of the cultural and technical rationale and advantages to offering culturally appropriate health services to indigenous women. This shows that universities—and in particular medical and nursing schools—need to modify their curricula to include cultural health studies. As one doctor at the hospital suggested, it would be beneficial to reach an agreement with universities and the Ministry of Health in order to teach ancestral practices at the medical schools. For example, the know-how of traditional midwifery could be included, and experienced *parteras* could play an active role in providing effective training for biomedical students and promoting the understanding of indigenous health beliefs and practices among future biomedical health care providers.

Overcoming the Existing Challenges

As highlighted by the *parteras* interviewed, one concern pertains to the issue of appropriate remuneration for *parteras* and how this could affect the sustainability of this initiative of intercultural health in the long term. The municipality of Otavalo only reimburses the *parteras* for their travel fees to go to the hospital, but the hospital does not provide any financial contribution to acknowledge the contribution of the *parteras* within the hospital.

A number of *parteras* explicitly stated that the lack of financial compensation made them feel that their work was not valued. Some of them also mentioned the difficult financial trade-off between working at the hospital versus in their community, because hospital work was unpaid. This needs to be taken into account as it could create conflicts within the health institution and affect the willingness of *parteras* to continue their collaboration at the hospital.

Another concern expressed by the interviewees was the ongoing power imbalance between biomedical health care providers and *parteras*. This is evident in the lack of an equal sharing of responsibilities between doctors, nurses, and *parteras*. The data show that *parteras* are still playing a limited role, their contributions mainly restricted to providing emotional and psychological support for the patients.

Although on certain occasions *parteras* played a more active role during the delivery, the definition of their professional role is rarely negotiated within the institutional setting at the hospital and is left to the discretion of the doctors. The unbalanced power relationship between indigenous medicine and biomedicine is also reflected by the fact that some traditional midwifery practices have been altered by the proximity of biomedical staff, notably those pertaining to the use of allopathic drugs. In contrast, medical staff, despite indicating interest in learning more about certain traditional practices such as vertical delivery, were nevertheless skeptical about or unreceptive to incorporating some of these practices, such as massage, into their techniques.

Conclusion

This study shows that, despite its challenges, the initiative of intercultural reproductive health implemented at the San Luis Hospital in Otavalo, Ecuador, represents an interesting model of cooperation between traditional midwifery and biomedicine. The data show that the contact between biomedical health staff and *parteras* can gradually help redefine the relationship and the involvement of the *parteras* both at the hospital and community levels. The presence of *parteras* at the hospital increased the patients' confidence in the local health care providers and facilitated a certain degree of exchange between the medical staff and the indigenous practitioners. The main challenge of this model is to improve health standards and overcome existing challenges, while at the same time replicating the experience in other health centres.

However, it is important to emphasize that the implementation of intercultural health itself does not necessarily provide an increased equality between indigenous and biomedical health systems. As long as inequality and discrimination vis-à-vis indigenous culture remain unchallenged, a truly respectful relationship between the biomedicine health care providers and traditional birth attendants will not develop. An effective intercultural reproductive health model needs to re-value traditional midwifery practices by enhancing the understanding of ancestral indigenous health practices and beliefs among health care providers, including the incorporation of such practices within the curriculum at academic institutions.

Due to the importance and topicality of intercultural reproductive health, the analysis of other case studies in Ecuador where these practices have been implemented is crucial in order to shed light on these pioneer initiatives in South America and move toward a more equitable and inclusive heath model for indigenous communities. Promoting intercultural health care practices in reproductive health through a mutual understanding and acceptance of differing views and practice in health between traditional medicine and biomedicine can help improve the cultural accessibility of health services in urban settings for indigenous women and thereby contribute to improving health outcomes for this population.

Acknowledgements

I am deeply grateful to the *parteras* and the women who participated in this research as well as the Jambi Wasi Clinic and the staff at the San Luis Hospital in Otavalo for facilitating this research.

Note

1. Article 363, paragraph 4 of the constitution of Ecuador states that "the state is responsible for ensuring health practices and alternative ancestral medicine by recognizing, respecting and promoting the use of their knowledge, medicines and instruments."

Critical Thinking Questions

1. What are the advantages of combining biomedicine and traditional midwifery practices in reproductive health? Do you think that these practices can make real improvements to the health of local communities?
2. What are the main obstacles to implementing sustainable and effective intercultural health care practices in the domain of reproductive health?
3. How can the initiative undertaken at San Luis Hospital in Otavalo be improved?

Glossary

Mestizo: A term used in Spanish-speaking America to mean a person of combined European and indigenous descent.

Parteras: A word used in many Latin American countries to indicate a traditional birth attendant.

Traditional birth attendants: A pregnancy and childbirth care provider who generally has not received formal education or training in health care provision. They often learn their trade through apprenticeship or are self-taught.

References

Alegria, M., Canino, G., & Shrout, P. (2008). Prevalence of mental illness in immigrant and non immigrant US Latino groups. *American Journal of Psychiatry, 1*(5), 359–369.

Athais, R. (2004). Indigenous traditional medicine among the Hupd'ah-Maku of Tiquie River (Brazil). *Indigenous peoples' rights to health conference and public meeting 2004* (pp. 44–52), London: London School of Hygiene & Tropical Medicine, Health Unlimited.

Bailey, P., de Bocaletti, E., Barrios, G., & de Cross, Y. (2005). Monitoring utilization and need for obstetric care in the highlands of Guatemala. *International Journal of Gynecology and Obstetrics, 8*(9), 209–217.

Bailey, P., Szaszdi, J., & Glover, L., (2002). Obstetric complications: Does training traditional birth attendants make a difference? *Pan American Journal of Public Health, 1*(1), 15–23.

Belliard, J., & Ramírez-Johnson, J. (2005). Medical pluralism in the life of a Mexican migrant woman. *Hispanic Journal of Behavioral Sciences, 2*(7), 267–285.

Brown, P. (2008). *Perspectives in medical sociology.* Long Grove, IL: Waveland Press.

Calvet-Mir, L., Reyes-Garcia, V., & Tanner, S. (2008). Is there a divide between local knowledge and western medicine? A case study among Native Amazonians in Bolivia. *Journal of Ethnobiology and Ethnomedicine, 18*(4), 18–32.

Cavender, A., & Albán, M. (2009). The use of magical plants by curanderos in the Ecuador highlands. *Journal of Ethnobiology and Ethnomedicine*, *5*(3), 1–9.

Cheung-Blunden, V., & Juang, L. (2008). Expanding acculturation theory: Are acculturation models and the adaptiveness of acculturation strategies generalizable in a colonial context? *International Journal of Behavioral Development*, *32*(1), 21–33.

Conrad, P. (2007). *The medicalization of society: On the transformation of human conditions into treatable disorders*. Baltimore, MD: Johns Hopkins University Press.

Cosminsky, S. (2001). Maya midwives of southern Mexico and Guatemala. In B.R. Huber & A.R. Sandstrom (Eds), *Mesoamerican healers* (pp. 179–210). Austin, TX: University of Texas Press.

Cujilema, M., & Ochoa Dávila, G. (2003). La salud indígena en Ecuador, mapa estratégico de la dirección nacional de salud de los pueblos indígenas. In D. Orellana Salvador (Ed.), *La salud en la globalización* (pp. 169–199). Quito, Ecuador: CIDES-Ecuador and Abya-Yala. Spanish.

Cunningham, M. (2002). *Etnia, cultura y salud: La experiencia de la salud intercultural como una herramienta para la equidad en las regiones autónomas de Nicaragua*. Ciencias Sociales Centroamericanas. Washington, DC: Organización Mundial de la Salud. Spanish.

Davis-Floyd, R. (2003). Home-birth emergencies in the US and Mexico: The trouble with transport. *Social Science & Medicine*, *5*(6), 1911–1931.

Doel, M., & Segrott, J. (2003). Beyond belief? Consumer culture, complementary medicine, and the disease of everyday life. *Environment and Planning*, *2*(1), 739–759.

Economic Commission on Latin America and the Caribbean (ECLAC). (2005). *The millenium development goals. A Latin American and Caribbean perspective*. Santiago, Chile: United Nations Publications.

Foster, J., Anderson, A., Houston, J., & Doe-Simkins, M. (2004). A midwifery model for training traditional midwives in Guatemala: A report from the field. *Midwifery*, *20*(3), 217–225.

Foucault, M. (1991). *Discipline and punish: The birth of a prison*. London: Penguin.

Ginsburg, F.D., & Rapp, R. (1995). *Conceiving the new world order: The global politics of reproduction*. Berkeley, CA: University of California Press.

Green, G., Bradby, H., Chan, A., & Lee, M. (2006). "We are not completely westernised": Dual medical systems and pathways to health care among Chinese migrant women in England. *Social Science and Medicine*, *6*(2), 1498–1507.

Green, L.B. (1989). Consensus and coercion: Primary health care and the Guatemalan State. *Medical Anthropology Quarterly*, *3*(3), 246–257.

Hahn, R.A., & Inhorn, M. (2010). *Anthropology and public health: Bridging differences in culture and society* (2nd ed.). Oxford: Oxford University Press.

Hollenberg, D., Zakus, D., Cook, T., & Xu, X. (2008/09). Re-positioning the role of traditional, complementary and alternative medicine as essential health knowledge in global health: Do they still have a role to play? *Journal of World Health and Population*, *10*(4), 62–75.

Janni, K.D., & Bastien, J.W. (2004). Special section on medicinal plants—exotic botanicals in the Kallawaya pharmacopoeia. *Economic Botany*, *58*(2), 274–282.

Jeffery, R.W. (2007). Indigenous struggle in Latin America: The perilous invisibility of capital and class. *Latin American Politics and Society, 49*(3), 191–203.

Lorentzen, J.M. (2008). "I know my own body": Power and resistance in women's experiences of medical interactions. *Body & Society, 14*(3), 49–79.

Marschke, M., Szablowski, D., & Vandergeest, P. (2008). Engaging indigeneity in development policy. *Development Policy Review, 26*(4), 483–500.

Ministerio de Salud Pública. (2008a). *Guia técnica para la atención del parto culturalmente adecuado.* Quito, Ecuador: Author. Spanish.

Ministerio de Salud Pública. (2008b). *Plan de reducción acelerada de la muerte materna.* Quito, Ecuador: Author. Spanish.

Ministerio de Salud Pública. (2011). *Informe nacional sobre la salud de los indígenas en Ecuador.* Quito, Ecuador. Spanish.

Mohan, A., & Kumar, R., (2015). Knowledge transfer: A basis for competitive advantage in organizations. *International Journal of Transformations in Business Management, 5*(3), 1–8.

Montenegro, R., & Stephens, C. (2006). Indigenous health in Latin America and the Caribbean. *The Lancet, 367,* 1859–1869.

Nigenda, G., Ruiz, J.A., Rosales, Y., & Bejerano, R. (2005). University-trained nurses in Mexico: an assessment of educational attrition and labor wastage. *Salud Publica de Mexico, 48*(1), 22–29.

Pan American Health Organization (PAHO). (2001). *Makewe-Pelale: Un estudio de caso en la complementriedad en salud.* Washington, DC: Author. Spanish.

Pan American Health Organization (PAHO). (2003). *Armonización de los sistemas de salud indígenas y el sistema de salud de las Américas. Lineamientos estratégicos para la incorporación de las perspectivas, medicinas y terapias indígenas en la atención primaria de la salud* (HSP/D#24). Washington, DC: Author. Spanish.

Rector, J.L. (2003). *The history of Chile.* Westport, CT: Greenwood Press.

Rodríguez, L. (2009). *Interculturalidad en salud reproductiva: Percepciones de las mujeres indígenas y prácticas de salud en el Hospital "San Luis de Otavalo," Ecuador* (Master's dissertation). Universidad Politécnica Salesiana, Quito, Ecuador. Spanish.

Salinas Mulder, S., Rance, S., Serrate Suárez, M., & Castro Condori, M. (2000).Unethical ethics? Reflections on intercultural research practices. *Reproductive Health Matters, 8*(15), 104–112.

Stake, R. (2005). Qualitative case studies. In N.K. Denzin & Y.S. Lincoln (Eds), *The SAGE handbook of qualitative research* (p. 456). Thousand Oaks, CA: SAGE.

Torres, J.M., & De Vries, R.G. (2009). Birthing ethics: What mothers, families, childbirth educators, nurses, and physicians should know about the ethics of childbirth. *The Journal of Perinatal Education, 18*(1), 2–24.

Turner, L. (2004). Bioethics in pluralistic societies. *Medicine, Health Care and Philosophy, 7*(2), 201–208.

Walsh, D., & Downe, S.M. (2004). Outcomes of free-standing, midwife led birth centres: A structured review. *Birth, 31*(3): 222–229.

CHAPTER 7

Giving Birth in the City of Cochabamba, Bolivia: Traditional Birth Attendants' Practices versus Biomedical Maternal Health Care

Costanza Torri, PhD
Department of Sociology, University of New Brunswick, Canada

Julie Laplante, PhD
Department of Sociology and Anthropology, University of Ottawa, Canada

Learning Objectives

1. To learn about indigenous birth practices in urban Bolivia.
2. To understand the motivations for giving birth at home versus in a hospital setting in urban areas.
3. To explore potential routes of dialogue between home and hospital birth practices.

Introduction

Bolivia is home to a culturally diverse population which, in 2009, was estimated at roughly 10,000,000 people (Instituto Nacional de Estadística [INE], 2012). The Aymaras and Quechuas, two indigenous groups in Latin America, make up the majority of the Bolivian population.

Bolivia still has the second-highest maternal and infant mortality rate, after Haiti, in Latin America (Pan American Health Organization [PAHO], 2009). In the case of Cochabamba, the fourth largest city in Bolivia with an approximate population of

1,938,401 according to the most recent census data (INE, 2012), the infant mortality in 2008 was 63 children per 1,000 live births, one of the highest rates in the country. This means that in 2008, more than 3,000 children in the district of Cochabamba died before their first birthday (United Nations Development Programme [UNDP], 2011).[1] In 2002, Bolivia developed a national social health insurance program directed toward improving maternal and infant health, known as Seguro Universal Materno Infantil (SUMI; in English: Universal Maternal and Infant Insurance). Despite the fact that the maternity services offered in the local hospitals are free, and despite geographic proximity to health services, approximately only one third of indigenous women continue to choose to give birth at a hospital. In the district of Cochabamba, 34,381 births were attended in hospital settings in 2009, which accounts for 68.4 percent of all births (INE, 2012).

This study analyzes multi-level factors that might help explain the lack of interest on the part of indigenous women living in the city of Cochabamba for locally available biomedical health care services for reproductive health. It explores the reasons why indigenous women tend to prefer giving birth at home with traditional birth attendants as opposed to in a hospital setting. Ways of touching bodies, of positioning the woman in labour, and of dealing with the **placenta**, among other matters, are viewed as sites of differentiation between traditional practices and newly offered biomedical practices. The chapter concludes by examining what can be changed to improve the dialogue between traditional medicine and biomedicine. The data collected in the field during the lead author's ethnographic research in the city of Cochabamba highlight the importance of promoting new ways of understanding birth that can represent an alternative to the biomedical model of giving birth.

Home versus Hospital Birth

Various researchers who begin with the premise that biomedical services should be used more frequently have focused on identifying barriers to delivery in hospitals or in other biomedical health centers (Ensor & Cooper, 2004; Ensor & Ronoh, 2005; Somanathan, 2005). The barriers identified by public health scholars and social scientists include poor geographic access (distance, poor road conditions, transportation problems, etc.) (Gohou, Ronsmans & Kacou, 2004; Graham et al., 2006), limited knowledge about the services available (Borghi, Ensor, Neupane & Tiwari, 2006; Kunst & Houweling, 2001; Lawn et al., 2004; Parkhurst, Danischevski & Balabanova, 2005), disrespectful attitudes of health care professionals (Nabukera et al., 2006), and feelings of psychological insecurity due to the fact that family members may not be present at the hospital (Hunt, Glantz & Halperin, 2002). Factors such as the quality, volume, and cost of services delivered by health care providers have also been acknowledged as important in determining willingness to access biomedical services during the delivery (Anderson et al., 2003; Kyomuhendo, 2003; Lai, 2004; Larsen et al., 2004).

The identification of barriers to the use of biomedical hospital services is, however, a limited approach for several reasons. First, it assumes that there are external barriers that can be identified and explained easily. Second, it promotes the idea that hospital births are the safest way to give birth rather than attempting to understand the reasons why many women prefer home birth. Third, it assumes that how and where one gives birth is an individual, "rational" decision. Anthropological approaches have increasingly drawn attention to the fact that, far from being an individual and rational decision, reproductive-related behaviour is embedded within a complexity of social relations and cultural institutions (Price & Thomas, 1999).

We argue that the mere examination of the financial or geographic barriers that hinder access to health care for pregnant women does not provide a complete explanation of why indigenous women prefer giving birth with the assistance of traditional birth attendants (*parteras*) rather than going to the hospital. Rather, beyond the possible "objective" barriers, it is also the detailed and "subjective" experiences of birth practices provided by women that might help us fully understand their preferred options for giving birth. By examining how pregnant women or those who have given birth describe their choices, we aim to understand and learn the practices they prefer during deliveries at home with traditional birth attendants.

Methodology

The fieldwork for this study was carried out by the lead author in the city of Cochabamba, Bolivia, between November 2009 and January 2010. Forty interviews were conducted, 10 with traditional birth attendants (*parteras*), 18 with pregnant women, and 12 with women who had recently given birth (i.e., within the two years of when the research was conducted). All of the women interviewed had delivered at least one of their children at home with a *partera*, or were planning to do so. Some of the women had also used the maternal health services available at governmental health facilities. The interviewees were selected through a purposive sample of reproductive-aged women (i.e., 18–45 years of age) residing in Cochabamba. Factors such as age, education, and average household income were considered in the selection process of the interviewees.

To understand why indigenous women in Cochabamba prefer traditional midwifery services to biomedical services, we interviewed a group of women who identified as belonging to the Quechua group, which is numerically the dominant ethnic group in the country. We addressed central questions such as the definition of ethnicity and "indigenous identity" by giving the participants the opportunity to define their own indigenous identity rather than ascribing it to them. During the selection process, participants were asked whether they considered themselves to be indigenous or non-indigenous. This approach is consistent with Denos and colleagues (2009), who assert that identities are unfinished and in process, and that people exert their agency to construct identities or reject imposed identities that position them in certain ways. We also avoided subscribing to a static notion of culture for the same reasons, understanding instead that culture is fluid and continuously negotiated and renegotiated. We furthermore did not equate culture with "belief," following the convincing arguments of Good (1994); we accepted that all practices, including biomedical ones, are culturally embedded and anchored in experiential knowledge. Hence, we embraced the idea that culture should be understood as a process that is continuously negotiated in practice, and that permeates both indigenous and biomedical practices.

The ages of the indigenous birth attendants interviewed ranged from 55 to 72 years, with an average age of 63 years. In terms of education, half of the participants had completed primary school, and half were illiterate. The *parteras* were selected with the help of SOBOMETRA, a local non-governmental organization, on the basis of their years of experience and popularity and social recognition within the community. We accept that this selection may be biased to the extent that our sample does not take into account *parteras* who are more marginalized or less popular in the community. Two thirds of the *parteras* interviewed were experienced traditional birth attendants with more than 30 years of practice. The interviews were semi-structured and mainly took place in the homes of the participants. All of the interviews were conducted in Spanish.

The themes discussed with the women who were pregnant or had recently given birth focused on their experiences with traditional birth attendants and maternal health services, their opinions of both kinds of services, and their motivations for choosing one service over the other. All responses were recorded with the permission of the participants and later transcribed. To ensure anonymity, names have been changed or omitted as appropriate.

Pre-natal Care and Delivery: Hospital versus Home

Interconnections between people and the environment are essential to understanding women's preference for home births. It is often stated by indigenous people that contact with medical staff in the hospital setting is "unhealthy," lacking "human touch" (literally and figuratively), and fails to consider particular ways of dealing with tangible and "material" objects, particularly with regards to the disposal of the placenta. Concerns about the hospital environment and its practices are thus a deterrent to giving birth in the hospital setting versus in a home setting.

Women mentioned the following main concerns, which will be discussed in more detail below:

- Poor medical attention received from medical staff and quality of health care
- Touching and delivery position
- Pregnancy care and massage
- Presence of the family and familiar environment during labour
- Presence of the family and familiar environment during delivery
- Hot and cold principles and the post-partum period
- The importance of rest and movement restriction after delivery
- The care of the placenta after delivery
- *Sobreparto* and confinement period after childbirth
- Controlling birth and use of contraceptives

Preferring to give birth at home may also be seen as a form of resistance by these women toward the hegemonic role of the biomedical staff over their bodies. The application of a feminist approach to medicine highlights how medical knowledge can be used as a form of power over women's bodies and how the apparently natural processes of reproduction and women's sexuality are defined as a medical condition requiring "expert" masculine knowledge, treatment, and intervention (Berenson, Miller & Findlay, 2009; Utz, 2011).

Poor Medical Attention Received from Medical Staff and Quality of Health Care

The majority of women interviewed said that poor medical attention at hospitals was the primary reason they preferred to deliver at home. It has been shown that indigenous women in hospital settings are subordinated to the biomedical health care providers (Canessa, 2006). The fact that many health care providers are middle- and upper-class men may further reinforce gender inequalities and ethnic discrimination in interactions with patients. More than two thirds of the participants (22 women) were reluctant to access or avoided accessing maternal health services due to what they perceived as impolite or inappropriate behaviour and attitudes of health care professionals. For instance, one woman stated, "if doctors were kind and paid careful attention to me, I would go to the health centre for the purpose of delivery. But as this is not the case, I will call a traditional midwife and deliver at home."

Thirteen of the women interviewed also identified financial affordability of care as a significant deterrent for indigenous women, in addition to their distrust of the medical system. As a 35-year-old woman put it: "Medicine is very expensive; it is like a business for doctors. Sometimes we only have money to pay the visit but not to buy the medicines. If you go to the hospital, medicines that are given for free are not effective, so you have to go to the chemist shop and get others for which you have to pay. I don't trust doctors and I avoid them as much as I can."

Women also noted that many indigenous people are not able to communicate fluently in Spanish and also cite the existence of language barriers resulting in poor communication between medical staff and indigenous patients. Women's lack of trust of biomedical staff is clearly summarized by one interviewee: "Doctors don't speak our language, don't know our customs and beliefs and despise us. If we go to health centres we are treated poorly and doctors don't explain too much or talk too much with us. They treat us as objects." Notwithstanding the issues of trust and understanding revealed in this woman's remark, it does reflect accurately one of the central principles of most biomedical practices, according to which bodies are treated as mere objects of intervention for health purposes and not complex entities connected to the emotional and spiritual spheres of an individual.

It should also be said that doctors are given very little specific training in indigenous practices, and are thus ill-prepared for the nuances of various communication skills, cultural beliefs/knowledge, and diversity. Our interviewees suggested that the time constraints of modern medical health care delivery may also limit doctors' ability to address the emotional needs of their patients.

Touching and Delivery Position

In indigenous practices, touching a pregnant woman's belly and talking about sexual relations and reproductive health are considered to be inappropriate, whereas biomedical health providers consider these practices to be fully normal. In one interviewee's words: "It was a humiliating experience indeed. Doctors were coming from time to time to see how dilated I was, they put their hand in my intimate parts and then called younger doctors to show them so that they could learn. I felt very embarrassed and humiliated."

Traditional birth attendants also touch the pregnant woman; however, they do not put their hand inside her vagina during labour to check the dilation of women's cervixes internally. As the labour progresses, the midwife takes the woman's pulse and feels her belly to determine the degree of descent of the baby or by doing abdominal palpation. This practice contrasts with the practices of traditional birth attendants in other places, who might perform vaginal examination in labour (Fronczak et al., 2007).

The majority of the indigenous women interviewed considered delivery position to be very important, preferring to give birth in a standing or vertical position which they found eased the delivery of the baby. As the interviewees explained, at the hospital women are obliged to give birth in a horizontal position. The procedure for giving birth in the hospital was designed to facilitate the doctor's task, so that the doctor is "giving birth," so to speak. The horizontal position allows the doctor to observe the delivery process, but it is not necessarily a position that ensures a comfortable delivery for the woman.

Pregnancy Care, Massage, and the Presence of the Family During Delivery

Some traditional practices are condemned by medical doctors but are widely accepted and practised among local traditional birth attendants. One of these is a traditional massage (*sobada*) administered to pregnant women by *parteras*.

The massage is used to determine the exact position of the baby, so that the *partera* can move it into an upright position for delivery. If the baby is lying across ("as a horizontal bridge"), the midwife rubs on both sides of the mother's belly so that the baby can return to the upright position. Problems are also identified through this massage, such as the case of a baby that is positioned "too low," making the woman unable to walk, or when the baby is "set too high," putting pressure on the woman's chest. The massage technique is performed by placing both hands on the woman's stomach, moving toward the centre from both sides. *Parteras* check the woman's pulse to assess her condition; based on this, a specific massage will be performed.

Although there is no scientific evidence that this practice is harmful, the *parteras* interviewed mentioned that nurses and doctors are skeptical about it, and in certain cases oppose it altogether. In fact, it is precisely because there is no scientific evidence supporting the effectiveness of this practice that it is deemed not useful and in some cases even harmful, if it is done too vigorously or in a prolonged way.

These findings are consistent with some ethnographies of pregnancy and delivery, such as those of Nyonator in Ghana and of Salim and Laplante in Brazil discussed in this book, which also point out the divergence that exists between the biomedical model that dominates the provision of formal health care and local beliefs and practices surrounding birth (Bailey, de Bocaletti, Barrios & de Cross, 2005; Lorentzen, 2008). This discrepancy is a matter of concern for public health professionals who fear that traditional culture may represent an obstacle to health, and for those who advocate interventions to replace existing beliefs with more accurate information derived from biomedicine. What is understated in this rationale is that biomedicine is not understood as also culturally embedded. This perhaps paradoxically creates a greater obstacle to health because it precludes the possibility of dialogue. Biomedical practices are, however, culturally embedded; acknowledging this would permit much richer interchanges to find the best ways to give birth incorporating both sets of practices. Our suggestion is thus to find ways to recognize that experiential skills are valuable in facilitating birth and that these kinds of skills should not be ignored or overlooked in health policies.

The women interviewed mentioned that they preferred delivering at home due to the presence of their family members. This priority highlights the benefits of physical and emotional proximity with the husband and other family members, as well as the reassurance of giving birth in a warm, private, and familiar space. However, maternity wards in hospitals and health clinics have transformed childbirth into a nearly public and technical act, where several strangers provide care and women feel uncomfortable in the impersonal labour rooms.

Hot and Cold Principles and the Post-partum Period

As the women's comments about their desired birthing environment have shown, concerns related to "warm" and "cold" are of pivotal importance. These include intimacy versus open spaces, human versus "medical" touch, and family versus strangers. The ways in which the experience of giving birth is organized are just as important in the post-partum period as they are in dealing with some complications that may occur after delivery. The concepts of warm and cold, both during and after delivery, are considered of great significance for indigenous women and *parteras*. Conversely, temperature during childbirth is disregarded in hospital settings. According to *parteras*, warm food and beverages are preferred before delivery, and the mother should be well covered in order to counteract the body's cold temperature, as well as avoid the cold in general.

According to indigenous humoral theory, the body, which becomes "hot" during the delivery process, passes into a state of "cold" after childbirth. When the baby is born, the uterus opens and allows cold air to enter, thus cooling the blood. Consequently, it is considered extremely important to keep the body warm during the post-partum period, especially those parts that are considered "open" and thus more exposed to the cold. For this reason, women are advised to wear gloves, socks, and a wool cap after childbirth. The ritual washing of the mother's body is done with water heated on a stove, to which warming herbs such as rosemary (*Rosmarinus officinalis*) or sage (*Salvia officinalis*) are added.

According to the *parteras* and the women interviewed, doctors are unable to assist pregnant women as they do not understand the importance of paying attention to the principles of "hot" and "cold." A 38-year-old woman stated: "A friend of mine went to give birth at the hospital. It was a very bad experience for her. Before giving birth they asked her to wear a light shirt and she felt cold all the time. This is why I don't want to give birth at the hospital and I prefer having my children at home with a *partera*."

The Importance of Rest and Movement Restriction After Delivery

The amount of rest needed, as well as the best position for resting after delivery, is also considered important. It is common for health care services to discharge women the same day as their delivery or on the following day. From the point of view of *parteras*, this is too dangerous for women, since women are very weak from loss of blood during the first three days after birth, so that catching cold could potentially make them very sick.

According to the indigenous women interviewed, the woman should lay down as much as possible after giving birth. They do not recommend remaining in a sitting position, as this clots the blood and makes it difficult for it to flow out in order to cleanse the body. The traditional period of rest after delivery is not fully understood by biomedical staff, who do not prescribe any movement restrictions to women after delivery. This was criticized by all the traditional birth attendants interviewed who recommended that a woman who has given birth should not leave the house for a week or two, and, in the meantime, should rest in bed and take herbal remedies to cleanse the blood.

The Care of the Placenta After Delivery

Because indigenous culture treats the expulsion of the placenta as another birth, the placenta and its symbolism of life and death are given special attention. Once the placenta is expelled, a placenta burial ritual (i.e., death ritual) is performed. Contrary to indigenous practices and beliefs, biomedical staff do not pay particular attention to the placenta during the delivery process, and it is disposed of as hospital medical waste. The idea that the placenta can be thrown away is extremely repugnant to members of traditional Andean cultures, and is understood as the equivalent of exposing a corpse (see box 7.1).

Box 7.1: The Placenta

Among the indigenous people of South America the placenta is generally burned after birth to neutralize it, and the remains are planted in the ground to protect it from evil spirits. The indigenous Bolivian Aymara and Quecha people recognize a spirit in the placenta. The placenta is considered to be a nursing mother with a life of her own. After delivery the placenta must leave the woman's body and return to the earth from whence it came. It is to be washed and buried by the husband in a secret place, normally close to the house. If this ritual is not performed properly, it is believed that the mother or baby may become ill or even die.

Sobreparto

The divide between beliefs/knowledge in how infection in the puerperal period (locally known as ***sobreparto***) is treated was also highlighted in the interviews. The period after delivery is considered risky by both traditional medicine and biomedicine. According to biomedicine, *sobreparto* is caused by an infection and should be treated primarily with antibiotics. In contrast, indigenous **ontology** attributes post-partum illnesses to increased vulnerability to evil spirits that may cause harm during this critical time. One of our respondents explained: "I don't go to the hospital because they don't understand indigenous culture. Doctors are unable to cure some women's health issues after delivery, such as *sobreparto*. When indigenous women try to explain the concept of *sobreparto* to doctors or nurses, they look at us in a strange way and they don't believe us. It does not make sense to them."

Controlling Birth and Use of Contraceptives

Two thirds of the women interviewed stated that they did not use "modern" contraceptive methods prescribed by doctors, despite having sources of information and access. Women also highlighted that the issue of contraception and what they perceived as an interference of the biomedical system in a personal and delicate sphere such as family planning was another reason why they were sometimes reluctant to approach biomedical health services for their reproductive health. Eight women stated that they preferred using "natural" methods to prevent pregnancy, such as abstinence or the pull-out method (*coitus interruptus*), because they believed that modern contraceptives have negative effects on the female body. One can wonder to what extent the women's opinions may be influenced by the views of their husbands, and how the men from indigenous communities feel about more modern contraceptive methods. The women interviewed thought that contraceptive injections can produce stomach pains and irregular bleeding.[2] In their view, doctors encourage the use of contraceptives without considering the side effects they may produce in women in the long term. Some of the women reported a popular belief that using contraceptive pills or injections may make a woman "crazy" because contraception can dramatically increase their sexual desire and lead them to promiscuity.

In one woman's words: "We should not go to the doctors because they want to prescribe us contraceptive pills or give us injections not to have children. These drugs can make us dizzy and make us become mad. [...] People say that contraceptive pills make women sick both physically and mentally. This is why I don't trust doctors and what they prescribe to us." It bears noting that most of the women interviewed were Catholic: one can wonder how their religious beliefs, as well as the role of traditional patriarchal views, may have shaped their attitudes toward the acceptability and risks of contraceptive use.

Although perceived negative experiences of biomedical interventions contribute to a woman's decision to avoid biomedical reproductive health care, another factor may be that the decision of whether or not to use contraceptives is made by men in most cases. Contraceptive use is played out in contexts of domestic violence, conflicted norms of masculinity, and limited socio-economic opportunities for women, and it is important to consider that personal health care and decision making take place in unequal socio-cultural contexts. If a woman does not want to get pregnant she must ask her husband's "permission" to use contraception. Many men do not grant this permission because they think it makes women unfaithful and that they might lose sexual control over their wives. One woman stated: "My mother wanted to go to see a doctor to have an injection not to have more children but my dad harassed her and prohibited her to go to the clinic. [...] Finally he forced her to have more children with him although she did not want to." This is consistent with existing literature showing how power over decisions—notably about health and health care—is distributed differentially by gender, thus contributing to gender inequalities and women's lack of capacity to make decisions about their health and their bodies (Armstrong, 2009; Curtis & Sutherland, 2004).

Conclusion

Listening to the voices of indigenous women in Cochabamba helps us understand why they choose to give birth at home. This birth choice is consistent with their views that giving birth in a more intimate way is healthier and safer for the mother and baby. While the hospital may be geographically close, in the minds of many women we interviewed it was associated with risks such as being exposed to dangerous cold and drafts, anonymity, and intimidation. For many women, giving birth at home follows other protocols meant to ensure the best way of giving birth, which clearly outweigh the disadvantages of foreign spaces and practices.

At the beginning of this chapter we cited data about maternal and infant mortality in Bolivia: listening to our participants gives insight on the alternatives chosen by women to ensure the safest way of giving birth as well as deal with death. Should complications arise, prompt transportation to the hospital—which generally deals effectively with emergency situations—should be organized. Data shows how the practices followed by the traditional birth attendants characterized by touch, proximity, warmth, and intimacy, are perceived by the women to be useful and effective. The women interviewed made it clear that they prefer the assistance of parteras in order to give birth in their homes. We learned from the indigenous women of Cochabamba that their preference for traditional home births is not only based on rational or practical considerations but is also thoroughly embodied. Their preferred space and organization in giving birth takes into account the interconnections of bodies in the world, and what is thought to be the ideal way to give birth. In their view, keeping the women's bodies warm, at home, and in gentle hands is the best way to ensure both maternal and infant health. It is in bracketing the "biological" as the sole way of knowing bodies that these practices can be recognized as legitimate. These interviews show that there is more to giving birth than the act of delivery and post-partum. During nine months or so, mother and child grow together in a particular world environment and will continue to do so afterwards. Although biomedical experts may suggest that it is safer for women to give birth in the hospital, the women interviewed expressed concern about the potential for harm resulting from the discomfort they felt in a hospital setting. Future research should explore the precise conditions surrounding maternal and infant mortality, ideally anchoring the enquiry in the intricacies of how these lives are lived and experienced as bodies-in-the-environment.

Acknowledgements

We are grateful to the *parteras* and traditional practitioners in Bolivia; the Consejo Departametal de Medicina Tradicional (Departmental Council for Traditional Medicine) in Cochabamba; and in particular to Jesus Gomez Paye, Vidal Montaño Roman, and Nidia Bustillos for all their support during the fieldwork in Cochabamba.

Notes

1. Bolivia is a unitary state consisting of nine departamentos, or provinces. These departamentos are the primary subdivisions of Bolivia, and possess certain rights under the Constitution of Bolivia.
2. The contraceptive injection contains a progestogen hormone. The progestogen is injected into a muscle or under the skin from where it is gradually released into the bloodstream.

Critical Thinking Questions

1. What do you think makes home births more appealing than hospital births for women in Cochabamba?
2. What is the importance of culture in making decisions about birth practices and behaviours?
3. In seeking to be open and to accept different ways of giving birth, how can the understanding of experiential practices provide a way forward for more effective reproductive health care?

Glossary

Ontology: The study of the nature of being, becoming, existence, or reality, as well as the basic categories of being and their relations.

Partera: Traditional birth attendant, normally without a formal medical education, in Bolivia and other Latin American countries.

Placenta: An organ that connects the developing fetus to the uterine wall to allow nutrient uptake, waste elimination, and gas exchange via the mother's blood supply.

Sobreparto: Local term used in Cochabamba to describe symptoms experienced by new mothers, such as weakness, general malaise, headaches, and body aches, which may persist for days after delivery.

References

Anderson, L., Scrimshaw, S., Fullilove, M., Fielding, J., & Normand, J. (2003). Culturally competent healthcare systems: A systematic review. *American Journal of Preventive Medicine, 24*(3), 68–79.

Armstrong, P. (2009). Public policy, gender, and health. In D. Raphael (Ed.), *Social determinants of health: Canadian perspectives* (2nd ed.) (pp. 350–361). Toronto: Canadian Scholars' Press, Inc.

Bailey, P., de Bocaletti, E., Barrios, G., & de Cross, Y. (2005). Monitoring utilization and need for obstetric care in the highlands of Guatemala. *International Journal of Gynecology and Obstetrics, 8*(9), 209–217.

Berenson, C., Miller, L., & Findlay, D. (2009). Through medical eyes: The medicalization of women's bodies and women's lives. In S. Bolaria & H. Dickinson (Eds), *Health, illness, and health care in Canada* (pp. 239–258). Toronto: Nelson Education.

Borghi, J., Ensor, T., Neupane, B., & Tiwari, S. (2006). Financial implications of skilled attendance at delivery: The case of Nepal. *Tropical Medicine International Health, 1*(1), 228–237.

Canessa, A. (2006). Todos somos indígenas: Towards a new language of national political identity. *Bulletin of Latin American Research, 25*(2), 241–263.

Carrillo, H. (2002). *The night is young: Sexuality in Mexico in the time of AIDS.* Chicago: University of Chicago Press.

Curtis, S.L., & Sutherland, E.G. (2004). Measuring sexual behaviour in the era of HIV/AIDS: The experience of demographic and health surveys and similar enquiries. *Sexually Transmitted Infections, 80*(2), 22–27.

Denos, C., Toohey, K., Neilson, K., & Waterstone, B. (2009). *Collaborative research in multilingual classrooms.* Bristol, UK: Multilingual Matters.

Ensor, T., & Cooper, S. (2004). Overcoming barriers to health service access: Influencing the demand side. *Health Policy Plan, 1*(9), 69–79.

Ensor, T., & Ronoh, J. (2005). Effective financing of maternal health services: A review of the literature. *Health Policy, 7*(5), 49–58.

Fronczak, N., Arifeen, S., Moran, A., Caulfield, L., & Baqui, A. (2007). Delivery practices of traditional birth attendants in Dhaka slums, Bangladesh. *Journal of Health Population and Nutrition, 25*(4), 479–487.

Gohou, V., Ronsmans, C., & Kacou, L. (2004). Responsiveness to life-threatening obstetric emergencies in two hospitals in Abidjan, Cote d'Ivoire. *Tropical Medicine International Health, 9*(2), 406–415.

Good, B.J. (1994). *Medicine, rationality, and experience. An anthropological perspective.* Cambridge: Cambridge University Press.

Graham, W.J., Cairns, J., Bhattacharya, S., Bullough, C.H.W., Quayyum, Z., & Khama, R. (2006). Maternal and perinatal conditions. In D.T. Jamison, J.G. Breman, A.R. Measham, et al. (Eds), *Disease control priorities for developing countries* (2nd ed.) (pp. 499–530). Washington, DC: World Bank.

Hunt, L.M., Glantz, N.M., & Halperin, D.C. (2002). Childbirth care-seeking behavior in Chiapas. *Health Care Women International, 23*(1), 98–118.

Instituto Nacional de Estadística (INE). (2012). *Censo Nacional de Población y Viviendas. Características de la población: autoidentificación* étnica. Vol. 4. La Paz, Bolivia: Author. Spanish.

Kunst, A.E., & Houweling, T. (2001). Inequalities in the utilisation of delivery care and other maternal health services. *Studies in Health Services Organization and Policy, 1*(7), 297–315.

Kyomuhendo, G.B. (2003). Low use of rural maternity services in Uganda: Impact of women's status, traditional beliefs and limited resources. *Reproductive Health Matters*, *11*(3), 16–26.

Lai, D. (2004). Impact of culture on depressive symptoms of elderly Chinese immigrants. *Canadian Journal of Psychiatry*, *49*(12), 820–827.

Larsen, G.L., Lupiwa, S., Kave, H.P., Gillieatt, S., & Alpers, M.P. (2004). Antenatal care in Goroka: Issues and perceptions Papua New Guinea. *Medical Journal*, *47*(4), 202–214.

Lawn, J.E., Cousens, S., Bhutta, Z.A., Darmstadt, G.L., Martines, J., Paul, V., ... Horton, R. (2004). Why are 4 million newborn babies dying each year? *The Lancet*, *364*, 399–401.

Lorentzen, J.M. (2008). "I know my own body": Power and resistance in women's experiences of medical interactions. *Body & Society*, *14*(49), 49–79.

Nabukera, S.K., Witte, K., Muchunguzi, C., Bajunirwe, F., Batwala, V.K., Mulogo, E.M., ... Salihu, H.M. (2006). Use of postpartum health services in rural Uganda: Knowledge, attitudes, and barriers. *Journal of Community Health*, *31*(2), 84–93.

Pan American Health Organization (PAHO). (2009). *Health Situation in the Americas: Basic Indicators 2009*. Washington, DC: Author.

Parkhurst, J.O., Danischevski, K., & Balabanova, D. (2005). International maternal health indicators and middle-income countries: Russia. *British Medical Journal*, *331*, 510–513.

Price, N.L. & Thomas, N. (1999). Continuity and change in the Gwembe Valley Tonga family and their relevance to demography's nucleation thesis. *Africa*, *69*(4), 510–548.

Somanathan, A. (2005). *Critical assessment of the extent and mechanisms by which maternal and newborn health care expenditure requirements exacerbate poverty*. Geneva: World Health Organization.

United Nations Development Programme (UNDP). (2011). *The road to development in Cochabamba*. La Paz, Bolivia.

Utz, R. (2011). Like mother, (not) like daughter: The social construction of menopause and aging. *Journal of Aging Studies*, *25*(2), 143–154.

CHAPTER 8

Women, *Jamu*, and Breast Feeding Practices in Indonesia

John Paul Nyonator, PhD candidate
Department of Sociology and Anthropology, University of Ottawa, Canada

Learning Objectives

1. To gain awareness of how women in Indonesia experience insufficient production of breast milk.
2. To understand how *jamu*, a traditional Indonesian medicine, is used by women in Central Java to improve their production of breast milk.

Introduction

Breast feeding is regarded as the optimal form of infant nutrition (American Academy of Pediatrics, 2012; World Health Organization [WHO], 2003). Public health and medical literature indicates that breast feeding has positive short- and long-term health benefits for both infant and mother (American Academy of Pediatrics, 2012; WHO, 2003). Exclusively breastfed infants have lower rates of gastrointestinal and respiratory infections (Howie et al., 1990); middle-ear infections (Jackson & Nazar, 2006; Scariati, Grummer-Strawn & Fein, 1997); diarrhea (Arifeen et al., 2001; Scariati, Grummer-Strawn & Fein, 1997); asthma (Golding, Emmett & Rogers, 1997; Oddy, de Klerk, Sly & Holt, 2002); eczema (Golding, Emmett & Rogers, 1997; Lawrence, 1995); and sudden infant death syndrome (Golding, 1993; Mitchell, 1992).

Box 8.1: Indonesia Health Law No. 36

The Indonesia Health Law No. 36 stipulates that every child has the right to be exclusively breastfed for the first six months of life, with a possibility for continuing breast feeding until the age of two years with complementary foods. During the period of breast feeding, the law requires that family, community, local government, and employers provide full support in terms of time and facilities for nursing mothers. Employers, for instance, are obliged to offer opportunities for working mothers to breastfeed and/or express breast milk during work hours. The penalty for failing to observe the law is a fine of up to 100 million rupiah (equivalent to $USD11,000) and a twelve-month jail sentence. The law also imposes rules on the use of infant formula.

They are also less likely to become obese as children and adolescents (Gillman et al., 2001; Grummer-Strawn & Mei, 2004), to develop type 1 or type 2 diabetes, or to suffer from inflammatory bowel disease, leukemia, or lymphoma (American Academy of Pediatrics, 2005). Breast feeding is also associated with increased bone density in childhood and adulthood (Gibson et al., 2000), lower blood pressure (Martin, Gunnell & Smith, 2005), and increased visual acuity (Markrides et al., 1995). Short-term health benefits for nursing mothers include less post-partum hemorrhage and greater weight loss; in the longer term, these women also have a lower risk of developing pre-menopausal breast cancer, ovarian cancer, osteoporosis, or hip fractures than women who have never breastfed (American Academy of Pediatrics, 2012; Dewey, Heinig & Nommsen, 1993; Labbok, 1999; Newcomb et al., 1994; Rosenblatt & Thomas, 1993). On the basis of these health considerations, the Indonesian government passed a law in 2011 that infants must be fed breast milk exclusively for the first six months of life (see box 8.1).

However, not every woman is able to breastfeed exclusively, and those who are unable must supplement or replace their milk with infant formula or donated breast milk, whether temporarily or as a long-term solution. The problem of insufficient milk supply, which is the most common reason given by mothers who stop breast feeding, has been well documented (Duong, 2011; Dykes, 2002, 2005; Greiner, Esterik & Latham, 2010; Hill & Humenick, 1989). Insufficient milk is conceptualized in the literature as a state in which a mother has or perceives that she has inadequate breast milk supply to satisfy the hunger of her child (Hill & Humenick, 1989). Gatti (2008) observes that perceived insufficient milk and insufficient milk supply are used interchangeably in the literature. She argues that perceived insufficient milk is based on maternal perceptions, while insufficient milk is actually measured by physiological factors and a variety of pathological conditions (obesity, ovarian cysts, elevated triglycerides, and adult-onset diabetes, etc.).

In a review of literature from 1996–2007, Gatti (2008) found that some women discontinue breast feeding during the first one to four weeks because of perceived insufficient milk supply. According to this author, approximately 35 percent of women who wean their children off breast milk early cite insufficient milk supply as the primary reason. Infant behaviours including crying after feeding and wakefulness, infant weight loss and the absence of heavily soiled diapers, and the mother herself not experiencing milk leakage from her breasts are typically regarded as indications that not enough milk is being produced (Gatti, 2008; McCarter-Spaulding & Kearney 2001; Sacco, Caulfield, Gittelsohn & Martinez, 2006). While these signs often do indicate insufficient milk supply, Gatti (2008) argues that the infant's behaviours may also be part of normal developmental variations. Scholars including McCarter-Spaulding and Kearney (2001) and Gatti (2008) have therefore called for women's milk production to be measured as part of identifying insufficient milk supply.

Since the publication of *Insufficient milk syndrome: A biocultural explanation* by Gussler and Briesemeister (1980), social, cultural, and physiological factors have been associated with perceived insufficient milk supply across many cultures. Gussler and Briesemeister (1980) hypothesize that perceived insufficient milk supply is a result of a lack of constant contact between mother and infant. By contrast, Greiner and colleagues (2010) propose that if constant mother-infant contact is a prerequisite for an adequate supply of breast milk, then societies whose child care patterns result in less mother-infant contact would appear doomed to a prevalence of insufficient milk. Researchers argue that mothers who do not initiate breast feeding or who stop breast feeding in the first three days because of perceived insufficient milk lack a basic understanding of normal infant breast feeding patterns (Dettwyler & Fishman, 1992; Greiner, Esterik & Latham, 2010). Furthermore, Dettwyler and Fishman (1992) argue that women use insufficient milk supply as culturally acceptable excuse for using formula, starting solid foods, or even terminating breast feeding for reasons of personal convenience.

Mothers who choose not to breastfeed at all often face criticism. Murphy (1999) found that mothers who formula-fed their babies were regarded as bad mothers who placed their needs, preference, or convenience above the welfare of their babies. Further, Barston (2012) argued that although breast feeding may be a beneficial act, it may not necessarily be the right choice for every mother and every child, whether for medical, psychological, or professional reasons. The concern for Barston (2012) and Murphy (1999) is the pressure on women to breastfeed even when they face difficulty in doing so. In drawing attention to this pressure, critics such as these do not oppose breast feeding entirely, but seek to advocate a supportive environment for all mothers.

That said, little attention has been paid to how women attempt to overcome the barrier of perceived insufficient milk supply. The few studies that have examined women's coping strategies indicate that mixed feeding with breast milk and formula is a common approach (Dykes, 2005; Sacco, Caulfield, Gittelsohn & Martinez, 2006). For example, Sacco and colleagues (2006) identified supplementation as the most common strategy used by women with insufficient breast milk production. To the best of my knowledge, there is no study that examines how women who achieve successful **exclusive breast feeding** for six months overcome problems with insufficient milk supply.

Accordingly, this study aims to contribute to the growing body of literature on insufficient breast milk by examining how nursing mothers in Yogyakarta, Indonesia, use the traditional medicine *jamu* to help them maintain adequate production of breast milk for their infants.

Traditional Medicine in Indonesia: *Jamu*

Jamu, as it is produced in the Indonesian province of Central Java where Yogyakarta is located, consists of herbal medicinal drinks made from mixtures of spices, roots, leaves, wood/bark, honey, palm sugar, and eggs. It is used to promote health and beauty. The roots, leaves, and spices are boiled, ground on a traditional stone, and filtered. Some of the ingredients are also pounded into powder. The exact ingredients of *jamu* depend on the condition it is being used to treat. *Jamu* is used to alleviate many health problems, ranging from the common cold to hypertension, diabetes, and chronic pain. Women in particular use *jamu* to treat a variety of reproductive and sexual health problems including menstrual irregularities, vaginal infections, sexually transmitted diseases, sexual enhancement, and breast milk production. In the past, *jamu* was exclusively prepared and sold by women, whose recipes were secret. Today in Yogyakarta, there are also men who prepare and sell *jamu* independently, as well as some who assist their wives in selling *jamu*. For example, the owner of Warung Jamu Ginggang café in the city is a man, and a *jamu* clinic known as Ir. R.M.H. Gembong Danudiningrat is owned and operated by Dr. Gembong, another man. Industrialists with substantial capital now manufacture instant *jamu* in the form of pills, tablets, and capsules. However, many Indonesians prefer fresh, homemade *jamu* because it does not contain any artificial chemicals. Women sell *jamu* on the streets, at marketplaces, and in shops. Some women also sell *jamu* door-to-door in their neighbourhoods. Most women carry plastic bottles of *jamu* in woven baskets on their backs as they travel on foot, but some have bicycles or motorcycles.

Methodology

Fieldwork was carried out during 2013–2014 in Yogyakarta, Central Java, Indonesia. I collected data through interviews with ten new nursing mothers, whom I recruited shortly after they had been discharged from hospital after giving birth. They were selected for the study because they were breast feeding at the time, lived in Yogyakarta, and were willing to discuss their experiences of breast feeding with me. Four of the mothers were recruited through personal networks and by referral from the initial recruits. Eventually, at the suggestion of my local research assistant, I made an appeal for participants on my assistant's Facebook page, and received expressions of interest from an additional 20 mothers. Because of time constraints, I recruited only six of these women on first-come-first-served basis.

All of the participants were in a heterosexual marriage, were Javanese Muslims, and resided in Yogyakarta. One mother lived and worked in Yogyakarta but her husband and child lived outside the city. Nearly all of the mothers were highly educated and employed. Two of the mothers had Master's degrees and two others were pursuing a Master's degree at the time. Five had undergraduate degrees, and the remaining two had secondary school certificates. In terms of employment, four of the mothers were government employees, one worked part-time as a university professor, two worked in the private sector, two were self-employed, one was not employed outside of the family home, and one was a student on leave from her studies for the purpose of nursing her son.

All interviews took place in the women's homes and lasted for roughly four to six hours with frequent interruptions as the women tended to their families. My aim was to encourage the women to talk about their experience of breast feeding and how they dealt with any issues of low milk supply. The formal portions of the interviews were tape-recorded with the permission of the mothers. Salient details from our informal conversations leading up to the interview proper were recorded in my field notes afterward.

In order to ensure confidentiality, I have replaced the women's names with pseudonyms. The interview recordings were transcribed and translated verbatim from Bahasa Indonesia (the official language of Indonesia) to English, and the transcripts were then imported into Nvivo software for analysis.

Results and Discussion: Women's Experiences of Insufficient Breast Milk Production

Insufficient breast milk production may be defined loosely as the state at which a mother has, or believes that she has, inadequate breast milk supply to satisfy her child's appetite (Hill & Humenick, 1989). Some of the interviewees reported that they had worried about having this problem even before they had given birth. First-time mother Fadila said that she had no breast milk for the first three days after giving birth. On the first day, she asked her cousin, who was nursing her own child at the time, to donate some breast milk for her daughter, Lily. Fadila expected that her milk supply would start on the second day but was disappointed again and resorted to feeding Lily with water. At the time of our conversation, Fadila remained optimistically determined to breastfeed Lily for the required six-month period in spite of her difficult experience. She was motivated by what she had learned from friends, Internet blogs, and the Indonesia Breastfeeding Mothers Association about the health benefits of breast milk, such as boosting the immune system and decreasing susceptibility to allergies and infections; she even resisted a midwife's efforts to persuade her to feed Lily with formula. Although the midwife who had attended her labour advised her not to take ***Jamu uyup-uyup*** (a type of *jamu* used for breast milk production) because its effects were not scientifically proven, Fadila's mother bought some from the market and insisted that Fadila drink a glass of it every morning and evening. Fadila's breast milk eventually came in and she became more confident that she had enough milk to feed Lily.

Like Fadila, several of the other mothers I spoke to reported that they had little or no milk production immediately after giving birth. In most cases, the women were immediately encouraged to drink *Jamu uyup-uyup* after their babies were born in order to stimulate their milk production. Wati, Rosada, and Ambar, all first-time mothers, told me about how their mothers and husbands persuaded them to drink *jamu* after the birth because they had little breast milk. Wati's mother, for example, was a door-to-door *jamu* seller in Yogyakarta, so as soon as Wati had given birth, she brought *Jamu uyup-uyup* for her to drink. Wati felt that the *jamu* did increase her breast milk production: "after drinking *jamu*, I feel my breasts always full of milk and my daughter Ella enjoys the taste of my breast milk." Rosada had no breast milk immediately after the birth of her daughter Lina and tried unsuccessfully to force milk out using an electric breast pump. Becoming worried that she could not breastfeed Lina, she resorted to drinking a soy-based beverage made for nursing mothers, and tried massaging her breasts to stimulate milk production. Rosada's breast milk finally came in on the third day after delivery, albeit in a very small amount. With her mother's encouragement, she drank *Jamu uyup-uyup* daily for the next four months to ensure that she had enough breast milk to feed her daughter. Rosada's experience of not having her breast milk come in within the first three days following delivery is a situation referred to as delayed milk arrival. Delayed milk arrival should not be considered an indication of insufficient milk supply because, as Segura-Millan, Dewey and Perez-Escamilla (1994) have observed, it may only be a transient situation lasting for the first few days immediately following the birth.

Ambar also had difficulty producing enough breast milk after birth. When Ambar and I met three months after she had given birth, she recalled that she could express only 20 millilitres of milk six weeks post-partum. Her son Jojo cried often, which alerted Ambar and her older sister Nur to the fact that he was not receiving enough breast milk to satisfy his hunger. Nur made *jamu* from turmeric and palm sugar for Ambar to drink at home and at work. Within a few weeks of starting this treatment, Ambar was producing enough milk to satisfy Jojo and had also noticed that her milk had a thicker, richer consistency.

In contrast to Fadila, Wati, Rosada, and Ambar, milk volume was not a problem for Darmi after she gave birth. She was able to express 500 millilitres of breast milk at a time. However, her mother-in-law bought *Jamu uyup-uyup* to help her sustain the quantity and the quality of her milk.

Even mothers with previous experience of breast feeding consumed *jamu* to stimulate the flow of their milk. Indah had two older children and was breast feeding a third child, Ida. Her husband wanted her to breastfeed Ida exclusively for six months, so he bought *Jamu uyup-uyup* from the street every day for Indah to ensure that Ida would have plenty of milk.

All of the mothers who participated in the study drank *Jamu uyup-uyup* regularly from the first month after delivery until the baby was between four and five months old. After the fifth month, the mothers only drank *jamu* occasionally, anticipating that they would start to give their babies solid food in the sixth month and would therefore need less breast milk. The mothers who continued to drink *jamu* after the five-month mark did so because their babies were unwell, or because they themselves were unwell and did not want to risk taking western drugs in case their residues were passed to the babies through the breast milk. For instance, Rosada reported that she drank ***Jamu watukan*** on behalf of her daughter Lina when she developed a common cold, cough, or flu. Another mother, Juleha, drank *Jamu jadem* (bitter plants boiled with water) whenever her son Aryo had diarrhea. It is common for mothers to drink *jamu* on behalf of their sick infants, in the belief that the healing effect would be transferred to the child through the breast milk. Infants were also nursed more than usual when they were ill.

Although, as was mentioned, the mothers regularly treated their own illnesses with *jamu*, they would take western medicines—at the lowest effective dosage—if the illness persisted. My interactions with the mothers I interviewed indicated that they were always careful in their use of western medicine. They expressed fear that taking the full dosages of western drugs could cause side effects in their breastfed babies. *Jamu* was preferred because it had no adverse effects and could even benefit the infant's health. The mothers knew that *jamu* contains no synthetic chemical compositions and works gradually on the body. Because the healing is gradual, *jamu* is believed to have longer efficacy compared with western medicine.

Not all of the mothers I interviewed drank *jamu* to help with breast milk production, however. Three of the 10 mothers were skeptical about the efficacy of *jamu*. One of those mothers was Putri, who stopped using *jamu* because she disliked the bitter leaves it was prepared from and how the *jamu* affected her baby. This issue came to light at the end of our conversation. When I asked Putri if she had ever tried *jamu* for breast milk enhancement, she replied: "I drank *jamu* for the first month after I gave birth to Rukia but I discontinued the use because Rukia reacted to the drink and had diarrhea." Putri felt that Rukia was too young and her stomach was sensitive to bitter herbs that were used to prepare *jamu*. She was also unconvinced that *jamu* was prepared in a sanitary way by the local women: "I don't even know if *jamu* is prepared under hygienic conditions or if the *jamu* seller washes her hands properly before preparing the drink." Siti, a mother of two, expressed doubt about the efficacy of *jamu* for breast milk production. She compared her previous experience of drinking *jamu* while breast feeding her first child with her current breast feeding without *jamu*:

> With my first child, I consumed *Jamu uyup-uyup* to increase my breast milk flow. For my second child, I did not consume *jamu*. But I don't see any difference in the quantity of my breast milk. [...] From my experience, I think the more you pump your breast or the baby suckle the breast, the more breast milk you produce. It is like the theory of demand and supply. [...] This works better than drinking *jamu* or eating a lot of vegetables to produce sufficient breast milk.

Siti's experience had taught her that expressing breast milk stimulated her milk supply the same as an infant's suckling would, and that the more she pumped her breasts, the more milk she would produce for her baby. This is consistent with other studies that have documented the connection between nipple stimulation (by suckling or pumping) and the production of the hormone prolactin, which triggers milk production (Greiner, Esterik & Latham, 2010).

Apart from *jamu* as a potential aid to breast milk production, the mothers I interviewed also mentioned that the food they ate affected the quantity and quality of their milk. According to the mothers' narratives, the infants derive nutrients from breast milk that promote good health and growth. Knowing the importance of breast milk, my participants told me that when they were pregnant, they were advised by their parents, friends, and older women in the community to eat healthy food so as to produce rich breast milk in sufficient quantities. The mothers increased their vegetable and fruit intake during the pre-natal and lactation period, consuming a range of produce including green beans, papaya leaf, ***daun katuk***, *kurma,* root of *kunyit,* banana, guava, mango, and apple. One participant, Nadja, observed that any time she ate junk food like instant noodles, she produced only a small amount of breast milk, which would also be watery; but whenever she ate the raw root of *kunyit,* her breast milk was not only more plentiful but also became thicker and tasted more appealing to her baby. Thick breast milk, to mothers, is indicative of the richness of the milk. Some of the participant mothers also reported drinking a commercial soy-based beverage for nursing mothers called Mama Soya, to stimulate the production of breast milk. Some mothers, however, did not feel the need to drink Mama Soya because they were confident that their balanced diet was sufficient to maintain ample breast milk production for their babies.

My discussions with these Yogya mothers about their dietary habits also addressed foods that they considered unsuitable for nursing mothers due to their potential effects on the baby's health. The main source of this information was grandmothers and older women in Yogya communities, who were passionate about transmitting their experience and knowledge to the younger women. They especially advised against consuming spicy foods and beverages containing coconut milk, which are believed to cause diarrhea in infants. Foods that are too cold or too hot are also to be avoided: cold foods (including ice) because they cool the breast milk, and hot foods because the heat might cause the quality and nutritional value of the breast milk to deteriorate.

Some new mothers, however, dismissed the advice of these grandmothers and older women. Rosada, for example, found the lack of scientific proof unconvincing: "I am advised not to take ice because my baby will get cold. From older mothers' experiences, these things do happen but I do not find any medical evidence on the Internet to support their claim." Wati also found that her experience contradicted her grandmother's advice: "I don't believe in my grandmother's advice. She says I should not consume food that contains coconut milk and that is spicy. I eat spicy foods and diets that contain coconut milk yet nothing happens to me and my baby." In a similar vein, Putri was reassured by her midwife's rejection of the traditional advice: "I don't believe in these traditional food safety measures because my midwife remarked there is no connection between mothers' diet and quality of breast milk." Above all, the main factor influencing the mothers' attitudes toward diet and breast feeding was whether their infants showed any signs of illness following nursing when they had consumed the so-called risky foods. To some degree, perceptions of infant well-being may depend on mother-child relationship; but in the age of the Internet, it is also easy for mothers to cross-check their grandmothers' knowledge with expert knowledge on breast feeding, and choose their own authority.

Conclusion

Nearly all of the mothers who participated in this study encountered the problem of insufficient breast milk production immediately after giving birth. None of them, however, was obliged to stop breast feeding because of this difficulty. Instead, they were strongly encouraged and supported by their mothers and husbands to drink *Jamu uyup-uyup*, a traditional medicine used to stimulate the production of breast milk. Their eventual nursing success was naturally credited to the *jamu*. The mother's narratives of their experiences highlight the role played by family in obtaining *jamu* for the women and motivating the first-time mothers in particular to use it, either to increase the quantity of their breast milk or to enhance its quality and flavour. *Jamu* is also regarded as a tonic to energize nursing mothers and protect both mother and infant from illness. The emphasis on a balanced diet including plenty of fruit and vegetables combined with drinking *jamu* is also consistent with Javanese cultural theories of health and illness. Mothers who have difficulty producing sufficient breast milk are thought to suffer from an imbalance in the body, which can be remedied by the intake of healthful fruit and vegetables along with *jamu*. Additional research is needed to understand what, if any, physiological effect *Jamu uyup-uyup* has on the production of breast milk, and what role Javanese women accord to traditional medicine with regard to breast feeding and milk production.

Critical Thinking Questions

1. How are perceptions and uses of *Jamu uyup-uyup* influenced by gender roles in Javanese society?
2. Should Indonesian health care providers prescribe *Jamu uyup-uyup* to women who are unable (or believe they are unable) to produce sufficient breast milk? Why or why not?

Glossary

Daun katuk: Leaf vegetable native to Southeast Asia (scientific name: *Sauropus adrogynus*). In addition to therapeutic applications in treatments for insufficient breast milk supply, it is also used to treat boils and fevers and to improve sexual vitality.

Exclusive breast feeding: Feeding infants solely on breast milk for the first six months of their lives.

Jamu uyup-uyup: Type of *jamu* used to stimulate and enhance breast milk production.

Jamu watukan: Type of *jamu* used to treat the common cold.

References

American Academy of Pediatrics. (2005). Policy statement: Breastfeeding and the use of human milk. *Pediatrics, 115*(2), 496–506.

American Academy of Pediatrics. (2012). Policy statement: Breastfeeding and the use of human milk. *Pediatrics, 129*(3), 827–841.

Arifeen, S., Black, R.E., Antelman, G., Baqui, A., Caulfield, L., & Becker S. (2001). Exclusive breastfeeding reduces acute respiratory infection and diarrhea deaths among infants in Dhaka slums. *Pediatrics, 108*(4), 167–171.

Barston, S. (2012). *Bottled up*. Berkeley, CA: University of California Press.

Dettwyler, K.A., & Fishman, C. (1992). Infant feeding practices and growth. *Annual Review of Anthropology, 21*, 171–204.

Dewey, K., Heinig, M.J., & Nommsen, L.A. (1993). Maternal weight loss patterns during prolonged lactation. *American Journal of Clinical Nutrition, 58*, 162–166.

Duong, D.V. (2011). Socio-cultural factors influencing infant feeding patterns within 6 months postpartum in rural Vietnam. In P. Liamputtong (Ed.), *Infant feeding practices: A cross-cultural perspective* (pp. 315–333). New York: Springer.

Dykes, F. (2002). Western marketing and medicine construction of an insufficient milk syndrome. *Health Care for Women International, 23*(5), 492–502.

Dykes, F. (2005). Supply and demand: Breastfeeding as labour. *Social Science & Medicine, 60*, 2283–2293.

Gatti, L. (2008). Maternal perceptions of insufficient milk supply in breastfeeding. *Journal of Nursing Scholarship, 40*(4), 355–363.

Gibson, J.H., Harries, M., Mitchell, A., Godfrey, R., Lunt, M., & Reeve, J. (2000). Determinants of bone density and prevalence of osteopenia among female runners in their second to seventh decades of age. *Bone, 26*, 591–598.

Gillman, M.W., Rifas-Shiman, S.L., Camargo, C.A., Berkey, C.S., Frazier, A.L., Rockett, H.R., ... Colditz, G.A. (2001). Risk of overweight among adolescents who were breastfed as infants. *Journal of American Medical Association, 285*(19), 2461–2467.

Golding, J. (1993). *Breastfeeding and sudden infant death syndrome: Report of the Chief Medical Officer's expert group on the sleeping position of infants and cot death.* London: Her Majesty's Stationery Office.

Golding, J., Emmett, P.M., & Rogers, I.S. (1997). Eczema, asthma and allergy. *Early Human Development, 49*, 121–130.

Greiner, T., Esterik, P., & Latham, M.C. (2010). Commentary: The insufficient milk syndrome: An alternative explanation. *Medical Anthropology: Cross-Cultural Studies in Health and Illness, 5*(2), 233–247.

Grummer-Strawn, L.M., & Mei, Z. (2004). Does breastfeeding protect against pediatric overweight? Analysis of longitudinal data from the Centers for Disease Control and Prevention Pediatric Nutrition Surveillance System. *Pediatrics, 113*(2), 81–86.

Gussler, J., & Briesemeister, L. (1980). The insufficient milk syndrome: A biocultural explanation. *Medical Anthropology, 4*(2), 145–174.

Hill, P.D., & Humenick, S.S. (1989). Insufficient milk supply. *Journal of Nursing Scholarship, 21*(3), 145–148.

Howie P.W., Forsyth, J.S., Ogsten, S.A., Clark, A., & Florey, C.D. (1990). Protective effect of breastfeeding against infection. *British Medical Journal, 300*(6716), 11–16.

Jackson, K.M., & Nazar, A.M. (2006). Breastfeeding, the immune response, and long-term health. *Journal of the American Osteopathic Association, 106*, 203–207.

Labbok, M.H. (1999). Health sequelae of breastfeeding for the mother. *Clinical Perinatology, 26*(2), 491–503.

Lawrence, R. (1995). The clinician's role in teaching proper infant feeding techniques. *Journal of Pediatrics, 126*(6), 112–117.

Makrides, M., Neumann, M., Simmer, K., Pater, J., & Gibson, R. (1995). Are long-chain polyunsaturated fatty acids essential nutrients in infancy? *Lancet, 345*, 1463–1468.

Martin, R.M., Gunnell, D., & Smith, G.D. (2005). Breastfeeding in infancy and blood pressure in later life: Systematic review and meta-analysis. *American Journal of Epidemiology, 161*, 15–26.

McCarter-Spaulding, D.E., & Kearney, M.H. (2001). Parenting self-efficacy and perception of insufficient breast milk. *Journal of Obstetric, Gynecologic and Neonatal Nursing, 30*(5), 515–522.

Mitchell, E.A. (1992). Four modifiable and other major risk factors for cot death: The New Zealand study. *Journal of Paediatrics and Child Health, 28*(1), 3–8.

Murphy, M. (1999). Breast is best: Infant feeding decisions and maternal deviance. *Sociology of Health and Illness, 21*(2), 187–208.

Newcomb, P.A., Storer, B.E., Longnecker, M.P., Mittendorf, R., Greenberg, E.R., Clapp, R.W., & MacMahon, B. (1994). Lactation & reduced risk of premenopausal breast cancer. *The New England Journal of Medicine, 330*(2), 81–87.

Oddy, W.H., de Klerk, N.H., Sly, P.D., & Holt, P.G. (2002). The effect of respiratory infections atopy, and breastfeeding on childhood asthma. *European Respiratory Journal, 19*(5), 899–905.

Rosenblatt, K.A., & Thomas, D.B. (1993). Lactation and the risk of epithelial ovarian cancer. *International Journal of Epidemiology, 22*(2), 192–197.

Sacco, L.M., Caulfield, L.E., Gittelsohn, J., & Martínez, H. (2006). The conceptualization of perceived insufficient milk among Mexican mothers. *Journal of Human Lactation, 22*(3), 277–286.

Scariati, P.D., Grummer-Strawn, L.M., & Fein, S.B. (1997). A longitudinal analysis of infant morbidity and the extent of breastfeeding in the United States. *Pediatrics, 99*(6), 1–5.

Segura-Millan, S., Dewey, K.G., & Perez-Escamilla, R. (1994). Factors associated with perceived insufficient milk in a low-income urban population in Mexico. *The Journal of Nutrition, 124*(2), 202–212.

World Health Organization (WHO). (2003). *Global strategy for infant and young child feeding*. Geneva: Author.

CHAPTER 9

Traditional Medicine and Reproductive Health, Conception, and Fertility in Turkey

Tamer Edirne, MD
Department of Family Medicine, University of Pamukkale, Turkey

Learning Objectives

1. To describe traditional medicine (TM) therapies used by infertile women in Turkey.
2. To discuss some spiritual healing methods used by infertile women in Turkey.
3. To understand how socio-cultural and religious contexts influence the use of TM among infertile women in Turkey.

Introduction

According to the World Health Organization (WHO), traditional medicine (TM) is becoming more popular globally, and more than three quarters of the world's population use TM or complementary and alternative medicine (CAM) for health care (WHO, 2002). TM includes a broad suite of resources that encompasses not only health systems, modalities, and practices, but also their accompanying theories and beliefs.

Factors influencing the use of TM for reproductive health differ geographically and culturally. Worldwide, women use TM for reproductive health, but different cultural beliefs and practices affect which TM modalities they choose. Regardless of their education or socio-economic background, women frequently combine two or more types of therapeutic treatments as a means of increasing the likelihood that their health complaint will be resolved (Daar & Merali, 2002; Vayena et al., 2002).

The aim of this chapter is to provide insight into how various TM practices, especially spiritual and religious practices, are used by Turkish women to enhance their fertility. Although the efficacy of these spiritual and religious interventions has not been demonstrated scientifically, religious healers continue to be a trusted source of help and are preferred to physicians by many Turkish people. The discussion begins with examples of TM methods used by infertile women in some rural regions of Turkey. As well, examples of spiritual and religious healing methods utilized by some Turkish people in the east and south of Turkey will be examined. The analysis will focus on the socio-cultural dimensions of fertility issues, paying particular attention to social perceptions of infertility in Turkey.

Socio-economic Status of Women in Turkey

Turkey straddles the divide between Europe and Asia, but most of its landmass is in Asia. Politically and culturally, it incorporates the divergent societal structures of the western and eastern values. This hybridization has yielded the only secular democratic country that also has a predominantly Muslim population (Cherry, 2002). At the beginning of the 20th century, Turkey was an underdeveloped agricultural country, in contrast to industrialized Europe. The traditional cultural heritage of Turkey dates back to the Ottoman Empire, which was mainly identified with Islam, where Turkish women were expected to give birth to as many children as possible and devote themselves to domestic work (Ayoob, 2004).

After the establishment of the republic in 1923, the Turkish state led by Kemal Ataturk initiated legal, educational, and social reforms that enhanced a rapid modernization, urbanization, and westernization of the country. A series of laws and reforms brought about an improvement in the legal status of women, beginning with the Turkish Civil Code in 1926, which outlawed polygamy. Turkey also removed **Sharia law**, the Islamic code that includes the segregation of the sexes and the existence of differential legal rights. Breaking with the Ottoman past, equal rights of divorce, child custody, and the vote were granted to Turkish women in 1934. In addition to their roles in the household, women were permitted to enter the public sphere for education or to work (Toktas & Cindoglu, 2006). This shift in gender ideology favoured the emancipation of women, who had previously been oppressed by religion through practices such as veiling, seclusion, and polygamy—all of which were common during the Ottoman Empire and under Islamic rules.

Although Turkish women have steadily enjoyed greater freedom and equality in recent decades, their social status is not uniform across the country: patriarchal structures (Edirne et al., 2010) are especially dominant in southern and eastern regions of the country. The avoidance of civil marriage in favour of the religious ceremony, the existence of polygamy, the marriage of teenaged girls, the demand of a bride-price by the husband's family, the denial of girls' right to education, and the emphasis on the importance of female fertility are signs of the uneven socio-economic status of women in these areas. Interesting social customs in traditional and patriarchal family systems like bride-price and dowry, where the families are forced to offer material goods and chattel to conduct the marriage, are known to result in female suicides and homicides due to harassment. Also, rates of female illiteracy are higher than those for men, and women's access to employment, political engagement, and health services are in general limited (see box 9.1) (Arat, 2000; Cosar & Onbasi, 2008; Tekeli, 1992).

Box 9.1

In the World Economic Forum (WEF) in 2010, Turkey ranked 126th out of 134 countries overall in terms of the Global Gender Gap Index. This extremely low rank is due primarily to the deficiencies that prevail in the domain of participation. In fact, Turkey's worst rank was in economic participation and equality of opportunity, where it came 131st out of 134. Above all, this is because the female labour force participation rate remains only around 25–30 percent. In terms of health access, Turkey was in a relatively better 61st place, but still occupies 109th position in education. Among the reasons for the low ranking of Turkey is the fact that there are approximately 4,000,000 illiterate adult women in Turkey and 500,000 girls who are prevented from participating in compulsory schooling (Isik, 2012).

The Importance of Motherhood and Children

In Turkey, as in some other Muslim societies, a moral preoccupation with female virginity exposes women to the risk of severe punishments—including so-called honour killings—if sexual misconduct is so much as suspected (Can & Edirne, 2011). There is significant literature in Turkey examining motherhood as a social and moral construct, and children are considered to be essential for the economic, social, and psychological well-being of a family. Children contribute to the family economy while young and represent an old-age security for their parents when they grow up. Thus, the child's economic and utilitarian value is important for parents, and high fertility is desirable because more children provide more support. In rural societies, there is a strong linkage between a family's wealth and well-being, and the number of children in the family. The psychological benefit of having children is represented by the joy, fun, companionship, pride, and the sense of accomplishment that parents gain from having children. The social benefits of having children stem from the social acceptance in the community a couple enjoys when they have children and the fact that children, especially sons, can continue the family name and the family traditions (Kagitcibasi, 1982; Kagitcibasi & Ataca, 2005; Saydam, 2003).

The Issue of Infertility and Its Consequences for Women

Infertility is generally defined as the inability to conceive a child after one year of having had unprotected sexual intercourse (Centers for Disease Control and Prevention, 2015). Although specific male and female conditions explain around 40 percent of all cases of infertility separately, in 20 percent of the cases the reason is never identified and remains unexplained (Centers for Disease Control and Prevention, 2015). Infertility affects approximately 80 million people worldwide—or, one in ten couples—and similar infertility rates are reported among Turkish married couples (Taşçı et al., 2008).

In patriarchal and pro-natal societies such as Turkey, women are often made to bear sole responsibility for infertility (Acıpayamlı, 1961; Kılıç, Apay & Beji, 2011; Taşçı & Özkan, 2007). In defining the status of women by their reproductive capacity along with cultural expectations that women will become mothers, infertile women are categorized as unhealthy, incomplete, and abnormal. This can have significant social consequences including stigmatization and isolation of these women, domestic violence, and divorce (Gijsels, Mgalla & Wambura, 2001; Giwa-Osagie, 2001; Kılıç, Apay & Beji, 2011). Infertility is considered an embarrassing condition and has been documented as a cause of anxiety, depression, frustration, grief, fear, guilt, and vulnerability for women (Cook, 2011; Hasanpoor-Azghdy, Simbar & Vedadhir, 2014; Lalos et al., 1986; Lechner, Bolman & van Dalen, 2007; van Balen & Inhorn, 2002; WHO, 2000). Male dominance in Turkey means that men can distance themselves from the stigma of impotence, and reject any responsibility for infertility. Men argue that the female body is the problem and in need of medical treatment, which in turn increases a woman's sense of embarrassment, guilt, and inadequacy and further accentuates her failure in social roles and identities (Letherby, 1999, 2002; Ulrich & Weatherall, 2000). Infertile women may experience life-threatening physical or psychological violence as a result of infertility, which leads to a desperate search for a viable pregnancy to improve their status in the family and society (Sahin & Sahin, 2003; Yildizhan et al., 2009).

Infertility and TM in Turkey

In Turkey, various traditional therapies, including spiritual therapies, are well known among local communities and are used extensively (Aydin et al., 2008; Gözüm, Tezel & Koc, 2003; Kav, Hanoglu & Algier, 2008; Tan, Uzun & Akçay, 2004). Local plants used for reproductive health have been documented in the literature (Edirne et al., 2010). These include European black pine (*Pinus nigra Arnold*), the resin of which is applied as a plaster to the woman's navel for at least three days; and wild daffodil (*Narcissus pseudonarcissus*) and heartsease (*Viola tricolor L.*, or Johnny Jump-up), the fresh leaves of which are compressed into a lozenge and inserted into the woman's vagina before sexual intercourse. Folk practices are also common, in addition to herbal remedies. One such treatment requires the woman to take two spoons of wheat oil twice a day and sit naked on hot ashes or hot bricks in order to stimulate her fertility. Perhaps not surprisingly, many women adopt a gentler version of this remedy by using thermal spas instead of hot ashes and bricks. Another folk remedy involves eating the uterus of a female rabbit before engaging in sexual intercourse.

Spiritual Practices

The spiritual therapies discussed below are prevalent in the east and south of Turkey, although occasional cases may be seen in other parts of the country, too. Many of the traditional therapeutic practices described here have existed for generations. This persistence is itself suggestive of a certain degree of efficacy. However, very few of these practices have been evaluated scientifically and there is no data that demonstrates their usefulness or safety.

Spiritual healing methods are regularly used by Turkish patients and are also common in other Muslim societies (Araz, Harlak & Meşe, 2007; Montazeri, Sajadian, Ebrahimi & Akbari 2005; Ni, Simile & Hardy, 2002). Following the basic precepts that Allah is the ultimate healer in whom all must seek refuge, and that the divine word expressed in the **Koran** has the power to heal body, mind, and soul, many Muslims utilize spiritual healing as part of their therapy.

There are several practices associated with spiritual healing therapies for infertility. In the first place, religion has a strong influence on people's beliefs about illness, and religious healing methods can exert positive influences on health by contributing to a sense of hope and helping the person cope with the stress of infertility (Roudsari, Allan & Smith, 2007). Within a specifically Muslim context, infertile women may seek a cure via a variety of practices including praying, reciting texts from the Koran, fasting, drinking holy water, or undertaking a pilgrimage to a holy place (e.g., the annual ***hajj*** pilgrimage to Mecca, or a pilgrimage to another holy site). Many of these practices are predicated on the notion that the infertility has been caused by a sin that must be atoned for. When the woman arrives at a holy site she may light candles or attach pieces of cloth to the trees while praying and expressing her desire for a child.

Many infertile women also visit a religious healer, called a ***hodja***, to pray for a cure, although this practice is most commonly associated with the treatment of critical illnesses such as cancer. The *hodja* is believed to have a special spiritual power that is inherited or earned through exceptional piety. The *hodja* communicates directly with Allah, and intercedes for his community. Among the variety of treatments that a *hodja* may offer, many involve the use of herbs and minerals. The *hodja* may also blow on the body of the patient to effect a cure (a therapy known as "**holy breath**"), or place water or food (e.g., rice) on the patient's body to be blessed and then consumed by the patient for therapeutic purposes and to enhance fertility. In day-to-day life, **amulets** (***tawiz***) containing verses from the Koran transcribed by a *hodja* are often worn around the neck as a defence against the **evil eye** (***nazaar***) or malicious spirits that might attack a woman and cause infertility. Chief among these spirits are ***jinn***, which many Muslims believe are spiritual beings, created from fire, that live on earth in a separate world from the one inhabited by humans. *Jinns* are able to possess the minds and bodies of humans and other beings, and force them to act against their will. Possession by *jinn* occurs for many reasons, and in some cases infertility is believed to be indicative of possession. If a woman's difficulty in conceiving is believed to have a spiritual cause, a *hodja* can diagnose possession by *jinn* and perform an ***exorcism*** to restore her fertility (for further reading, see Edirne et al., 2010).

Generally, these interventions are offered to patients with the promise that they can cure multiple diseases and health conditions, including infertility. However, enigmatic forms of spiritual healing, such as "holy breath," may be confusing or intimidating for the recipient, whereas more intensive interventions such as exorcisms may also have a devastating effect on the psychological health of women affected by infertility, who then have the added psychological pressure that malevolent spirits possess them (Edirne et al., 2010). It should be emphasized that these treatments are directed at vulnerable individuals who are desperate to have children.

Conclusion

As shown in this chapter, the pressure to have children means that many infertile women in Turkey turn to home remedies and consultation with traditional and religious healers in their communities in an effort to conceive. Low success rates and high prices for modern medical infertility treatments also lead many women to choose these practices for infertility.

Many patients access TM therapies outside the context of biomedical care; pay for such therapies out of pocket; do not consult with their physicians regarding such care; and use CAM therapies as part of a healing process that involves meaning and is attentive to the illness experience and perceptions of risk and vulnerability (Eisenberg et al., 1998). Some of these therapies may focus less on the kind of physiological results but may be rather associated with therapies at the borderland of psychological and spiritual care.

Cultural norms put pressure on women to use any means to produce a viable pregnancy; however, this is even more complicated when women enter into the biomedical health system. The stress of being on a waiting list for infertility treatment, the embarrassment of having her reproductive system scrutinized by a (male) doctor, the ethical and economic constraints of some modern treatment methods, and uncertainty about the outcome contribute to women seeking alternative methods to become pregnant (Benyamini, Gozlan & Kokia, 2005; Fido & Zahid, 2004; Nene, Coyaji & Apte, 2005; Widge, 2005).

This is especially evident in countries such as Turkey where there is an expectation that women have large numbers of children, divorce due to inability to bear children is prevalent, and traditional health practices are socially and culturally accepted along with biomedical treatment (Acıpayamlı, 1961; Koçyiğit, 2012). What infertility means to a woman and her family is highly influenced by a cultural context. In order to understand traditional reproductive health beliefs and practices and the use of TM for infertility, the values and reasons attached to having children must be evaluated and understood.

Critical Thinking Questions

1. Why are traditional health practices used in the treatment of infertility in Turkey?
2. What are some important socio-cultural factors responsible for the utilization of traditional health practices in Turkey? Can you suggest cross-cultural interventions to modify local attitudes?
3. How can we ensure that health care providers are able to meet the reproductive needs of women affected by infertility in a culturally sensitive way?

Glossary

Amulet: An object with powers to protect its owner from danger and harm. Many Muslims wear amulets containing verses of the Koran written by *hodjas*.

Evil eye: Many Muslims believe that so-called "evil eye," which originates as a jealous look or remark about the fortune of a person, may cause an adverse event for another person. The evil eye may cause physical problems, mental illnesses, or failure in relationships or business.

Exorcism: The practice of purging demons or other spiritual entities from a person who is believed to be possessed. Islamic exorcism is used to remove evil *jinn* (spiritual entities) from a possessed person by placing a hand on the person and reciting verses from the Koran.

Hajj: An Islamic pilgrimage to the holy city of Mecca, in Saudi Arabia. It is one of the five pillars of Islam, and a religious duty which must be carried out at least once in lifetime by every adult Muslim who is physically and financially capable.

Hodja: A religious leader who uses knowledge from the Koran to heal the body, mind, and soul of Muslim patients.

Holy breath: The *hodja* is believed to transmit the healing power of the divine word by blowing his breath in the name of Allah onto objects or food and drinks which are carried or consumed by the recipient to dispel evil influences or cure illnesses.

Jinn: Supernatural creatures in Islamic mythology that are also mentioned in the Koran. They are believed to be invisible spirits with free will that may inhabit, possess, or influence individuals in a positive or negative way. Muslims may believe that mental illnesses or difficulties in life are caused by evil *jinn* and may consult a hodja to exorcise the *jinn*.

Koran: The central religious text of Islam, which Muslims believe to be a revelation from Allah.

Nazaar: An amulet of stone or glass which is believed to protect against evil eye. Also called evil eye stone.

Sharia: The moral code and religious laws of the prophet Muhammad. The Islamic law consists of the precepts set forth in the Koranic verses and the example set by the Islamic prophet Muhammad.

Tawiz: A locket usually containing verses from the Koran worn with the belief that it will remove the owner of any evil or affliction put on them through black magic, keep them safe, and also bring good luck.

References

Acıpayamlı, O. (1961). Türkiye'de Doğumla İlgili Adet ve İnanmaların Etnolojik Etüdü. Ankara: Atatürk University Press.

Arat, Y. (2000). From emancipation to liberation. The changing role of women in Turkey's public realm. *Journal of International Affairs, 54*(1), 107–123.

Araz, A., Harlak, H., & Meşe, G. (2007). [Health behaviors and alternative medicine use]. *TAF Preventative Medicine Bulletin, 6*(2), 112–122. Turkish.

Aydin, S., Bozyaka, A.O., Mazicioglu, M., Gemalmaz, A., Ozcakir, A., & Ozturk, A. (2008). What influences herbal medicine use?—prevalence and related factors. *Turkish Journal of Medical Sciences, 38*(5), 455–463.

Ayoob, M. (2004). Turkey's multiple paradoxes. *Orbis, 48*(3), 451–463.

Benyamini, Y., Gozlan, M., & Kokia, E. (2005). Variability in the difficulties experienced by women undergoing infertility treatments. *Fertility and Sterility, 83*(2), 275–283.

Can, M., & Edirne, T. (2011). Beliefs and attitudes of final-year nursing students on honour crimes: A cross-sectional study. *Journal of Psychiatric and Mental Health Nursing, 18*(8), 736–743.

Centers for Disease Control and Prevention. (2015). *Reproductive health*. Retrieved May 18, 2015 from www.cdc.gov/reproductivehealth/Infertility/Index.htm#aa

Cherry, M. (2002). When a Muslim nation embraces secularism. *The Humanist, 62*(3), 21–23.

Cook, E.P. (2011). Characteristics of the biopsychosocial crisis of infertility. *Journal of Counselling & Development, 65*(9), 465–470.

Cosar, S., & Onbasi, F.G. (2008). Women's movement in Turkey at a crossroads: From women's rights advocacy to feminism. *South European Society and Politics, 13*(3) 325–344.

Daar, A., & Merali, Z. (2002). Infertility and social suffering: The case of ART in developing countries. In E. Vayena, P.J. Rowe & P.D. Griffin (Eds), *Current practices and controversies in assisted reproduction. Report of a WHO meeting on "Medical, Ethical and Social Aspects of Assisted Reproduction"* (pp. 15–21). Geneva: World Health Organization.

Edirne, T., Gunher, A.S., Gucuk, S., Yildizhan, R., Kolusari, A., Adali, E., & Can, M. (2010). Use of complementary and alternative medicines for fertility enhancement by a sample of Turkish women: A descriptive study. *BMC Complementary and Alternative Medicine, 10*, 11.

Eisenberg, D.M., David, R.B., Ettner, S.L., Appel, S., Wilkey, S., Van Rompay, M., & Kessler, R.C. (1998). Trends in alternative medicine use in the United States, 1990–1997: Results of a follow-up national survey. *Journal of the American Medical Association, 280*(18), 1569–1575.

Fido, A., & Zahid, M.A. (2004). Coping with infertility among Kuwaiti women: Cultural perspectives. *The International Journal of Social Psychiatry, 50*(4), 294–300.

Gijsels, M., Mgalla, Z., & Wambura, L. (2001). "No child to send": Context and consequences of female infertility in northwest Tanzania. In J.T. Boerma & Z. Mgalla (Eds), *Women and infertility in sub-Saharan Africa* (pp. 204–221). Amsterdam: Royal Tropical Institute/KIT Publishers.

Giwa-Osagie, O.F. (2001). Social and ethical aspects of assisted conception in Anglophone sub-Saharan Africa. In E. Vayena, P.J. Rowe & P.D. Griffin (Eds), *Current practices and controversies in assisted reproduction. Report of a WHO meeting on "Medical, Ethical and Social Aspects of Assisted Reproduction"* (pp. 50–54). Geneva: World Health Organization.

Gözüm, S., Tezel, A., & Koc, M. (2003). Complementary alternative treatments used by patients with cancer in eastern Turkey. *Cancer Nursing, 26*(3), 230–236.

Hasanpoor-Azghdy, S.B., Simbar, M., & Vedadhir, A. (2014). The emotional-psychological consequences of infertility among infertile women seeking treatment: Results of a qualitative study. *Iranian Journal of Reproductive Medicine, 12*(2), 131–138.

Isik, S.N. (2012, October). The future of women in Turkey: What are the prospects? *Reflections Turkey*. Retrieved from www.reflectionsturkey.com/?p=795

Kagitcibasi, C. (1982). Old-age security value of children: Cross-national socio-economic evidence. *Journal of Cross-Cultural Psychology, 13*(1), 29–42.

Kagitcibasi, C., & Ataca, B. (2005). Value of children and family change: A three-decade portrait from Turkey. *Applied Psychology, 54*(3), 317–337.

Kav, S., Hanoglu, Z., & Algier, L. (2008). [Use of complementary and alternative medicine by cancer patients in Turkey: A literature review]. *International Journal of Hematology and Oncology, 18*(1), 32–38. Turkish.

Kılıç, M., Apay, S.E., & Beji, N.K. (2011). Infertility and culture. İstanbul Üniversitesi Florence Nightingale Hemşirelik Dergisi, *19*(2), 109–115.

Koçyiğit, O.T. (2012). [Infertility and its socio-cultural impacts]. *Insanbilim Dergisi, 1*(1), 27–38. Turkish.

Lalos, A., Lalos, O., Jacobsson, L., & Von Schoulta, B. (1986). Depression, guilt and isolation among infertile women and their partners. *Journal of Psychosomatic Obstetrics & Gynecology, 5*(3), 197–206.

Lechner, L., Bolman, C., & van Dalen, A. (2007). Definite involuntary childlessness: Associations between coping, social support and psychological distress. *Human Reproduction, 22*(1), 288–294.

Letherby, G. (1999). Other than mother and mothers as others: The experience of motherhood and non-motherhood in relation to infertility and involuntary childlessness. *Women's Studies International Forum, 22*(3), 359–372.

Letherby, G. (2002). Challenging dominant discourses: Identity and change and the experience of "infertility" and "involuntary childlessness". *Journal of Gender Studies, 11*(3), 277–288.

Montazeri, A., Sajadian, A., Ebrahimi, M., & Akbari, M.E. (2005). Depression and the use of complementary medicine among breast cancer patients. *Support Care Cancer, 13*(5), 339–342.

Nene, U.A., Coyaji, K., & Apte, H. (2005). Infertility: A label of choice in the case of sexually dysfunctional couples. *Patient Education and Counselling, 59*(3), 234–238.

Ni, H., Simile, C., & Hardy, A.M. (2002). Utilization of complementary and alternative medicine by United States adults: Results from the 1999 national health interview survey. *Medical Care, 40*(4), 353–358.

Roudsari, R.L., Allan, H.T., & Smith, P.A. (2007). Looking at infertility through the lens of religion and spirituality: A review of the literature. *Human Fertility, 10*(3), 141–149.

Sahin, H.A, & Sahin, G.H. (2003). An unaddressed issue: Domestic violence and unplanned pregnancies among pregnant women in Turkey. *European Journal of Contraception & Reproductive Health Care, 8*(2), 93–98.

Saydam, B.K. (2003). Türk toplumunda infertil kadınların statüsü [The status of infertile women in Turkish population]. *Saglık ve Toplum, 13*(1), 30–34. Turkish.

Tan, M., Uzun, O., & Akçay, F. (2004). Trends in complementary and alternative medicine in eastern Turkey. *Journal of Alternative and Complementary Medicine, 10*(5), 861–865.

Taşçı, E., Bolsoy, N., Kavlak, O., & Yücesoy, F. (2008). İnfertil Kadınlarda Evlilik Uyumu [Marital adjustment in infertile women]. *Journal of the Turkish Society of Obstetrics and Gynecology, 5*(2), 105–110. Turkish.

Taşçı, K.D., & Özkan, S. (2007). University school for health sciences students' opinions about infertility. *TAF Preventive Medicine Bulletin, 6*(3), 187–192.

Tekeli, S. (1992). Europe, European feminism, and women in Turkey. *Women's Studies International Forum, 15*(1), 139–143.

Toktas, S., & Cindoglu, D. (2006). Modernisation and gender: A study of girls' technical education in Turkey since 1927. *Women's History Review, 15*(5), 737–749.

Ulrich, M., & Weatherall, A. (2000). Motherhood and infertility: Viewing motherhood through the lens of infertility. *Feminism and Psychology, 10*(3), 323–336.

van Balen, F., & Inhorn, M.C. (2002). Interpreting infertility: A view from the social sciences. In M.C. Inhorn & F. van Balen (Eds), *Infertility around the globe: New thinking on childlessness, gender, and reproductive technologies* (pp. 3–32). Berkeley: University of California Press.

Vayena, E., Rowe, P., Griffin, D., Van Look, P., & Turmen, T. (2002). Foreward. In E. Vayena, P.J. Rowe, P.D. Griffin (Eds), *Current practices and controversies in assisted reproduction. Report of a WHO meeting on "Medical, Ethical and Social Aspects of Assisted Reproduction"* (pp. xv–xvii). Geneva: World Health Organization.

Widge, A. (2005). Seeking conception: Experiences of urban Indian women with in vitro fertilization. *Patient Education and Counselling, 59*(3), 226–233.

World Health Organization (WHO). (2000). *Women's mental health: An evidence based review.* Geneva: Author.

WHO. (2002, May 16). *WHO launches the first global strategy on traditional and alternative medicine* [media release]. Retrieved May 18, 2015 from www.who.int/mediacentre/news/releases/release38/en/

Yildizhan, R., Adali, E., Kolusari, A., Kurdoglu, M., Yildizhan, B., & Sahin, G. (2009). Domestic violence against infertile women in a Turkish setting. *International Journal of Gynaecology and Obstetrics, 104*(2), 110–112.

CHAPTER 10

Birth from the Peripheries: Local Realities in Dzodze, Ghana

John Paul Nyonator, PhD Candidate
Department of Sociology and Anthropology, University of Ottawa, Canada

Learning Objectives

1. To learn about birth practices used by local traditional birth attendants (TBAs) in Dzodze, Ghana.
2. To understand the relationships that exist between traditional birth attendants and biomedical practitioners.
3. To learn about the training of traditional birth attendants in Dzodze, Ghana.

Introduction

In 2011 in Ghana, nearly one in three births (31 percent) occurred at home (Ghana Statistical Service, 2012). Among women who gave birth at home, 50 percent had babies who were delivered by traditional birth attendants (TBAs), while 36 percent had babies who were delivered by family members and friends (Ghana Statistical Service, 2012). In the Volta region, where this research took place, approximately 36 percent of babies were delivered at home (Ghana Statistical Service, 2012). It is often taken for granted by the government, public health experts, and international health organizations that pregnant women will choose to give birth in a hospital rather than at home, so long as obstacles of transportation, distance, cost, health personnel, and cultural factors can be overcome. However, I suspect that this is not entirely the case, and that it is not necessarily desirable for all women to give birth in a hospital setting. Drawing on anthropological theories of knowing and experience, this chapter focuses on giving birth in rural areas in Ghana. I explore the local context in which TBAs operate in Dzodze, Ghana, and how they are trained. I also consider how TBA-assisted home births take place; the relationships that exist between TBAs, hospital midwives, and doctors; and the support that TBAs receive from the government and larger community.

Theoretical Approach

The theoretical approach adopted in this ethnographic study of birth practices is the theory of knowing and experience. I chose this approach because it allows understanding of the complexities of birth practices from the perspective of traditional birth attendants. Here I draw from the work of Farquhar (1994), Ingold (2012), and Merleau-Ponty (1962), in particular.

In her book *Knowing practice*, Farquhar (1994) provides an ethnographic and textual account of "knowing" in the context of Chinese medicine, by observing diagnosis and treatment by doctors from the insider perspective of a scholar. She contrasts "knowing Chinese medicine" with "knowledge of Chinese medicine" and defines "knowing" as "knowing practice." In a similar vein, Ingold (2012) offers a persuasive approach to "knowing from the inside." He argues that knowing is not transmitted across generations as a ready-made *corpus* of information, but instead goes through a continual process in which learners engage practically with their environment. Further, he points out that the only way one can really know things is from the very inside of one's being—not from the mere accumulation of information in one's mind. A phenomenological stance is one that eliminates a level of abstraction according to which the mind comes first. Knowing, therefore, implies an active engagement in the world. Active engagement in the world is learned through doing, what Ingold calls "skill." So, in doing, one can be more or less skillful with time and practice. Doing is already knowing, and it is done through attuned attention in the world. When Ingold (2000) speaks about skills, he is not talking about skills as "techniques of the body," but rather "the capabilities of action and perception of the whole organic being (indissolubly mind and body) situated in a richly structured environment" (p. 5). Skills, for Ingold (2000), are not transmitted intergenerationally. On the contrary, they are integrated into the way of functioning of human organisms through training and experience in the performance of particular activities. Farquhar's (1994) and Ingold's (2012) understandings of "knowing" therefore challenge the positivists' claim that we come to know reality through a scientific method that is objective and detached from experience and that is far from the particularity of the knower and his or her specific cultural context.

In Ghana, the traditional birth attendants, who are locally called ***afeme vixelawo***, do not acquire their skills through formal education but through experience and regular assistance at births. For the *afeme vixelawo*, knowing is a process that takes place in a practical context, and over a period of time through assisting a number of women in the delivery processes.

The notion of knowing relies on human perception and experience, what Merleau-Ponty (1962) calls phenomenology of perception. For Merleau-Ponty (1962), the body is central to what we come to know in the world. According to Merleau-Ponty (1964), the body is much more than an instrument or object: it is not just a vehicle or container from which we come to experience the world, but rather it is through the body that we come to see the world, understand it, and be seen as part of it. For Merleau-Ponty, the body is actively implicated in the process of learning and it is not a passive object receiving information—the body is a meaning-making entity in itself. Since the body is actively implicated in the world, it is the point from which we embody things and relate to objects in the world. So the relationship between the body and the world that it inhabits is fluid and continuously transformed according to embodied experience.

Local Context—Dzodze

Dzodze is a town located southeast of the Volta region, in the Ketu North District of Ghana. Dzodze has a population of approximately 22,862 people (Ghana Statistical Service, 2014) and is mainly inhabited by the ethnic group of the Ewes. The major economic activities practised in the region are farming, livestock husbandry, and small-scale trade. I chose Dzodze as the setting for this study because of my practical knowledge of the area: I grew up near Dzodze and some of my relatives were delivered at home by TBAs.

In Dzodze, children are either born at home with the assistance of a TBA or at a hospital with the guidance of a registered midwife. Traditional and hospital services can also be combined. For instance, a pregnant woman may attend pre-natal care services at a hospital but deliver at home with the assistance of a TBA, or she might receive pre-natal health care from a TBA but go to a health care facility for the birth itself. According to my interviews, the main reason that women sought pre-natal care from a TBA but chose to give birth at a hospital was fear of certain cultural practices of the TBAs, such as the cutting of the umbilical cord with an unsterilized blade. On the other hand, women who attended pre-natal care at a hospital but chose to give birth at home with the assistance of a TBA generally did so because they feared having a caesarian section or because they felt pressured by their husbands or extended family to deliver at home. As well, the TBAs offer incentives to women to give birth at home. They claim to be able to prevent severe labour pain and facilitate an easy delivery by administering herbal enemas in the final months of pregnancy. They also tell women considering a hospital birth that the midwives will shout at them throughout their labour and not reassure them during the process—the opposite of the care provided by TBAs. Additionally, TBAs reported that some women choose deliver at home because of anxiety about their babies being stolen or exchanged with another woman's child at the hospital.

St. Anthony's Hospital is the only hospital in Dzodze. Its patients come from surrounding villages and towns including Denu, Keta, Akatsi, and sometimes from the neighbouring Republic of Togo. The hospital has a bed capacity of 166 with 173 employees (St. Anthony's Hospital, 2008). Its medical staff numbers four Ghanaian physicians, 16 expatriate physicians, 53 nurses and midwives, two medical assistants, and two anaesthetists (St. Anthony's Hospital, 2008). The main reasons patients are admitted at the hospital include malaria, anemia, hernia, road accidents, and retention of urine (St. Anthony's Hospital, 2008). Apart from the hospital's goal of providing biomedical health care to the poor and marginalized in society, St. Anthony's also brings healing to the patients through the use of holy water, anointed oil, and prayers.

There are also traditional healers in Dzodze. They are commonly known as ***bokɔ***, and treat patients using plant-based therapies. The plants used in traditional medicine are not considered to be effective in curing diseases due to their phytotherapeutic properties alone, but due to the spiritual power of the healers who invoke ancestral spirits before using them (Bierlich, 1999; Twumasi, 2005). The healers are well-respected members of the community because of their knowledge in the healing process and their ability to provide possible explanations of misfortunes (Nyonator, 2010).

Methods

My fieldwork was conducted between September and December 2009 in Dzodze, to understand the local realities of child birth, how TBAs learn their profession, and the nature of current relationships between TBAs and registered midwives. In order to learn the experiential and bodily knowledge about local childbirth, I contacted the public health units of Dzodze hospital to get the names and locations of TBAs that work in Dzodze. At the time of recruitment, there were only nine TBAs registered with the public health units. I contacted all nine TBAs but only seven of them were recruited into the study; I was unable to interview the other two TBAs because they had relocated to another community. I also recruited two midwives for the study because of their specific roles as liaison with the public health unit to oversee activities of the TBAs in Dzodze. The TBAs who took part in the study were between 30 and 80 years of age and had been delivering children for between 12 and 20 years. None of the TBAs had any formal education, and delivering children was not their full-time job: the majority of the TBAs were market traders, farmers, or potters in order to earn a living income.

I conducted four 30-minute interviews with each of the TBAs. The midwives were interviewed only once. The interviews were recorded, transcribed verbatim, and translated from Ewe into English. I read through the transcribed text several times and extracted relevant themes by compiling informative quotations under various subject headings. This helped me to see trends, similarities, and contradictions in the material gathered. I also used direct quotations from the interviews to illuminate the experiences of TBAs. Ethical approval was obtained from University of Ottawa Ethics Board.

Bodily Practices of Traditional Birth Attendants

According to the TBAs I interviewed, "pregnancy is not a disease but God's gift," and as such needs to be nurtured and taken care of. In other words, childbirth is understood by TBAs as a natural life event rather than a pathological condition that requires tending in a hospital setting. Although much of the literature suggests that TBAs receive training through apprenticeship alone (Ofili & Okojie, 2005; Twumasi, 2005), my fieldwork indicated that the TBAs must first receive a "calling" from the ancestors before advancing to the apprenticeship. TBAs explained their vocation as a "family thing" that one inherits. It is only through inheritance that one can understand and know the skills and the techniques involved in the delivery process. As an older TBA, Mama Klenam (the honorific title "**Mama**" is commonly used to refer to older women in Ghana) put it, "the [i.e., any] person can be trained in traditional midwifery but she will never be an expert in it. The person cannot determine accurately the extent of the presentation of the fetus and cervical dilatation using her fingers." This statement highlights the importance of ancestral calling and kinship for TBAs, and explains why they are often hesitant to share their knowledge with people who are not part of a designated descent line but are simply interested in local midwifery.

Another reason cited by TBAs for their reluctance to transfer knowledge to others centres on the fact that their profession deals with blood and that many young girls are afraid of blood. There were instances of fainting as a result of contact with and sight of exceptional blood loss during a delivery. Females who can stand the sight of blood and are interested in child delivery practices can be trained by the TBAs, but it is believed that they cannot be really experts in midwifery since they were not called by the ancestors. I met Mama Adzo, who explained to me how she was called into midwifery:

> Let me say that child delivery is inheritance from our mothers in the family. My mother had not learned it from anybody. When she was in her final stages of life, a pregnant woman came to her for delivery but she asked me to deliver for the pregnant woman on her behalf. I took the pregnant woman to the delivery room but had no knowledge on what to do. So, I quickly took the pregnant woman to the hospital for delivery. After the death of my mother, I was called by the spirit of my mother among my other siblings to take over her midwifery career. I took up the job and delivered many babies for people in Kuli and its surrounding villages. I have children but I have not taught any of them how to deliver babies for pregnant women. Since it is a family inheritance, if I join my ancestor one day, I am sure that I will also transfer my knowledge in midwifery to one of my children.

Even though Mama Klenam and Mama Adzo believed that they had inherited their midwifery skills from their ancestors, they also wanted certificates in midwifery to show that they were recognized as experts like their counterparts in the hospital. For these TBAs, a certificate in midwifery is important because it legitimatizes their knowledge and status in the community. As Mama Adzo clearly indicated in her interview, "I only want the certificate to prove that this is the work I do."

Three of the TBAs said that they had received the ancestral calling but also took two weeks of training from registered midwives at the hospital in Dzodze. According to these TBAs, hospital training was given to them because the political regime in 1998 believed that TBAs killed many babies during delivery. The TBAs were taught not to assist women in cases of **breech birth** (when the baby's feet or buttocks enter the birth canal first) but to refer these cases to the hospital. However, TBAs encounter many problems when they refer women to the hospital, including lack of transportation, distance, and, in some cases, husbands' refusal for their wives to be sent to the hospital. These circumstances sometimes forced TBAs to assist women in complicated births in order to save the life of the mother and child (see box 10.1).

Local Birth Practices in Dzodze

When a woman in labour is brought to a TBA, the TBA examines her by the use of the human senses. From the western perspective, the senses refer to the five senses (taste, smell, touch, hearing, and sight) identified by Aristotle (Goody, 2002). This

Box 10.1: Maternal Mortality Ratio

According to Ghana Millennium Development Goals Report (2015), the maternal mortality ratio (MMR) in Ghana has improved from 780 maternal deaths per 100,000 live births in 1990 to 380 maternal deaths per 100,000 live births in 2013. Based on this trend, it was projected that maternal mortality would be 358 maternal deaths per 100,000 live births by 2015, which is higher than the MDG target of 190 deaths per 100,000 live births. The rate of mortality for children under five years of age was 60 deaths per 1,000 live births in 2014 compared to the MDG target of 40 deaths per 1,000 live births (Ghana Millennium Development Goals Report 2015).

Although Ghana has made improvements in its MMR, it appears that reaching Millennium Development Goals 4 & 5 in 2015 will be a challenge.[1] According to the United Nations Development Programme (2012), the interventions that have been implemented in Ghana to reduce the MMR include the provision of free maternal health services, increased national school enrollment of registered midwives to 13 percent, increasing the knowledge of registered midwives about using the **partograph** (a printout record that is used to monitor the stages of labour), improvements in emergency obstetric and neonatal care, and increased anti-malaria programs for pregnant women.

It is widely assumed that supervised delivery decreases the risks of labour complications and reduces maternal deaths. In this regard, skilled birth attendants are seen as an important intervention for safe motherhood. Nevertheless, the number of registered midwives in Ghana is low. In 2008, there were an estimated 3,780 midwives, nurse-midwives, and nurses with midwifery competencies (United Nations Population Fund [UNPF], 2011). That number increased only marginally to 4,185 midwives in 2012 (UNPF, 2014). Again, there is no equitable distribution of registered midwives in rural and urban settings in Ghana. These challenges of the health system in Ghana as well as the strengths of TBAs—such as cultural competence, empathy, and psychosocial support for women—make TBAs an important asset to pregnant women in rural areas.

is a narrower definition of the senses according to local TBAs, as among the Ewes there are more than five senses. For example, in addition to Aristotle's five senses, the TBAs use the sense of humour, rhythm, and ***seselelame*** (feeling in the body) during childbirth. The sense of humour is used when the woman is in severe pain. The senses of rhythm and *seselelame* are used to listen to the heartbeat of the baby. The senses are channels of communication, operating at both cultural and physiological levels (Goody, 2002). The senses of touch, sight, and hearing are also used by the TBAs during childbirth. This consists of touching the pregnant woman, visually observing whether or not contractions are taking place, and listening to the heartbeat of the baby in the uterus.

According to the TBAs, three conditions must be met for a woman to deliver her baby: the contractions have started, the amniotic sac has broken, and the baby has moved. They insert the middle finger of their left hand into the woman's vagina to gauge whether her cervix is dilated and the baby has positioned itself correctly (i.e., head first) or not. As Mama Enyo told me, "we are old women who had experiences of child birth. So we know where the uterus is located." When the finger touches the head of the baby, it indicates that the baby is correctly positioned for delivery. On the other hand, the baby may also show its foot or buttocks at the entrance of the cervix (known as the "breech position"). When this happens, the TBAs who have received training from the hospital refer the woman to the hospital. They are taught not to attempt to turn the baby manually because that can result in the death of the pregnant woman.

Interestingly, TBAs who follow traditional practices use other mechanisms to turn and reverse the feet or the buttocks for delivery. For instance, Mama Klenam reported that she rubs shea butter in her two palms to palpate the baby and turn the baby if in the breech position. She also inserts shea butter into the vagina during labour to stimulate full cervical dilatation. She buys the shea butter from the market and takes it to a healer who invokes an ancestral spirit on it before it is used. She sends the shea butter to the healer because there is a general belief in Dzodze that enemies or witches could delay or prevent a woman from giving birth. Post-term pregnancies are often associated with the work of witchcraft. It is believed that witches can hold the baby in the uterus until the woman dies along with her unborn child. Dela, another TBA, reported that she gives soapy water to women to drink when they are in labour so that the baby can easily detach from the uterus. Further, when the cervix is not fully dilated, pounded okra mixed with saltpeter is given to the pregnant woman to drink. The belief is that the pounded okra—a vegetable with slimy secretions that is often used to thicken soups—stimulates the production of mucus in the woman and makes the fetus slippery for delivery.

The TBAs may ask women to assume various physical positions during delivery. These include what are called the "kneel down position," the "sit down position," and the "lay flat position." For the kneel down position, the pregnant woman kneels down, holds her knees, sits on her heels, and opens her thighs. Her heels support her buttocks, and the position facilitates the descent of the fetus. The second method is the sit down position. Here, old cloths are laid on a mat for the pregnant woman to sit on with her legs extended forward and spread apart. The TBA sits facing the pregnant woman, braces her own legs between the pregnant woman's thighs and waits patiently for the baby to be pushed for her to receive. It is important to note that the woman in labour is not forced to push during contractions. The lay flat position is what the biomedical practitioners refer to as the dorsal recumbent position. The TBAs appropriated this form of knowledge from the biomedical practitioners in order to modernize their practices. Here, the pregnant woman lays on her back with her knees flexed and thighs apart.

After the baby is born, the next step consists of the removal of the placenta and the cutting of the umbilical cord. The cutting of the umbilical cord and the ritual burial of the placenta form an essential part of the culture of Dzodze. During the removal of the placenta, shallots (local name: *afe sabala*) are given to the woman to chew and swallow with water. Some TBAs also give the woman an empty beer bottle to blow into, as it is believed that this can reduce her pain levels. The placenta is buried outside the compound of the house. Traditionally, it is believed that when a placenta is not properly buried with herbs it can result in mental health problems for the child and make the woman infertile. It is customary for the TBAs to bury the placenta, but the family may bury it on their own if they wish. In the past, once the TBA had cut the umbilical cord, she would apply a mixture of salt, sand, herbs, and *soot* (the black powder that surrounds cobwebs) to the stub of the cord. However, TBAs themselves observed that this practice often led to convulsions and subsequently resulted in the death of the baby. Currently, they dress the stub of the cord with a mixture of salt and chalk for three days. Once the cord is detached from the baby, they clean the wound with warm water and dry gin. After delivery, if the new mother complains of abdominal pains, none of the TBAs I interviewed prescribed herbal concoctions to her. One might expect TBAs to use herbal remedies to treat abdominal pains, but instead they prescribe acetaminophen tablets. The dosage is two tablets in the morning after breakfast and two in the evening after dinner. The mother stops taking the tablets as soon as she no longer experiences the abdominal pains. When a woman bleeds excessively during delivery, milk is given to her. The idea is that milk will make up for the lost blood, and make the woman healthy once again. Sometimes, the milk is mixed with tomato paste or ***Malta***, a commercial soft drink made with barley. The woman is also advised to eat plenty of green vegetables, such as spinach, to replenish her blood.

TBAs do not charge their clients a set fee. They believe that helping women to deliver is a humanitarian job; therefore, work should be put before money. As Mama Akorfa put it, "since God in heaven knows that I have worked for them, He will bless me." Those who do not have money to pay for a TBA's services are not charged. A word of thanks from the family of the new mother is appreciated a great deal by the TBAs, who value this recognition of their work. On the other hand, clients who have the means are asked to pay for the materials used during the delivery and to give a token payment for the TBA's services.

Relationship between Local Midwives and Hospital Practitioners

Presently, the relationship between TBAs and registered midwives can be described as cordial, yet it is also characterized by economic and political tension because of the unequal treatment that TBAs receive from the government. All of the TBAs I interviewed felt that their work was not recognized by the state. They felt that they contributed significantly to improving reproductive health and reducing maternal mortality in their communities, but without being rewarded financially or symbolically by the state. In the words of Mama Adzo:

> The current relationship existing between us and the hospital is good because it helps us as health workers to save the life of mothers and new born babies but it is not beneficial to us. We deliver for mothers and sometimes, under critical conditions, we use our own money to transport pregnant women to the hospital for a caesarean section. But for all these lifesaving jobs we do, government do not pay us any money for our services. Our counterparts at the hospitals are paid every month for the same child delivery job. We know that we do not have the certificate to take a sum of money with the midwives at the hospital but government should be fair to give us some allowance since we also do child delivery and contribute to the health care in Ghana.

The hospital records the names of TBAs who reside in the community, and occasionally organizes workshops to educate them on safe motherhood, safe delivery, family planning, and nutrition. However, the hospital midwives never consult TBAs about their skills in attending birth—so no official recognition of their expertise is seen here. Sometimes, mosquito nets are given to the TBAs to sell to nursing mothers. Rarely, working kits such as cotton, gloves, and methylated spirits are distributed to the TBAs to use at deliveries. Each month, TBAs send reports to the public health unit on the number of children they delivered. The report contains the date of birth of the newborn and the names of the mother and father. This helps to improve the birth and death registration system in Ghana. Babies delivered by the TBAs are also referred by them to the hospital for immunization. One observation that I made in the field was that some TBAs asked nurses from the hospital to give pain-relief injections to pregnant women. While this practice may promote relationships between TBAs and nurses on an individual level, it is not to be encouraged because the non-steroidal anti-inflammatory drugs that are typically used are associated with an increased incidence of fetal heart defects if administered to the mother in the late stages of pregnancy (Koren et al., 2006).

Some TBAs do not want to refer their clients to the hospital because they feel that this undermines their credibility, considering their experience with and expertise in childbirth. Other TBAs are reluctant to refer women to the hospital because of previous interactions with hostile, rude, or arrogant registered midwives. While TBAs make an important contribution to the provision of health care in Ghana, the fact that their work and knowledge are not considered legitimate inhibits effective collaboration. What is particularly lacking in the relationship between TBAs and registered midwives is trust. Registered midwives criticize TBAs for their lack of understanding of the anatomy and physiology of the human body, and their involvement in dangerous practices that may risk the lives of mothers and babies. For example, registered midwives accuse TBAs of using unsterilized blades to cut the umbilical cord, which risks exposing the newborn to infection. TBAs, on the other hand, suspect public health nurses of wanting to encourage hospital referrals on account of the TBA's lack of formal education; each referral represents one less client for the TBA. This mistrust hinders collaboration between the TBAs and registered midwives. If we are to improve maternal and child mortality rates, we need to appreciate that both TBAs and registered midwives have different skills that can be coordinated beneficially to help more women in many more situations.

Assistance to Traditional Birth Attendants

Following the Declaration of Alma Ata in 1978, the Ministry of Health of Ghana, in collaboration with the WHO, UNFPA, and UNICEF, began to provide training for TBAs. The declaration called for urgent action by all governments to promote and protect the health of all people. The official recognition of TBAs was a direct response to the declaration, which identified TBAs as a valuable medical resource that could be integrated into primary health care in developing countries. In Dzodze, TBAs now receive some two weeks of training from western health care providers, the object of which is to improve the skills of the TBAs and enhance the relationship among TBAs, the hospital, and the larger community. However, it appears that there have not been any initiatives to improve collaboration between TBAs and registered midwives and other health care workers. TBAs should be valued both for their knowing practices as well as their contextual knowledge. In my interviews with registered midwives, I was told emphatically that midwives supervised some activities of trained TBAs. My field observation, however, revealed that this supervision is very limited because the TBAs practise in remote rural areas. When supervision did take place, it focused on the number of babies the TBAs had delivered, and also encouraged TBAs to refer women to the hospital.

Untrained TBAs do not receive any working kits from the government, but must supply their own equipment or ask the pregnant woman or her family to purchase materials. Hospital-trained TBAs do receive working kits during their training but are thereafter obliged to replenish them themselves, ideally with funds from their clients. Some TBAs complained that this put a financial burden on them if their clients were unable to contribute toward their costs.

In order to facilitate the work of the TBAs, certain things need to be done. (1) TBAs should be supplied with working kits by the government to enable them to do their work. (2) Mobile phones should be provided to TBAs to facilitate access to emergency services during complicated deliveries. This will boost the confidence of TBAs to work harder in reducing neonatal and maternal death in rural areas. (3) Communities should help build maternity centres for TBAs so that local women can give birth in a hygienic and safer environment. (4) TBAs should be given hospital privileges to assist women who want their services in labour wards, under the supervision of registered midwives. This will enhance trust between TBAs and health care workers. (5) Incentives in the form of a monthly allowance should be given to TBAs in recognition of their work and contribution toward improving reproductive health. This money can also serve as a contingency fund to pay for the transport of pregnant women when there are obstetric emergencies. For these goals to be realized, however, the work of TBAs as useful knowing practices must be understood. Perhaps registered midwives, too, could be trained on experiential and bodily knowledge in traditional obstetric practices and the reasons underlying the practices.

Conclusion

This chapter has described local birth practices of TBAs and the relationships that exist between TBAs and registered midwives in Dzodze, Ghana. I have suggested that TBAs are valuable medical assets to women, especially in rural communities and among the urban poor. The ultimate aim of TBAs and registered midwives is to assist women to give birth in a safe and healthy way. If this aim is to be achieved, then it is necessary for TBAs, registered midwives, and doctors to reach a mutual understanding and work together for their shared goal of reducing maternal, neonatal, and infant mortality. However, the relationship between the TBAs and registered midwives is complicated by a lack of recognition of the TBAs' knowledge and practices. Because TBAs have no formal education, registered midwives, doctors, and other medical professionals often assume that they cannot offer legitimate assistance to women in childbirth. TBAs are often blamed for engaging in high-risk and unsafe birth practices that expose mothers and infants to infections and possible death. Many registered midwives and doctors find it difficult to accept and work with TBAs. Even those registered midwives and doctors who have accepted TBAs still regard them as inferior because of their lack of formal education in midwifery.

I suggest that one way to foster co-operation and mutual respect between the TBAs and registered midwives is to encourage registered midwives to learn about the TBAs' traditional obstetric practices, the logic behind the practices, and their benefits. Further, paying TBAs a monthly allowance and thus making them waged employees of the state may also help to remove barriers to collaboration and camaraderie.

Note

1. The Millennium Development Goal 4 aims at reducing mortality rates for children under five years of age by two thirds by 2015 (based on mortality rates in 1990).

Critical Thinking Questions

1. With the limited health facilities and human resources for health crisis (doctors, midwives, and nurses), especially in rural areas in Ghana, how can TBAs effectively be integrated into the health care system to improve maternal-child health?
2. Do you think that a system of hospital referral would be enough to improve the health of pregnant women?
3. How can we recognize the work of TBAs in the rural communities as useful knowing practices?

Glossary

Afeme vixelawo: Local name for traditional birth attendants in the Ewe language.

Bokɔ: Traditional Ghanaian healers who use plant-based therapies. A *bokɔ* may also be a diviner.

Breech birth: When the baby's feet or buttocks enter the birth canal first, in contrast to the typical head-first birth presentation.

Malta: Soft drink made with barley. Produced by Guinness Ghana Limited.

Mama: Honorific title bestowed to elderly women in Ghanaian society.

Partograph: A printout graphical record that plots key maternal and fetal data (e.g., vital signs) against time during the labour process.

Seselelame: An Anlo-Ewe word meaning "feelings in the body."

References

Bierlich, B. (1999). Sacrifice, plants and Western pharmaceutical. Money and health care in Northern Ghana. *Medical Anthropology Quarterly, 13*(3), 316–337.

Farquhar, J. (1994). *Knowing practice: The clinical encounter of Chinese medicine*. Boulder, CO: Westview Press.

Ghana Millennium Development Goals Report. (2015). *Ghana Millennium Development Goals Report*. Accra, Ghana.

Ghana Statistical Service. (2012). *Ghana multiple indicator cluster survey with an enhanced malaria module and biomarker 2011: Monitoring the situation of children and women in Ghana.* Accra, Ghana: Author.

Ghana Statistical Service. (2014). *2010 population and housing census: District analytical report, Ketu North District.* Accra, Ghana: Author.

Goody, J. (2002). The anthropology of the senses and sensation. *La Ricerca Folklorica, 45*, 17–28.

Ingold, T. (2000). *The perception of the environment. Essays on livelihood, dwelling, and skills.* London & New York: Routledge.

Ingold, T. (2012). *Making: Anthropology, archaeology, art, and architecture.* New York: Routledge.

Koren, G., Florescu, A., Costei, A.M., Boskovic, R., & Moretti, M.E. (2006). Nonsteroidal antiinflammatory drugs during third trimester and the risk of premature closure of the ductus arteriosus: A meta-analysis. *The Annals of Pharmacotherapy, 40*(5), 824–829.

Merleau-Ponty, M. (1962). *Phenomenology of perception.* (C. Smith, Trans.). New York: Routledge.

Merleau-Ponty, M. (1964). *The primacy of perception and other essays on phenomenological psychology, the philosophy of art, history, and politics.* (J.M. Edie, Trans.). Evanston, IL: Northwestern University Press.

Nyonator, J.P. (2010). *Informal medicine and biomedicine: Ghanaian assemblage.* Mauritius: VDM Publishing House.

Ofili, A.N., & Okojie, O.H. (2005). Assessment of the role of traditional birth attendants in maternal health care in Oredo Local Government Area, Edo State, Nigeria. *Journal of Community Medicine and Primary Health Care, 17*(1), 55–60.

St. Anthony's Hospital. (2008). *Annual hospital report.* Dzodze, Ghana: Author.

Twumasi, P.A. (2005). *Medical system in Ghana.* Accra, Ghana: Ghana Publishing Corporation.

United Nations Development Programme. (2012). *2010 Ghana millennium development goals reports.* Accra, Ghana: Author.

United Nations Population Fund (UNPF). (2011). *The state of the world's midwifery: Delivering health, saving lives.* New York: UNFPA.

United Nations Population Fund. (2014). *The state of the world's midwifery: Delivering health, saving lives.* New York, NY: UNFPA.

PART III

GLOBAL NORTH

The third part of this book analyzes how CAM is used in the Global North for women's reproductive health, and the processes by which the therapeutic practices and concepts are translated into these non-traditional socio-cultural settings. It thus emphasizes the importance of disease, healing, and the body as sites of cross-cultural negotiation.

As the introduction clarified, the label *traditional medicine* (TM) is used to indicate a health practice that has developed over time within a particular culture. When health care practices are not part of the tradition of a specific country and are not fully integrated into the dominant local health care system, they are defined as "complementary" or "alternative." This section explores how the different systems of TM have been incorporated into western cultures, and how they are utilized to support women's reproductive health in the Global North. It asks how this can be done in a manner that permits TM therapies to contribute to the biomedical understanding of health and disease while at the same time retaining their cultural integrity.

Emerging scholarship on the interconnections between biomedicine and CAM emphasizes medical pluralism and integrative medicine, not in terms of discrete cultural systems set in opposition to one another (e.g., traditional medicine versus biomedicine), but rather as an open system of dynamic relations between institutions and patients. As the following chapters demonstrate, women in search of treatment for their reproductive health in the Global North frequently access multiple health care providers of both CAM/TM and biomedical treatments, sometimes trying out different therapies simultaneously.

Two chapters explore the influence of socio-demographic factors (such as age, education, income, and marital status) on how women find out about CAM and the extent to which they use it, whether on its own or in conjunction with biomedical therapies. Chapter 12 focuses on important gaps in the research on Australian women of reproductive age and their use of CAM for reproductive health, such as motivations for using CAM and sources of information about CAM for reproductive health problems. Chapter 14 describes the types of CAM that are commonly used by women with breast cancer, including natural products, mind and body medicine, manipulative and body-based practices, and other therapies, as well as how these women find the sources of information about CAM. The decision-making process regarding CAM use among breast cancer patients and the role of health care professionals in integrating CAM into biomedicine are also explored in this chapter.

The important issue of TM adaptation as CAM and cultural appropriation is addressed in the other two chapters. In chapter 11, CAM approaches to perimenopausal relief (including western phytotherapy, traditional Chinese medicine (TCM), and Ayurvedic medicine) are the backdrop to a discussion of how colonization and cultural appropriation of TM continue to imbue today's globalized health care landscape. Chapter 13 examines how practitioners of TCM in the Canadian provinces of British Columbia and Ontario construct evidence of effectiveness and safety of their practices in the area of reproductive health. TCM has become reinvented as preventative medicine in transnational encounters with the Global North. By combining "hard" (bioscientific) and "soft" (experiential) evidence bases, the TCM practitioners interviewed illuminate the scope for a symmetrical and fully integrative health care system in which the contributions of different epistemologies meet diverse health care needs.

CHAPTER 11

A Post-colonial Feminist Analysis of Two Popular Complementary Medicine Hot Flash Remedies

Nadine E. Ijaz, MSc, PhD Candidate
University of Toronto, Toronto, Canada

Learning Objectives

1. To incorporate feminist, post-colonial theoretical perspectives into an analysis of complementary and alternative medicine therapies.
2. To illustrate the concepts of paradigm appropriation and assimilation in relation to two specific complementary and alternative medicine remedies for menopause-associated hot flashes: black cohosh and soy isoflavones.

Introduction

Many complementary and alternative medicine (CAM) therapies originate from non-western or indigenous systems of medicine (Hollenberg & Muzzin, 2010). Positioning CAM usage in a global context, Keshet and Simchai (2014) have distinguished between nations in the Global North, where CAM usage represents "privileged health care for privileged" (that is, affluent white) women and men, and the Global South, where women "are generally forced to use folk/traditional medicine ... as a cheap alternative instead of biomedicine" (p. 84). Scholars such as Harding (1998) and Shiva (1999) have engaged **post-colonial** critiques of biomedicine. Such critics problematize the racist, colonial dominance that biomedical scientists have historically exerted over many non-European, traditional/indigenous systems of medicine worldwide.[1] Hollenberg and Muzzin (2010) have extended such an anti-colonial analysis to the CAM phenomenon, as is discussed below.

Indeed, such historically contextual perspectives are increasingly entering the global conversation around therapies originating in traditional/indigenous health care systems. Two recent United Nations reports recommended that nations take steps to address and prevent **misappropriation** of traditional/indigenous medical knowledges (World Health Organization [WHO], World Intellectual Property Organization & World Trade Organization, 2013). Several nations in the Global South, including India and China, have created multilingual digital repositories to prevent further patents being placed on their nations' traditional herbal formulations (WHO et al., 2013)—a **neo-colonial** phenomenon referred to as "biopiracy" (Shiva, 1999). However, relatively little scholarship has examined the sociological dynamics of CAM usage in the Global North using a post-colonial lens; Hollenberg and Muzzin's 2010 work is an important exception.

With reference to the CAM phenomenon, Hollenberg and Muzzin (2010) have theorized two key mechanisms by which misappropriation of traditional/indigenous knowledges may take place: paradigm appropriation and paradigm assimilation. "In paradigm appropriation," they write, "biomedicine appropriates certain aspects from other healing systems or traditions without fully acknowledging the paradigmatic worldview from which the particular treatment aspect was taken" (Hollenberg & Muzzin, 2010, p. 48). Paradigm assimilation implies that "one paradigm not only appropriates or takes over another entire healing paradigm or system, but re-interprets it" (Hollenberg & Muzzin, 2010, p. 49). As a result, non-biomedical therapies become reframed and validated (or invalidated) in relation to how well they may (or may not) fit into the biomedical paradigm.

Aside from Hollenberg and Muzzin's original work, there are few applied illustrations of this theoretical perspective available to scholars and students. My aim in this work is to contribute to filling this gap by illustrating how two popular CAM remedies used in treating hot flashes associated with the menopause transition—black cohosh herbal extracts and soy isoflavone products—exemplify both paradigm appropriation and paradigm assimilation. By highlighting these products' historical origins, the context of their contemporary usage, and marketing and scholarly discourses surrounding them, I demonstrate key mechanisms through which paradigm appropriation and assimilation ultimately take place.

In order to situate this analysis appropriately alongside existing critical sociological scholarship around perimenopausal therapies, I contextualize my discussion in what follows within the parameters of **feminist** scholars' critiques of biomedicine's contemporary conceptions of menopause. This intersectional approach demonstrates the ways in which patriarchal and neo-colonial impulses may closely intersect in contemporary health care. Ultimately I aim to disrupt the characterization of two popular CAM treatments as "alternatives" to biomedical care by showing ways in which the historical emergence and therapeutic composition of black cohosh and soy isoflavone products, as well as marketing and scholarly discourses surrounding them, both reproduce and reinforce biomedicine's neo-colonial, patriarchal underpinnings.

Black Cohosh, Soy Isoflavones, and Biomedicine's Menopause Construct

Over the last decades, an increasing proportion of women in Europe and North America have been seeking out so-called "natural" or CAM treatments to address health concerns (such as hot flashes) associated with the menopausal transition; reports range from 22–80 percent of women surveyed (see Kupferer, Dormire & Becker, 2009; Pitkin, 2012).[2] The two most extensively researched CAM approaches for this problem are black cohosh and soy isoflavone products: plant-derived remedies marketed as alternatives to conventional hormone replacement therapies (HRT). In 2005, black cohosh products—used primarily for menopausal concerns—represented the eighth most popular herbal/dietary supplement sold in the United States, generating sales of over $USD9.7 million in that country alone (Zimmermann et al., 2010).

This trend may be partially understood in light of increased public demand for "safer" as well as non-hormonal treatment options for menopause-related concerns, which increased after 2002, when the American Women's Health Initiative (WHI) clinical trial was halted and its results were made public (Burger, MacLennan, Huang & Castelo-Brano, 2012). WHI associated use of a particular HRT, the drug Premarin, with serious potential negative effects, including increased breast cancer, stroke, heart disease, and pulmonary embolisms. Global HRT usage subsequently dropped 40–80 percent (Burger, MacLennan, Huang & Castelo-Brano, 2012), a dramatic shift given that Premarin had previously been one of the five most commonly used drugs in the United States (MacPherson, 1981). Pharmaceutical researchers and companies have since developed a new range of seemingly safer HRT therapies (Panay, 2012), yet the demand for "natural" menopause treatments has concurrently risen.

However, this marketplace diversification should also be viewed in light of feminist critiques of biomedicine's "perimenopause construct."[3] Feminist scholars have for many years problematized biomedicine's definition of women's natural menstrual cessation as a diagnosable hormone deficiency condition (Murtagh & Hepworth, 2003). Such scholars have argued that this conception—which emerged in the 1930s (Erol, 2009)—fails to differentiate between "natural life events" and "illnesses requiring regular medical attention," effectively paternalizing women into excessive pharmaceutical care (Gannon, 1998, p. 295). The widespread historical usage of HRT is indeed remarkable given that just 6–20 percent of perimenopausal women are reported to find hot flashes bothersome (Pimenta, Leal, Maroco & Ramos, 2011). Feminist researchers have also demonstrated that perimenopausal hot flashes are not universal, but vary intergenerationally (Utz, 2011), as well as across social strata (Murtagh & Hepworth, 2003) and across cultures (Chirawatkul & Manderson, 1994). Owing largely to such critiques, an increased emphasis on informed choice has in recent years entered the sphere of women's health care, replacing the former climate of pre-emptive treatment (Kuhlmann, 2009).

Overall, the improved safety profile of widely available perimenopausal treatments and the emergent culture of informed choice within aging women's health care may be seen—at least tentatively—as an advance. The increased popularity of CAM therapies such as black cohosh and soy isoflavone products arguably represent a relatively effective and safe choice within women's options. A considerable body of biomedical clinical evidence has supported the utility of both black cohosh (Betz et al., 2009; Shams et al., 2010; Villaseca, 2012) and soy isoflavone products (Kurzer, 2008; Taku et al., 2012; Usui, 2006; Villaseca, 2012) in a low to modest reduction of perimenopausal hot flash symptoms. Furthermore, both black cohosh and soy isoflavone products have been shown to be relatively safe.[4]

Regardless, feminist scholars Murtagh and Hepworth (2003, p. 1651) argue that the "discourse of prevention" and "choice" that has recently emerged in women's health care ultimately reinforces the perimenopause construct, by building for women a binary set of choices "to take or not to take hormone replacement therapy." Engaging this analytic framework, a closer examination of popular marketing discourses around black cohosh and soy isoflavone products suggests that these "alternative" products may not after all deeply contest the "relations of power that produce menopause in medical and popular discourse" (Murtagh & Hepworth, 2003, p. 1651). Indeed, although marketing materials (as illustrated below) both feature linguistic slogans reflecting feminist critiques of biomedicine's perimenopause construct and appear to position themselves in contrast to biomedicine in other strategic ways, marketers ultimately rely heavily on biomedical concepts and evidentiary frameworks to promote their products.

Marketing materials for black cohosh and soy isoflavone products commonly engage language that contests the notion of menopause as disease, producing counter-narratives that reflect feminist critiques of the perimenopause construct. One black cohosh product website, for example, states that "once treated by mainstream medicine as a disease, menopause is a normal transition in a woman's life from an age of fertility to one of wisdom" (Sisu, 2015). Such emancipatory discourses aim to position the product as representing worldviews distinct from conventional biomedicine. Marketers further aim to distinguish black cohosh and soy isoflavone products from biomedical therapies by characterizing them as "natural" and safer than conventional HRT. One soy isoflavone product, for instance, apparently "balances hormones naturally, without side effects" (Organika, 2015).

However, despite the use of sophisticated discursive strategies aiming to position these products outside of biomedicine's perimenopause construct, marketing materials ultimately tend to reproduce the construct's conceptual parameters. For instance, a substantial portion of the website for Remifemin, a popular black cohosh extract, is devoted to the symptoms, diagnosis, and treatment of perimenopause and menopause (Enzymatic Therapy, 2008). Furthermore, many marketing materials make use of biomedical evidence to support the remedies' clinical efficacy and safety in treating menopause-related symptoms: "studies have shown that premium isoflavone supplementation helps alleviate menopausal symptoms" (Nature's Way, 2015).

While feminist-style marketing discourses surrounding these products may imply that their composition and usage would disrupt biomedical conceptual notions of perimenopause and menopause, I suggest that these remedies fall squarely into Murtagh and Hepworth's binary framework ("to take or *not to take* HRT," emphasis added) without deeply disrupting the patriarchal biomedical, conceptual notions of perimenopause that feminists have long critiqued.

What calls for further unpacking, however, is the repeated discursive allusion to black cohosh and soy isoflavones' traditional/indigenous origins in both product marketing materials and scholarly accounts. For instance: "black cohosh ... was used by the American Indians, and later by the colonists, to relieve menstrual cramps and symptoms of menopause" (Sisu, 2015). Situating biomedicine's cultural construction of menopause within a globalized framework, and referencing the Turkish context (where many affluent women embrace menopause's biomedicalization as a symbol of empowered modernity), Erol (2009) argues that feminist-inspired, choice-based health care frameworks have contributed to a progressive abandonment of traditional cultural perspectives on the aging process. Chirawatkul and Manderson (1994, p. 1552) have similarly documented an adoption of "western technological approaches over village understandings and values" around menopause in Thailand. That said, how might we interpret aging women's increasing adoption, in the Global North, of so-called CAM remedies—which in the case of black cohosh and soy isoflavones originate in traditional herbal and dietary practices, respectively?

It is important at this point to acknowledge I am undertaking two levels of analysis of the black cohosh/soy isoflavone phenomenon in this work. The first level engages feminist theory as a conceptual overlay to women's motivations for using complementary medicine in the Global North. The second level engages post-colonial theories of misappropriation to engage a critical, structural analysis of particular complementary medicine remedies. Having made this clear, I propose that representing a subversion of—or alternative to—biomedicine's longstanding, neo-colonial global dominance, which has historically denigrated the value of traditional health care approaches (Hollenberg & Muzzin, 2010), contemporary usage of black cohosh and soy isoflavone hot flash remedies may be understood as implying a profound misappropriation of traditional/indigenous knowledges. This becomes clear by examining the historical origins, material composition, and discursive worlds surrounding these products, using Hollenberg and Muzzin's twin concepts of paradigm appropriation and assimilation (2010).

Neo-colonial CAM? Two Exemplars

It is clear that contemporary black cohosh and soy isoflavone usage may be historically tracked to traditional cultural uses in North America and eastern Asia respectively. However, modern CAM usages of these plant extracts are profoundly different from the traditional/indigenous uses that preceded them both in material terms, and in relation to the paradigms that inform their respective composition. These differences—and the way they are depicted in contemporary marketing and scholarly accounts surrounding both remedies—offer a clear illustration of the ways in which such CAM remedies can exemplify neo-colonialism in contemporary health care.

How Traditional?

Black cohosh (*Actaea racemosa)* is a plant endemic to eastern North America, with a traditional history of use by Indigenous peoples (including Iroquois, Cherokee, Algonquian, and Mi'kmaq Nations) (Foster, 1999). Ethnobotanical literature unfortunately provides little detail on the healing paradigms that may have informed such usage, though it is clear that traditional uses included both ceremonial as well therapeutic applications for ailments that today might be characterized as rheumatic, urinary, respiratory, reproductive, and musculoskeletal. In most uses, the plant's root and rhizome would have been extracted into boiling water (Foster, 1999).

The domesticated soybean (*Glycine max*) has been used across eastern Asia as both food (Munro et al., 2003) and medicine (Lu, 1986) going back several millennia. Therapeutic soybean preparations have been used since the third century BCE in traditional Chinese medicine (TCM) (Lu, 1986). Like other medicinal plants in TCM, soy preparations are traditionally characterized in terms of their thermal qualities ("cooling"), flavours ("neutral and sweet"), and effects within specific bodily systems ("moistening") (Lu, 1986). Various preparations of the plant are traditionally described as producing distinct therapeutic effects (e.g., tofu for periodic diarrhea and pink eye, soybean sprouts for coughs with yellow phlegm) (Bensky, Clavey, Stoeger & Gamble, 2004).

However, contemporary usage of black cohosh and soy for menopause-related hot flashes is considerably dissimilar to traditional indications for both plants. While Indigenous North American black cohosh usage related to women's reproductive functioning has indeed been historically reported, including promotion of menses and post-partum milk flows, hot flashes do not appear amongst the concerns treated. Similarly, while classical Chinese medical texts describe traditional usage of numerous plants and plant combinations for treating hot flashes (Bensky, Clavey, Stoeger & Gamble, 2004), soy foods are not among these, and the hot flashes mentioned are not associated exclusively with menopause. There is furthermore no ethnobotanical indication that traditional East Asian soy food consumption had as its particular aim the prevention of hot flashes amongst middle-aged women. Rather, the specific use of both plant extracts for menopause-related symptoms emerged relatively recently.

Black cohosh usage for menopause-associated symptoms emerged around the mid-19th century, after American "eclectic" physicians—a group of herbal medicine practitioners in the United States who had learned about black cohosh usage from Indigenous peoples—began to emphasize the plant's varied reproductive applications (Foster, 1999). It is unclear to what degree this emphasis reflected the traditional indications that Indigenous North American people had shared with the eclectics. Reports of the eclectics' clinical successes reached Germany in the late 19th century, which progressively gave rise to considerable biomedical research on the plant's utility in treating aging women's hot flashes in particular (Foster, 1999).

The development of soybean extracts for perimenopausal women took place much more recently, in the 1990s. In 1991, the *Lancet* medical journal published anthropologist Margaret Lock's feminist critique of menopause's biomedicalization, which, in reporting significantly lower rates of hot flash reports from Japanese as compared with Canadian women aged 45–55, contested the presumed universality of biomedicine's perimenopause construct (Lock, 1991). A group of scientists responded by suggesting that the estrogen-like activity of a biochemical constituent known as "isoflavones," consumed by Japanese women in traditional soy foods, may account for the apparent cross-cultural hot flash differential (Adlercreutz, Hamalainen, Gorbach & Goldin, 1992). This suggestion gave rise to dozens of subsequent studies that demonstrated the viability of this hypothesis (Messina, 2010).

Regardless of these two remedies' current characterization as CAM therapies, the contemporary adoption of a traditional herbal treatment—black cohosh—and a traditional dietary practice—soy food consumption—into biomedically informed health care clearly exemplifies what Hollenberg and Muzzin (2010) have termed "paradigm appropriation." The hallmark of such appropriation, they write, is "the separation of technique from healing paradigm" (Hollenberg & Muzzin, 2010, p. 49), demonstrated in these cases by the decontextualization of each remedy from its traditional cultural context. Although (as will be illustrated further on) both marketing and biomedical research discourses surrounding the two remedies do indeed refer repeatedly to their traditional cultural origins, the underlying cultural contexts and worldviews that informed each plant's traditional usage are rarely addressed.

Rather, traditional usages—frequently cited in discursive accounts—have been significantly reinterpreted within the biomedical paradigm, exemplifying Hollenberg and Muzzin's concept of paradigm assimilation. In paradigm assimilation, a non-biomedical healing system or approach is completely reinterpreted in biomedical terms. Two key mechanisms through which such paradigm assimilation takes place become apparent upon closer examination. Deeply informed by Hollenberg and Muzzin's theoretical work, I term these mechanisms "erasure/negation" and "recomposition/privileging."

Erasure/Negation

Erasure/negation refers to the systematic exclusion of important aspects of a given remedy's traditional context of usage, achieved by reframing that remedy to suit the biomedical paradigm. In both marketing and scholarly accounts, it is apparent that reference to black cohosh's traditional usage attributes particular weight to the plant's historically reported reproductive uses (which may not in fact have even included hot flashes). In this process, the plant's diverse traditional ceremonial and medicinal uses become implicitly negated in favour of an emphasis on exclusively physical, menopause-related applications. A biomedical journal excerpt, for example, reads: "black cohosh was originally used by Native American peoples in the treatment of many conditions, *especially gynecologic disorders*" (Kligler, 2003; emphasis added).

Similarly, diverse discursive accounts reinterpret the nutritional and socio-cultural importance of traditional soy food consumption in East Asian countries from within the biomedical worldview. The following passage, from a biomedical review of the "effects of soy consumption on menopausal symptoms" (Kurzer, 2008, p. 227), provides a useful illustration:

> It has been estimated that hot flash incidence is far lower in Asian countries than in the West. [...] Given the fact that the soybean, typically consumed in the Asian diet, contains the phytoestrogen isoflavones, it has been suggested that soy consumption may be responsible for this difference in symptoms. Recent data suggest that average consumption of isoflavones in Japan is between 15–30 mg/day, while in the United States and Europe, it is 1–2 mg/day. It has thus been suggested that soy consumption may be an effective substitute for postmenopausal hormone replacement therapy.

In this passage, the full range of traditional East Asian soy foods—diverse in their preparation, distinct in their nutritional profiles and cultural histories—are as a whole subsumed and reframed in terms of their hot flash preventative action. This newly constructed meaning gains its power only with reference to non-East Asian women who have presumably not yet "benefitted" from the possible therapeutic action of soy, but may now—with the help of biomedical understanding—do so. Such a reframing profoundly erases and negates the cultural wisdom underpinning traditional soy food preparation and consumption, thoroughly assimilating such into the biomedical paradigm.

Recomposition/Privileging

Paradigm assimilation is furthermore evident in relation to the material composition of black cohosh and soy isoflavone products in widespread usage for hot flash reduction. The preparations of these plants used in contemporary research—and widely marketed for menopause-related applications—differ considerably from Indigenous North American black cohosh teas, and traditional East Asian soy foods such as tofu and tempeh. Far from reflecting minor variations to the traditional/indigenous approaches from which they originate, these novel products may be seen as cultural artifacts bearing the clear mark of the biomedical paradigm. More specifically, commercial preparations of black cohosh and soy isoflavones researched and marketed for hot flash reduction are commonly characterized by three related biomedical practices: constituent isolation, compound standardization, and constituent synthesis.

In constituent isolation, biomedical researchers begin by identifying, segregating, and researching a particular biochemical constituent in relation to a specific therapeutic application. This approach fundamentally reflects biomedicine's reductionist notion that singular "active constituents" in medicinal plants act as "silver bullets" (Duke & Bodenschutz-Godwin, 1999) for particular therapeutic effects (Williamson, 2001). This culturally specific biomedical notion is antithetical to more holistic conceptualizations of plant medicines typical of traditional/indigenous medical paradigms (Hollenberg & Muzzin, 2010), wherein multiple components of a plant are understood as acting synergistically (Barsh, 1997; Williamson, 2001).

In contrast to traditional soy foods such as tempeh, natto, or miso, which are prepared from the whole intact soybean, soy isoflavone products are largely composed as isolates of individual constituent extracts (e.g., the isoflavones genestein, daidzein, and glyceitein) or as protein-isolate extracts (Kurzer, Morgan & Greaves, 2004), clearly exemplifying the principle of constituent isolation. The (biomedical) assumption informing such contemporary products is that the isolated constituent is therapeutically equivalent to the original whole plant preparation. Despite such a theoretical conjecture's problematic character even from within the biomedical paradigm,[5] this assumption is often repeated in scholarly accounts: "consumption of 30 mg/day of soy isoflavones (or at least 15 mg genistein) reduces hot flashes by up to 50% [...]. The greatest benefit may be realized when the isoflavone-rich *food or supplement* is taken" (Kurzer 2008, p. 227; emphasis added).

A process related to constituent isolation involves compound standardization, as is exemplified by the black cohosh extract marketed as Remifemin: a proprietary alcohol-based extract studied in two thirds of perimenopause-related black cohosh research trials (Betz et al., 2009). In compound standardization, a plant extract is industrially compounded to contain a standard, calibrated proportion of one or more plant constituents characterized as "active ingredients." In the case of Remifemin, the standardized constituents are known as terpene glycosides and are currently considered by many biomedical researchers to be the so-called active constituents involved in black cohosh's hot flash reducing effect (Kligler, 2003). In addition to being scientifically contestable,[6] it is clear that such a perspective did not underpin Indigenous black cohosh usage. Biomedicine's signature silver bullet principle—the reification of the isolated constituent over holistic synergism—is again apparent in the paradigmatic reinterpretation of a traditional herbal medicine.

A third process reflective of paradigm assimilation—constituent synthesis—takes the silver bullet principle one step further: a previously isolated biochemical compound is now chemically synthesized, producing a non-plant sourced extract with similar characteristics. An increasing number of soy isoflavone products are synthetically produced rather than extracted from beans (Taku et al., 2012). Marketing materials and biomedical studies commonly treat the synthetic and plant-sourced extracts as equivalent, such as in a recent meta-analysis of soy isoflavone products' clinical efficacy for hot flashes (Taku et al., 2012); this study explicitly evaluates isoflavone products from both synthetic and "natural" (soy) sources as though they are identical. Contrary to the intrinsic and often spiritual value ascribed to whole plant medicines across many traditional/indigenous healing paradigms (Hollenberg & Muzzin, 2010), constituent synthesis exemplifies a paradigm that considers the plant itself as non-essential to the therapeutic process (see box 11.1).

Box 11.1: Distinguishing CAM from Conventional Care

Aside from their relative marginality, it remains unclear what traits objectively distinguish CAM therapies from conventional care. Though CAM treatments are commonly characterized as more "natural" than pharmaceutical drugs, some such products (such as soy isoflavones) may be synthetically produced. Conversely, some hormone replacement therapies (such as Premarin) are sourced from seemingly natural materials (e.g., urine of pregnant mares) (MacPherson, 1981).

Rather, as a relatively inefficient vehicle for particular medicinal ingredients, the source plant may be altogether dispensed with in favour of a synthetic replica of the "active" constituent.

What is perhaps most notable in light of these three widespread mechanisms of paradigm appropriation—isolation, standardization, and synthesis—is that in many cases, very little biomedical research exists to examine the traditional remedies or dietary practices from which novel therapies have been innovated. For example, virtually no published studies have directly examined the impact of traditional soy food consumption on menopause-associated hot flashes,[7] implicitly conveying a presumed inferiority of such foods as compared to modern isolates. Biomedicalized novel products are moreover frequently characterized as explicitly superior to their traditional antecedents. For example, a 2003 biomedical review of black cohosh therapies recommends only those extracts "standardized *properly* to the terpene glycoside fraction" (Kligler, 2003; emphasis added). A popular soy isoflavone product website similarly ascribes shortcomings to soy foods as compared to industrially produced isolates: "it is clear that *many soy foods fall short* when it comes to delivering the full isoflavone benefits. Unless you are eating multiple servings per day, these products simply do not provide enough soy isoflavones some experts think might be needed for the full health benefits" (Revival Products, 2014; emphasis added).

Box 11.2: Kun Bao Wan

CAM therapies do not all equally exemplify the misappropriation of traditional/indigenous health care knowledges into the biomedical paradigm. For example, the traditional Chinese herbal formulation Kun Bao Wan has been evidenced as comparably effective to HRT in treating perimenopausal hot flashes (Azizi et al., 2011). Notably, the clinical trial designs incorporate Chinese medicine-based diagnostic parameters in addition to patients' "perimenopausal status," as such giving importance to the traditional paradigm from which the intervention originates.

Such an implicit and explicit privileging of biomedical innovations over traditional health care approaches, characterizing them as more advanced is—as Hollenberg and Muzzin (2010) have previously pointed out—an important dimension of paradigm assimilation (see box 11.2).

Conclusion

It is ultimately not difficult to discern a clear qualitative distinction between a boiled tea of black cohosh root, and a standardized, commercially patented, alcohol-based extract pressed into tablets with various binders and flavours. Neither is much imagination needed to distinguish between East Asia's diverse and tasty traditional soy foods, and powdered isolates from uncooked soybeans or synthetic versions of the same. To invoke traditional/indigenous usage of these two plants in scholarly and marketing discourses surrounding the use of contemporary black cohosh and soy isoflavones products for menopause-associated hot flashes is to profoundly misrepresent these medicines' cultural and historical origins.

Black cohosh and soybeans are plants in widespread cultivation worldwide in service of diverse, lucrative industries. Yet the traditional frameworks within which these plants have been used for millennia are increasingly threatened, lending additional significance to the misappropriation described in this work. Wild black cohosh has been identified as a species at risk (United Plant Savers, 2013). While industrially processed, genetically engineered[8] soy-based isolates and foods are becoming increasingly popular (North American Menopause Society, 2011), consumption of traditional soy foods in Eastern Asia is on the decline (Munro et al., 2003).

Consumers seeking out CAM therapies commonly do so due to a preference for "natural" over synthetic medicines, generally believing the former to be safer than the latter (Bubela, Boon & Caulfield, 2008). Black cohosh and soy isoflavones may indeed be safer options than some conventional hormone replacement therapies for reducing menopause-associated hot flashes. Studies of CAM usage also indicate that its overall appeal arises from patients' critique of and dissatisfaction with conventional biomedical care as authoritarian, mechanistic, and reductionist (Keshet & Simchai, 2014)—characteristics also common within feminist critiques of biomedicine. As noted earlier, however, black cohosh and soy isoflavone products—as currently marketed and researched—do not appear to contest deeply the patriarchal foundations of biomedicine's perimenopause construct, long critiqued by feminists.

Many CAM users furthermore align with a holistic worldview (Keshet & Simchai, 2014) that may include a dimension of spirituality and a belief in a "vitalistic" life force (Kaptchuk & Eisenberg, 1998)—values arguably common to many traditional/indigenous health care paradigms (Hollenberg & Muzzin, 2010). However, as demonstrated in this chapter, the profound cultural misappropriation expressed in the product composition, research, and marketing surrounding black cohosh and soy isoflavones as hot flash remedies fails to represent such CAM users' articulated values. Additional scholarly work (see Adams, Hollenberg, Lui & Broom, 2009) is clearly needed to examine ways in which such so-called alternative, as well as emancipatory feminist, anti-colonial values may—or may not—ultimately be integrated into mainstream health care.

Notes

1. Although I am aware that much North American scholarship uses the term *Indigenous* to refer primarily to the continent's First Peoples, I adopt Hollenberg and Muzzin's broadened conception of "indigenous medicine" as a "formal knowledge system comprised of local medicines and healing knowledges, originating from an Indigenous community and/or country with an Indigenous population. Examples include traditional Chinese medicine, Ayurvedic medicine, and First Nations/Aboriginal Medicine" (2010, p. 35).
2. Kupferer, Dormire & Becker, 2009. As part of the aging process, most women experience a permanent cessation of their menstrual periods (menopause) during their late 40s or early 50s.
3. The time leading up to the menopause is referred to in conventional western biomedicine as perimenopause, and characterized in that system by "reduced secretion of the ovarian hormones oestrogen and progesterone" (Nelson, 2008). Within biomedicine, hot flashes are considered a diagnosable and treatable symptom of perimenopause (MacPherson, 1981).
4. Despite ongoing concerns about pre-market adulteration of some black cohosh products (Teschke, 2010), previous reports about black cohosh-induced liver toxicity have been largely discounted (Firenzuoli, Gori & di Sarsina, 2011; Naser et al., 2011; Teschke, 2010;

Teschke et al., 2011). Soy isoflavones may however produce increased gastrointestinal disturbances (Taku et al., 2012), increase the risk of hypothyroidism (Sathyapalan et al., 2011), and aggravate pre-existing breast cancers (Munro et al., 2003).

5. Biomedical researchers increasingly recognize a "synergy among the components of intact soy protein" (Usui, 2006, p. 12), wherein single versus multiple/combined isoflavones produce notably different effects in the body. It is also increasingly clear that the fermentation processes characteristic of many traditional East Asian soy foods significantly alters isoflavone concentrations, enhances nutrient absorption, and produces additional nutritional compounds not typically formed in human digestion (North American Menopause Society, 2011).
6. Ruhlen and colleagues (2008) have demonstrated that black cohosh's effectiveness in alleviating menopausal hot flashes does not in fact appear to arise from triterpene glycosides alone, but rather from a complex series of synergistic pathways between the whole root/rhizome extract and human tissues.
7. The rare biomedical studies examining the therapeutic potential of soy foods typically examine the clinical utility of contemporary innovations such as muffins prepared with soy flour (Kurzer 2008; Kurzer et al., 2004) rather than traditional soy foods.
8. Of American-grown soybeans, 93 percent are likely to be genetically engineered (United States Department of Agriculture, 2012).

Critical Thinking Questions

1. Can you identify other traditional/indigenous dietary or medicinal practices that have been biomedically appropriated or assimilated as so-called CAM therapies?
2. What challenges might be associated with undertaking scholarly research on traditional/indigenous health care approaches in ways that incorporate the paradigms from which such therapies originate?

Glossary

Feminist: A feminist stance recognizes the globalized, historical, and contemporary subjugation of women within male-dominated (patriarchal) socio-political and economic structures, and aims toward more egalitarian power relations.

Misappropriation: A phenomenon in which a dominant cultural group extracts and disembeds particular cultural knowledges or practices from a more marginal cultural group, usually producing economic or social harm.

Neo-colonial: A contemporary, ongoing manifestation of European colonialism.

Post-colonial: A post-colonial stance centralizes the voices, histories, and knowledge systems of peoples affected by European colonialism in its various manifestations, actively contesting the presumed superiority of Euro-centric worldviews.

References

Adams, J., Hollenberg, D., Lui, C., & Broom, A. (2009). Contextualizing integration: A critical social science approach to integrative health care. *Journal of Manipulative Physiological Therapeutics, 32*, 792–798.

Adlercreutz, H., Hamalainen, E., Gorbach, S., & Goldin, B. (1992). Dietary phyto-oestrogens and the menopause in Japan. *Lancet, 338*(8803), 1233.

Azizi, H., Liu, Y.F., Du, L., Wang, C.H., Brahrami-Taghanaki, H., Esmaily, H.O., & Xue, X.O. (2011). Menopause-related symptoms: Traditional Chinese medicine vs. hormone therapy. *Alternative Therapies in Health and Medicine, 17*(4), 48–53.

Barsh, R. (1997). The epistemology of traditional healing systems. *Human Organization, 56*(1), 27–37.

Bensky, D., Clavey, S., Stoeger, E., & Gamble, A. (2004). *Chinese herbal medicine: Materia Medica* (3rd ed.). Vista, CA: Eastland.

Betz, J.M., Anderson, L., Avigan, M.I., Barnes, J., Farnsworth, N.R., Gerden, B., ... Senior, J.R. (2009). Black cohosh: Considerations of safety and benefit. *Nutrition Today, 44*(4), 155–162.

Bubela, T., Boon, H., & Caulfield, T. (2008). Herbal remedy clinical trials in the media: A comparison with the coverage of conventional pharmaceuticals. *BMC Medicine, 6*(35). doi:10.1186/1741-7015-6-35 or www.biomedcentral.com/1741-7015/6/35

Burger, H.G., MacLennan, A.H., Huang, K.E., & Castelo-Brano, C. (2012). Evidence-based assessment of the impact of the WHI on women's health. *Climacteric, 15*(3), 281–287.

Chirawatkul, S., & Manderson, L. (1994). Perceptions of menopause in Northeast Thailand: Contested meaning and practice. *Social Science & Medicine, 39*(11), 1545–1554.

Duke, J.A., & Bodenschutz-Godwin, M.J. (1999). The synergy principle in plants, pathogens, insects, herbivores and humans. In P.B. Kaufmann, L.J. Cseke, S. Warber, J.A. Duke & H.L. Brielmann (Eds), *Natural products from plants* (pp. 475–502). New York: CRC Press.

Enzymatic Therapy. (2008). *Natural black cohosh*. Retrieved August 3, 2014 from www.remifemin.com/About-Remifemin/Natural-Black-Cohosh.aspx

Erol, M. (2009). Tales of the second spring: Menopause in Turkey through the narratives of menopausal women and gynecologists. *Medical Anthropology, 28*(4), 368–396.

Firenzuoli, F., Gori, L., & di Sarsina, P.R. (2011). Black cohosh hepatic safety: Follow-up of 107 patients consuming a special *Cimicifuga racemosa* rhizome herbal extract and review of literature. *Evidence-based Complementary and Alternative Medicine*. doi:10.1093/ecam/nen009

Foster, S. (1999). Black cohosh: A literature review. *HerbalGram, 45*, 35–50.

Gannon, L. (1998). The impact of medical and sexual politics on women's health. *Feminism & Psychology, 8*(3), 285–302.

Harding, S. (1998). *Is science multicultural? Postcolonialisms, feminisms and epistemologies*. Bloomington, IN: Indiana University Press.

Hollenberg, D., & Muzzin, L. (2010). Epistemological challenges to integrative medicine: An anti-colonial perspective on the combination of complementary/alternative medicine with biomedicine. *Health Sociology Review, 19*(1), 34–56.

Kaptchuk, T., & Eisenberg, D. (1998). The persuasive appeal of alternative medicine. *Annals of Internal Medicine, 129*, 1061–1065.

Keshet, Y., & Simchai, D. (2014). The "gender puzzle" of alternative medicine and holistic spirituality: A literature review. *Social Science and Medicine, 113*, 77–86.

Kligler, B. (2003). Black cohosh. *American Family Physician, 68*(1), 114–116.

Kuhlmann, E. (2009). From women's health to gender mainstreaming and back again: Linking feminist agendas and new governance in healthcare. *Current Sociology, 57*(2), 135–154.

Kupferer, R., Dormire, S.L., & Becker, H. (2009). Complementary and alternative medicine use for vasomotor symptoms among women who have discontinued hormone therapy. *Journal of Obstetric, Gynecologic, and Neonatal Nursing, 38*, 50–59.

Kurzer, M. S. (2008). Soy consumption for reduction of menopausal symptoms. *Inflammopharmacology, 16*, 227–229.

Kurzer, M.S., Morgan, T., & Greaves, K. (2004). Soy isoflavones decrease hot flash frequency:

A meta-analysis of studies examining soy protein, soy foods, and soy isoflavones. *Journal of Nutrition, 134*(5), 1246S.

Lock, M. (1991). Contested meanings of the menopause. *Lancet, 337*, 1270–1272.

Lu, H. (1986). *Chinese system of food cures*. New York: Sterling.

MacPherson, K.I. (1981). Menopause as disease: The social construction of a metaphor. *Advances in Nursing Science, 3*(2), 95–113.

Messina, M. (2010). A brief historical overview of the past two decades of soy and isoflavone research. *Journal of Nutrition, 140*(7), 1350S–1354S.

Munro, I.C., Harwood, M., Slywka, J.J., Stephen, A.M., Doull, J., Flamm, W.G., & Adlercreutz, H. (2003). Soy isoflavones: A safety review. *Nutrition Reviews, 61*(1), 1–33.

Murtagh, M., & Hepworth, J. (2003). Feminist ethics and menopause: Autonomy and decision-making in primary medical care. *Social Science & Medicine, 56*(8), 1643–1652.

Naser, B., Schnitker, J., Minkin, M.J., de Arriba, S.G., Nolte, K.-U., & Osmers, R. (2011). Suspected black cohosh hepatotoxicity: No evidence by meta-analysis of randomized controlled clinic trials for isopropanolic black cohost extract. *Menopause, 18*(4), 366–375.

Nature's Way. (2015). *Nature's way soy isoflavones—standardized extracts—60 caps*. Retrieved June 10, 2015 from http://astronutrition.com/nature-s-way-soy-isoflavones-standardized-extracts-60-caps.html?___landing=canada&gclid=CLOVoMOohcYCFQ6OaQod-oIA8w

Nelson, H. (2008). Menopause. *Lancet, 371*, 760–770.

North American Menopause Society. (2011). NAMS 2011 isoflavones report: The role of soy isoflavones in menopausal health: Report of the North American menopause Society/Wulf H. Utian translational science symposium in Chicago, IL (October 2010). *Menopause, 18*(7), 732–753.

Organika. (2015). *Organika soy isoflavones 50 mg, 90 capsules*. Retrieved June 10, 2015 from www.vitamart.ca/organika-soy-isoflavones-50mg.html?gclid=CLPMgbCahcYCFYI7aQodgCMABQ

Panay, N. (2012). Body-identical hormone replacement. *Climacteric, 15*(No. S1), 1–2.

Pimenta, F., Leal, I., Maroco, J., & Ramos, C. (2011). Perceived control, lifestyle, health, socio-demographic factors and menopause: Impact on hot flashes and night sweats. *Maturitas, 69*, 338–342.

Pitkin, J. (2012). Alternative and complementary therapies for the menopause. *Menopause International, 18*, 20–27.

Revival Products (Soy.com). (2014). *Our products: Naturally concentrated*. Retrieved October 17, 2014 from www.soy.com/Naturally-Concentrated_ep_66-1.html

Ruhlen, R.L., Sun, G.Y., & Sauter, E.R. (2008). Black cohosh: Insights into its mechanism(s) of action. *Integrative Medicine Insights, 3*, 21–32.

Sathyapalan, T., Manuchehri, A.M., Thatcher, N.J., Rigby, A.S., Chapmen, T., Kilpatrick, E.S., & Atkin, S.L. (2011). The effect of soy phytoestrogen supplementation on thyroid status and cardiovascular risk markers in patients with subclinical hypothyroidism: A randomized, double-blind, crossover study. *Journal of Clinical Endocrinology and Metabolism, 96*(5), 1442–1449.

Shams, T., Setia, M.S., Hemmings, R., McCusker, J., Sewitch, M., & Ciampi, A. (2010). Efficacy of black cohosh-containing preparations on menopausal symptoms: A meta-analysis. *Alternative Therapies in Health and Medicine, 16*(1), 36–44.

Shiva, V. (1999). *Biopiracy: The plunder of nature and knowledge*. Brooklyn: South End Press.

Sisu. (2015). *Black cohosh—60 caps*. Retrieved June 10, 2015 from www.nationalnutrition.ca/detail.aspx?ID=1356

Taku, K., Melby, M.K., Kronenberg, F., Kurzer, M.S., & Messina, M. (2012). Extracted or synthesized soybean isoflavones reduce menopausal hot flash frequency and severity: Systematic review and meta-analysis of randomized controlled trials. *Menopause, 19*(7), 776–790.

Teschke, R. (2010). Black cohosh and suspected hepatotoxicity: Inconsistencies confounding variables, and prospective use of a diagnostic causality algorithm. A critical review. *Menopause, 17*(2), 426–440.

Teschke, R., Schwarzenboeck, A., Schmidt-Taenzer, W., Wolff, A., & Hennermann, K.-H. (2011). Herb induced liver injury presumably caused by black cohosh: A survey of initially purported cases and herbal quality specifications. *Annals of Hepatology, 11*(3), 249–259.

United Plant Savers. (2013, June 4). *Species at-risk: Black cohosh*. Retrieved October 17, 2014, from www.unitedplantsavers.org/content.php/432-Black-Cohosh

United States Department of Agriculture. (2012). Adoption of genetically engineered crops in the U.S. Retrieved March 29, 2013 from www.ers.usda.gov/data-products/adoption-of-genetically-engineered-crops-in-the-us.aspx-.UVSLvxfMCSo

Usui, T. (2006). Pharmaceutical prospects of phytoestrogens. *Endocrine Journal, 53*, 7–20.

Utz, R. (2011). Like mother, (not) like daughter: The social construction of menopause and aging. *Journal of Aging Studies, 25*, 143–154.

Villaseca, P. (2012). Non-estrogen conventional and phytochemical treatments for vasomotor symptoms: What needs to be known for practice. *Climacteric, 15*(2), 115–124.

Williamson, E. (2001). Synergy and other interactions in phytomedicines. *Phytomedicine, 8*(5), 401–409.

World Health Organization (WHO), World Intellectual Property Organization & World Trade Organization. (2013). Promoting access to medical technologies and innovation: Intersections between public health, intellectual property and trade. Geneva: World Health Organization.

Zimmermann, R., Witte, A., Voll, R.E., Strobel, J., & Frieser, M. (2010). Coagulation activation and fluid retention associated with the use of black cohosh: A case study. *Climacteric, 13*(2), 187–191.

CHAPTER 12

The Use of Complementary and Alternative Medicine by Australian Women for Infertility

Jo-Anne Rayner, PhD
College of Science, Health, and Engineering, La Trobe University, Australia

Karen Willis, PhD
Faculty of Health Sciences, Australian Catholic University, Australia

Learning Objectives

1. To describe the patterns of use of complementary and alternative medicine among Australian women for reproductive health, especially for infertility.
2. To evaluate critically the reasons why women choose to use complementary and alternative medicine for reproductive health care, particularly to treat infertility.
3. To explain some of the social and demographic factors that impact on women's use of complementary and alternative medicine for infertility.

Introduction

> I have a view that I'll try anything [to become pregnant] no matter how kind of crazy it seems. Sometimes my husband just rolls his eyes when I say, "I'm going to see a hypnotherapist or kinesiologist" or "I've snuck a couple of crystals into my handbag" or something like that. If someone suggested that I should sit in my back garden and howl at the moon, I would do it. (As quoted in Rayner, McLachlan, Forster & Cramer, 2009, p. 52)

Consider this quotation from Carole, describing her quest to achieve motherhood. Interviewed for a study carried out in 2008 (Rayner, McLachlan, Forster & Cramer, 2008; Rayner, McLachlan, Forster & Cramer, 2009), Carole is a 42-year-old Australian working full-time in a professional role. At the time of interview she was using biomedical treatments as well as complementary and alternative medicine (CAM) in an effort to become pregnant. Carole's words give a sense of the pressure that women experience when they encounter problems trying to conceive. The quotation also conveys the idea that using CAM is somewhat bizarre, somehow outside mainstream therapeutic acts. We do not know whether Carole's strategies were successful, whether she achieved her goal of pregnancy and a live birth. However, we do know that increasingly, Australian women turn to CAM to assist with reproductive health events and issues, including infertility. How can we explain this, especially given the scientific advances in biomedicine such as the use of **assisted reproductive technologies (ART)** such as **in vitro fertilization (IVF)** in diagnosing and treating infertility?[1] Why are women willing to pay out-of-pocket expenses when the cost of biomedical infertility treatments is partially subsidized by the Australian universal health care scheme **Medicare** and the **Pharmaceutical Benefits Scheme (PBS)**?[2] Most importantly, what drives Australian women to use such a diverse range of alternative medicines and therapies at the same time as they use mainstream biomedicine treatments?

In this chapter, we address some of these questions. In particular, focusing on infertility and drawing on data from previous studies, we will examine the patterns of CAM use by Australian women for reproductive health; the profile of women most likely to use CAM; some of the reasons and predictors of their CAM use; and women's experiences of using CAM as a health care option. This analysis is important because the use of—and expenditure on—CAM as health care has increased in Australia over the past two decades, despite little evidence to support its safety and efficacy. Even more importantly, the primary users of CAM in Australia are women of reproductive age (Xue et al., 2007). They are well-educated, living in metropolitan cities, working in paid employment earning higher than average incomes, and have private health insurance coverage (Frawley et al., 2013; Rayner et al., 2009). While Australian women's use of CAM during pregnancy is well documented (Frawley et al., 2013), important gaps in women's use of CAM for reproductive health remain, in particular the use of CAM for infertility (Rayner, Willis & Burgess, 2011). Although no Australian population-based studies exist, smaller studies suggest the use of CAM by women with fertility problems is high (Rayner et al., 2009; Rayner, Willis & Dennis, 2012; Reid & Alfred, 2013; Stankiewicz, Smith, Alvino & Norman, 2007).

Australian Women's Use of CAM for Reproductive Health

Australians are some of the largest consumers of CAM worldwide (Armstrong, Thiebout, Brown & Nepal, 2011; Harris, Cooper, Relton & Thomas, 2012; Xue et al., 2007). As in other industrialized countries (Esmail, 2007; Harris, Cooper, Relton & Thomas, 2012), Australians use CAM as a preventative approach to maintain health and well-being, and to treat chronic conditions, highlighting a growing trend for individuals to take responsibility for their health and show an active commitment to wellness and illness prevention (Crawford, 2006). In the latest Australian population-based survey, 69 percent of adults reported using CAM in 2005 (Xue et al., 2007), a 20 percent increase since 1993 (MacLennan, Wilson & Taylor, 1996). The survey noted that 44 percent of Australians consulted a CAM therapist, representing almost the same number of annual visits to biomedical practitioners (Xue et al., 2007); additionally, 40 percent used CAM on a daily basis (Swift, Stollznow & Pirotta, 2007). In 2009, Australian women spent $AUD349 per annum on self-prescribed CAM and an average of $AUD416 on consultations with CAM therapists[3] This amount was significantly higher among women living in major cities compared to women in rural areas (Adams et al., 2011).

The characteristics of Australian women who use CAM during pregnancy (Adams et al., 2011; Frawley et al., 2013) are similar to that of women who use CAM during pregnancy in other countries (Bishop, Northstone, Green & Thompson, 2011; Stouss et al., 2014). These women are in their 30s, have university qualifications, are employed with a disposable income, and live in urban areas. In addition, they have previously or habitually used CAM. In terms of their reproductive health, they are more likely than non-users of CAM to suffer from fatigue and back pain in pregnancy, and are planning a natural birth (Steel et al., 2014). The demographic profile of Australian women who use CAM for infertility (Rayner et al., 2009; Rayner et al., 2012) and during breast feeding (Sim et al., 2013) is similar to those who use it during pregnancy, although women using CAM for infertility are often older (Rayner et al., 2009; Rayner et al., 2012; Stankiewicz, Smith, Alvino & Norman, 2007).

CAM Therapies Used by Australian Women

What CAM do Australian women use for their reproductive health care needs? The answer is an unequivocal "all of them." The various types of therapies and modalities described as CAM is demonstrated in a review of the literature on CAM used for infertility (Rayner, Willis & Burgess, 2011). The therapies and modalities used in this review to assist fertility or treat infertility included nutritional advice, vitamin and mineral supplements (both self-prescribed and prescribed by a therapist), **western herbal medicine** and herbal products, herbal teas, **acupuncture**, **reflexology**, **traditional Chinese medicine (TCM)**, traditional faith healers, spiritual healings, religious interventions and prayer, meditation, **hypnosis**, yoga, exercise, **naturopathy**, **kinesiology**, mind-body techniques, counselling, support groups, and **chiropractic treatments**.

As in the general population, Australian women's use of CAM for reproductive health is dominated by self-prescription of vitamin and mineral supplements (Frawley at al., 2013; Smith, Bateson & Weisberg, 2013) and herbal medicines (Sim et al., 2013) purchased over-the-counter in pharmacies, supermarkets, and health-food stores, or via the Internet (Zhang et al., 2008). Among women attending an infertility clinic in South Australia, 62 percent used self-prescribed vitamins, minerals, and herbal medicines (Stankiewicz, Smith, Alvino & Norman, 2007); and 60 percent of western Australian women reported using self-prescribed herbal medicines to support breast feeding (Sim et al., 2013). Australian women do not use CAM for reproductive health at the exclusion of mainstream biomedicine, or because they want to avoid consulting doctors; rather, CAM is used in combination with biomedical treatments (Frawley et al., 2013; Rayner et al., 2009). Women who are high users of CAM for reproductive health (self-prescribed and consultations with therapists) also consult biomedical and allied health practitioners more frequently than women who do not use CAM (Sibbritt, Adams & Lui, 2011). In this sense, CAM can be viewed as complementary to biomedical treatments for reproductive health, rather than as a substitute (Gaffney & Smith, 2004). This was particularly evident in the research undertaken into women's use of CAM for infertility. All of the women interviewed by Rayner and colleagues (2009) used CAM as well as biomedical treatments to treat their infertility. Furthermore, an audit of new clients of a CAM practice in metropolitan Melbourne revealed that 63 percent of women consulting a naturopath or acupuncturist for fertility assistance were also using biomedical infertility treatments (Rayner et al., 2012). Australian CAM therapists also report that their services are used to supplement biomedical infertility treatments, particularly among older women (Rayner et al., 2009; Rayner et al., 2012), as the following quotations from therapists indicate:

> I've been practising for about seven years as a naturopath and for this last year as an acupuncturist. I suppose 70 to 80 percent of the people I see are probably women seeking assistance with fertility and increasingly so using ART. (Acupuncturist and naturopath, as quoted in Rayner et al., 2009, p. 5)

> Women come in for various reasons. Some want to get fit and healthy before they get pregnant and some have already got fertility problems. Others have been trying for over ten years. They are various ages but more the 30- and 40-year-olds. (Naturopath, as quoted in Rayner et al., 2009, p. 5)

> I'm an acupuncturist and 90 percent of the clients that I see are coming in for fertility-related issues. More than half of those are doing ART and have quite a detailed history of infertility related problems or a history of using IVF. (Acupuncturist, as quoted in Rayner et al., 2009, p. 5)

In addition to combining self-prescribed CAM and biomedical treatments for reproductive health, Australian women are also more likely to consult CAM therapists (Steel et al., 2014), and to use multiple CAM therapies simultaneously (Frawley et al., 2013). In the study conducted by Rayner and colleagues (2009), the women interviewed reported using up to 17 different types of CAM to assist with infertility. Some of these were prescribed or delivered by CAM therapists, but many were self-prescribed. The following quotations from Debra, Anna, and Bernadette (not their real names) are illustrative of this simultaneous use of multiple CAM modalities:

> I do masses of different therapies which I've kind of found along the way. [Besides Chinese medicine] I take this naturopathic liquid for anxiety and I started "breathe work," which was amazing. I found a magazine article on this woman who does Brazilian work for fertility and she's really good at specialising with older women and with husbands whose sperms [sic] weren't so great. So now I do both [TCM and Brazilian] and she also does pulse therapy. (Debra, aged 44 years, as quoted in Rayner et al., 2009, p. 5)

> I saw everyone at "[CAM practice]." I go for both naturopathy and acupuncture and I do herbal medicines on the side. (Anna, aged 34 years, as quoted in Rayner et al., 2009, p. 5)

> I had a lot of trouble due to damaged fallopian tubes so natural conception isn't an option for me. We've been trying IVF [for] about 18 months and I've been coupling that with acupuncture and naturopathy, and herbal medications, also the good old multivitamins (Bernadette, aged 40 years, from Rayner et al., 2008, unpublished quotation)

Australian women who use CAM for reproductive health do not always disclose their CAM use to the biomedical practitioners they also consult. The reasons they report for not doing this includes their concern about receiving a negative response about this use from biomedical practitioners; but many women also reported that their doctors did not ask them about their CAM use (Rayner et al., 2009; Sim, Hattingh, Sherrif & Tee, 2014).

While we understand the demographic profile of women who use CAM for reproductive health (Frawley et al., 2013; Rayner et al., 2009; Rayner et al., 2012; Sim et al., 2013), recent research by Steel and colleagues (2014) has identified potential external predictors for women consulting CAM therapists during pregnancy. These include the referral patterns of private biomedical practitioners; the positive attitudes to CAM use by attending midwives; women's confidence in accessing information to assist them with reproductive health problems; women's access to CAM therapists (there are fewer services available in rural and regional areas of Australia); and the types of services offered in private hospitals (some offer acupuncture and massage, which can be partially subsidized by private health insurance).

Some of these are also predictors for women's use of CAM for infertility. Some of the women interviewed about their use of CAM for infertility (Rayner et al., 2009) were referred to a CAM therapist by a biomedical doctor, usually a fertility specialist. The therapists to whom women are most likely to be referred are acupuncturists and massage therapists. Acupuncture has become more acceptable in biomedicine as adjunct therapy for the treatment of infertility (Rayner et al., 2010), as it is perceived to pose few risks especially if undertaken by a biomedically trained practitioner (Rayner, Willis & Pirotta, 2011; Smith, Armour & Betts, 2014). The following quotations from Fran, who has been combining CAM and IVF, and from one CAM therapist, suggest that some biomedical practitioners are happy for women using biomedical treatments for infertility to complement these with specific CAM therapies:

> My medical practitioner [a private fertility specialist] did suggest trying acupuncture in combination with the 2nd stimulated cycle. (Fran, aged 38 years, as quoted in Rayner et al., 2009, p. 6)

> I've been working since 1978. In the last 10–15 years, [I] got into treating a lot more women for infertility mostly because of referrals. Principally I work on a referral basis with some of the specialists in this area and use herbal medicine and supplements. (Herbalist and naturopath, from Rayner et al., 2008, unpublished quotation)

There is little support for the use of other CAM among medical practitioners. The lack of evidence to support the use of CAM has generated considerable debate among the medical community about using or referring to CAM more generally (Dwyer, 2011), with concerns raised about CAM use in pregnancy (Sibbritt et al., 2014) and for infertility (Rayner et al., 2010). Most of the CAM therapists interviewed by Rayner and colleagues (2009) reported reluctance and even contempt by biomedical doctors to refer to or even acknowledge CAM therapists:

> There are some people who are just out and out rude, and they're not a lot of fun to deal with. (Herbalist and naturopath, as quoted in Rayner et al., 2009, p. 6)

Motivations of Australian Women for Using CAM

A review by Hall and colleagues (2011) summarized women's reported motivations for using CAM during pregnancy. These included the belief that CAM therapies provided safe alternatives to pharmaceutical drugs; an appreciation of the holistic potential afforded by CAM therapies; and the desire to have control and satisfaction in their pregnancy experience. The literature supports the argument that Australian women who use CAM for reproductive health believe it to be "natural" and therefore safe (Pedersen, 2013). Women using CAM therapies and modalities during pregnancy and for infertility report similar sentiments about the "naturalness" of CAM and this association with safety (Gaffney & Smith, 2004; Rayner et al., 2009). Similarly, women who use herbal medicines to support breast feeding consider them safer to use than pharmaceutical drugs, as the following anonymous quotations show:

> I really didn't want to take anything harsh that could affect my baby's health. I would say that because I was breastfeeding, I was more cautious over what I take and what I eat, and I think that using natural herbs would be safer than using chemicals. (As quoted in Sim et al., 2014, p. 5)

> I think if you can avoid taking chemical pharmaceutical drugs, then I would exhaust every single herbal option before I go near any pharmaceutical … the herbal options are usually much safer. (As quoted in Sim et al., 2014, p. 5)

A belief in **holism** seems to be a strong motivator for Australian women to use CAM for reproductive health (Gaffney & Smith, 2004; Rayner et al., 2009). Women interviewed about their use of CAM for infertility (Rayner et al., 2009) described holism as "a whole of body approach," "a beginning as opposed to an ending," "making a difference to your psyche," and "a more general rather than specific effect." The findings that Australian women who use CAM for infertility and during pregnancy desire to take a more proactive role in their health care and a belief in the holistic nature of most CAM modalities has also been found in research conducted in other countries as a motivation for using CAM (O'Reilly, Sevigny, Sabarre & Phillips, 2014; Sirois, 2008; Sointu, 2006; Strouss et al., 2014).

Another factor explaining women's use of CAM for reproductive health care is the personalized nature of the interaction with CAM therapists, who are usually female, the length of consultations, and the use of individually tailored interventions (Rayner et al., 2009). Australian women using CAM for reproductive health report a strong sense of emotional support from the CAM therapists they consult and a feeling of empowerment and control in making the decision to use CAM (de Lacey, Smith & Paterson, 2009; Rayner et al., 2009; Reid & Alfred, 2013; Steel et al., 2014). This is particularly the case in the use of CAM for infertility. In Australia, women's use of CAM to assist with infertility operates along a continuum that ranges from women trying to optimize their physical health whilst trying to conceive to their "desperate" endeavours to achieve and maintain a pregnancy when all biomedical options are failing (Willis & Rayner, 2015). In Australia, the social and political milieu activity supports the family and the desire for parenthood remains high among the majority of men and women (Gray et al., 2008), despite the growing tendency to delay childbearing (Li, Zeki, Hilder & Sullivan, 2013). Analysis of data from the Australian Longitudinal Study of Women's Health showed that over a decade (1996–2006) one in six Australian women who had ever tried to conceive reported problems with infertility. Three quarters of these women sought medical advice, and half used ART (Herbert, Lucke & Dobson, 2009). Over the past 30 years, Australian couples have used ART for infertility; however, the use of ART is accompanied by significant psychological and physical side effects, as well as being expensive, all of which have been linked to the discontinuation of treatment (Dawson, Diedrich & Felberbaum, 2005). Women interviewed by Rayner and colleagues (2009) described ART, particularly if unsuccessful, as "gruelling," "stressful," "damaging," "humiliating," and "destructive." By way of contrast, women using CAM therapies for infertility, even in combination with ART, report a sense of "wellness" derived from the therapies and satisfaction with the CAM therapists. They described the experience as "positive" and "affirming," enhancing "self-care" and associated with feelings of "empowerment" and "control." The following quotations from women in different studies using different forms of CAM for infertility are illustrative of these feelings:

> The TCM practitioner looks at your whole body. She is not overly interested in one specific area, whereas at the gynaecologist it's very specific. (Anonymous woman, aged 38 years, as quoted in Reid & Alfred, 2013. p. 7)

> You feel [you're] not in control through the whole IVF process. You've handed your body over to someone else. Doing acupuncture was what I'd chosen to do and I felt some control. (Debra, aged 44 years, as quoted in Rayner et al., 2009, p. 6)

> Actually, doing acupuncture was something that I'd chosen to do and I felt some control as a result. (Fran, aged 38 years, as quoted in Rayner et al., 2009, p. 7)

Of particular importance to women was the therapeutic relationship they established with the CAM therapists they consulted for infertility. The following quotations from interviews with women who use CAM for infertility remark on the importance of this relationship:

> The difference between going from that experience [ART] to going to the naturopath and sitting down and chatting with a lovely woman who talks about when I'm pregnant, is a radical shift in the way you perceive what you're doing and how you relate to your body. Profoundly different and that was a huge benefit, a blessing for me. (Gai, aged 40 years, as quoted in Rayner et al., 2009, p. 7)

> I think it's the system to an extent. Perhaps complementary therapies are slightly outside that system and don't have those constraints and give you the opportunity to develop relationships a little bit more. It's a lot about the person and you're gelling with the person as well. (Gai, aged 40 years, as quoted in Rayner et al., 2009, p. 7)

Australian women who consult CAM therapists for other reproductive health issues have reported similar feelings. Steel and colleagues (2014) report that women who consulted CAM therapists during pregnancy often did so because they felt they received more empathy and support from these therapists, and had more control over their health and body than they did from the biomedical practitioners they consulted. These women found the CAM therapists easier to talk to, and provided longer consultations, a result also reported by women using CAM for infertility (Rayner et al., 2009; Reid & Alfred, 2013). Steel and colleagues (2014) speculate whether women's consultations with some CAM therapists during pregnancy, in particular naturopaths, compensates for perceived deficits in the care provided by their biomedical practitioners, a conjecture supported by reports from Australian women about their experiences with using CAM for infertility (Rayner et al., 2009; Reid & Alfred, 2013; Smith et al., 2011). The following anonymous quotations from women participating in a trial of acupuncture to support infertility related stress commented on the support they received from the acupuncturist:

> I found her [acupuncturist] really easy to talk to in that regard, so that was good. What I found really positive was talking to [her] before the treatment; that was really great. (As quoted in Smith et al., 2011, p. 927)

> I think there is a benefit in having someone to talk to as well as the actual acupuncture. It was an unexpected opportunity to talk to someone about the situation who you knew was going to be private. (As quoted in Smith et al., 2011, p. 927)

The majority of the women who used acupuncture to support infertility-related stress had university qualifications, were working full-time, had previously used acupuncture, and were older (Smith et al., 2011). Age also seems to be a motivating factor for women's use of CAM to assist with infertility in Australia (Rayner et al., 2009; Rayner et al., 2012; Read et al., 2014) and in other countries (O'Reilly, Sevigny, Sabarre & Phillips, 2014; Read et al., 2014; Smith et al., 2010). Australian women are delaying childbearing and having children at older ages (Li, Zeki, Hilder & Sullivan, 2013) and women who use ART tend to be older again (Hilder et al., 2014; Macaldowie, Wang, Chambers & Sullivan, 2013;). Their age-related declining fertility may provide the impetus to use all assistance available, including CAM. The following quotations from women and CAM therapists provide some support for this:

> Having hit 40 [years] and I'm feeling desperate, absolutely desperate [to conceive], I would try anything and everything. (Bernadette, aged 40 years, as quoted in Rayner et al., 2009, p. 5)

> When things weren't working I started to become desperate so I started exploring other avenues and so I started naturopathics [sic]. (Debra, aged 44 years, from Rayner et al., 2008, unpublished quotation)

> I do all of those natural things, I go to a lot of different natural therapists. I think my age is the issue and IVF does nothing to make your eggs younger. (Carole, aged 42 years, as quoted in Rayner et al., 2009, p. 5)

> There are some IVF specialists who sort of specialize in the older woman, who have women going for what I think it is a ridiculous amount of time, referring women to us who are 46 years old for their first pregnancy, and you think "oh, please..."(Herbalist, from Rayner et al., 2008, unpublished quotation)

While Steel and colleagues (2014) found the costs of CAM to be a disincentive to use by women during pregnancy, the strong desire to achieve motherhood among the women interviewed by Rayner and colleagues (2009) meant they often paid large amounts of money out-of-pocket for both ART and CAM infertility treatments. Although all of the women interviewed received rebates from their private health insurance and Medicare for their biomedical treatments and a little from private health insurance for their CAM consultations, this had little impact on their decision to use CAM, the frequency with which they consulted practitioners, or the number of modalities they employed, even if it was a struggle at times. Anna, who spent $AUD14,000 in the previous year on fertility treatments, explains:

> The cost is a really huge factor for us. We don't have the backup funds. I said to my husband "How much money do we spend? Do we take another mortgage out on our house? How far do you go?" and there's no answer for that. It depends how desperate you want a child. I'll keep going and I'd be going weekly if I had the funds. (Anna, aged 34 years, from Rayner et al., 2008, unpublished quotation)

Women using CAM for infertility indicated that they would continue to use it even if they did not have private health insurance because of the value they placed on the relationships with CAM therapists and the control they gain from this choice.

Sources of Information for CAM Therapies

Australian women commonly obtain information about CAM from informal sources, most notably from family and friends, the media and increasingly via the internet. Fran and Carole, who were interviewed about their use of CAM for infertility, describe how they sourced the CAM therapists they consulted, and CAM therapists report friends and the internet as a referral source:

> I basically did a Yellow Pages web search on acupuncture and fertility as my key words in the CBD, because I work in the CBD, and then looked at websites and picked the one that looked the most professional. (Fran, aged 38 years, from Rayner et al., 2008, unpublished quotation)

> I kept on Googling things like fertility and infertility on the net, and I found "[Name of CAM fertility clinic]" because they've got a web page. I had no recommendations or anything, so I just came here for the naturopathy and acupuncture. (Carole, aged 42 years, from Rayner et al., 2008, unpublished quotation)

> There's a huge percentage [of referrals] that I see that are self-referred or friends. I think women listen to friends. (Naturopath, from Rayner et al., 2008, unpublished quotation)

> Word of mouth is huge I think and when you look at the research on what women take in pregnancy, a lot of it is self-prescribed or what friends say they should take, and the Web. (Acupuncturist and naturopath, from Rayner et al., 2008, unpublished quotation)

There has been a sharp increase in the use of the Internet for medical or health information in Australia, and women report using the Internet as both a source of information about CAM and for the supply of CAM products for reproductive health (Rayner et al., 2009; Sim et al., 2014; Steel et al., 2014). Unpublished findings from a study undertaken by the authors (Rayner, Willis & Thorpe, 2011) exploring women's discussions on an infertility Internet chat room emphasize the importance of informal information channels about reproductive health and the use of CAM. Talking with "friends" online across geographic and social divides, these women shared early pregnancy symptoms and how they dealt with some that were problematic. This often included using CAM, such as treating morning sickness with herbal tea or acupuncture, and eating a healthy diet to treat constipation. There was also an emphasis on the use of vitamins. The following quotations are indicative of these women's informal discussions of CAM online:

> I have had no morning sickness either. In fact since I have been treated for nausea with acupuncture my nausea has gone!! I have been having acupuncture the whole time. I do think it helped me get a BFP [big fat positive-pregnant] the first time round but I read that acupuncture cannot stop a miscarriage. (28-year-old woman pregnant after second round of IVF, as quoted in Rayner, Willis & Thorpe, 2011)

> Glad acupuncture is working for your morning sickness! Might have to give it a try if mine gets bad. (26-year-old woman, pregnant with twins after six ART cycles, as quoted in Rayner, Willis & Thorpe, 2011)

> Psyllium husks are good and natural [for constipation] and you can sprinkle these onto cereal if you have that. I haven't had as many issues so far this time. (39-year-old woman, pregnant after ART, as quoted in Rayner, Willis & Thorpe, 2011)

Other sources of information about the use of CAM for reproductive health included conventional health care professionals such as fertility specialists, general practitioners (GPs), midwives, and pharmacists, as well as referrals from CAM practitioners (Frawley et al., 2013; Rayner et al., 2009; Sim et al., 2014; Steel et al., 2014) as the following quotations suggest:

> Obstetricians who may not be doing IVF but who are doing some of the three IVF kind of assisted stuff, ovulation induction and that kind of stuff. (Acupuncturist and birth attendant, from Rayner et al., 2008, unpublished quotation)

> You do get a few GPs saying "I suggest you see a naturopath," maybe if they're younger. (Naturopath and herbalist, as quoted in Rayner et al., 2009, p. 6)

Conclusion

In this chapter, we have provided examples of Australian women's use of CAM for reproductive health, in particular for infertility. The literature suggests that Australian women critically negotiate the management of their reproductive health care and actively work to address their individual needs. They make decisions about the types of health care they will use, including the use of CAM, that are relevant to the individual social, situational, and reproductive context, even if this means ignoring medical advice to avoid CAM. Australian women integrate both CAM and biomedical treatments to maximise the desired outcome, whether this is achieving a viable pregnancy, alleviating problems during pregnancy or pain during labour, or to increase breast milk supply.

The proliferation of CAM use for reproductive health has occurred because women want natural solutions for their reproductive health needs. Furthermore, they want to remain in control of some aspects of their health and well-being. They also value the relational aspects that they report are part of their encounters with CAM therapists. Research suggests that empathy (Mercer & Reilly, 2004) and trust (Rowe & Calnan, 2006) in one's health care provider is integral in the face of uncertainty. Many of the reproductive events for which women use CAM involve uncertainty, such as being pregnant or breast feeding for the first time. For infertile women particularly, the need for a trusting relationship may be heightened. They have experienced a loss of certainty in their body, and may also have experienced stressful biomedical encounters that do not result in guaranteed outcomes. The relationship with a CAM therapist may therefore represent an integral way of regaining trust in one's body and the therapeutic encounter.

Notes

1. In Australia since 1990, assisted reproductive technologies (ART) have been reimbursed through Medicare, and associated drug therapies for infertility are funded under the Pharmaceutical Benefits Scheme (PBS). Despite this government subsidy the out-of-pocket expenses remain high. ART is now mainstream biomedical treatment for infertility in Australia. The use of ART by Australians grew steadily until 2009, as the number of initiated treatments increased by over 10 percent per year between 2002 and 2008, although in 2010 Australia recorded a decline in the use of ART for the first time in three decades. This was attributed to a reduction in government subsidies for fertility treatments through Medicare, resulting in an increase in the average out-of-pocket expenses of consumers. In 2013, use of ART in Australia increased by 1.9 percent from 2012 and 4 percent of all Australian women who gave birth in in 2012 received some form of ART treatment. The rate of live births following the use of ART continues to remain at less than 20 percent. The average age of Australia women using ART continues to increase; however, the majority of births occur in women aged under 30 years. The majority of Australian ART clinics are situated in more populated and affluent metropolitan areas, which anecdotally appears to be the case for CAM practices specializing in fertility treatment.
2. The Australian health care system is a complex set of arrangements between the public and private sectors, and the national and state governments. National government policy includes the provision of tax-financed medical services (Medicare), medicines (PBS) and acute health care (universal access to public hospital treatment with no fees), as well as support for the private sector through measures that encourage the uptake of private health insurance. The national government is responsible for funding Medicare and the PBS. The six state and territory governments are responsible for funding public hospitals. Consumers can choose their own medical practitioner except when they are a patient in a public hospital. Most medical services are provided by private practitioners, paid by fee-for-service with a fixed rate (85 percent) of reimbursement. The government has no control over the fees charged by medical practitioners but "recommends" fees through a Medical Benefits Schedule (MBS). Medical services provided in a private hospital are reimbursed at a lower (75 percent) fee-for-service rate. Out-of-pocket expenses are covered by private health insurance and the patient. Private health insurance premiums depend on extent of coverage chosen. Insurance covers private medical/surgical treatment in a hospital

(private/public) and cost of some ancillary services. Insurance companies must accept all purchasers without discrimination and all increases in premiums must have government approval. Private health insurance provides limited rebates for some CAM services but not medicines.

3. Australians spent a total of $AUD4.13 billion on CAM as health care (visits and over-the-counter purchases) in 2005, more than twice as much as was spent in 2000; and expenditure on CAM products accounted for almost half the expenditure on all non-subsidized health care products. A large proportion of the CAM consumed by Australians is self-prescribed, including vitamins and mineral supplements as a form of clinical nutrition and herbal remedies.

Critical Thinking Questions

1. Recall the first example in this chapter of Carole and her quest to "try anything" to get pregnant. What advice would you give her? How would your advice differ if you were chatting with Carole on an online support group, if you were her naturopath, or if you were a nurse or midwife at a fertility clinic?
2. Do you think that CAM for reproductive health or for infertility should be fully subsidized by government or private health insurers? Why, or why not? What are the implications of your answer for women who lack the economic resources to pay for CAM?
3. How important is the therapeutic relationship with CAM providers, even if the therapies used have limited evidence of benefit? Give reasons for your answers.

Glossary

Acupuncture: The stimulation of specific points along the skin of the body involving various methods such as the application of heat, pressure, or laser, or penetration with thin needles. Stimulating specific acupuncture points corrects imbalances in the flow of *qi* through channels known as meridians.

Assisted reproductive technology (ART): The application of laboratory or clinical technologies to gametes (human egg or sperm) and/or embryos for the purposes of reproduction.

Chiropractic treatments: A specific type of manipulation called an adjustment to improve many health problems that are related to the skeletal and muscular system. The basic principle is that changes to the normal structure and function of the skeleton and the muscles can produce effects not only in those areas, but also in other areas of the body and health in general.

Holism: The idea that natural systems and their properties should be viewed as wholes, not as collections of parts. In health care, the term "holistic" is used to describe approaches that take into account the social, spiritual, psychological, and physical aspects of an individual's health and well-being.

Hypnosis: A form of psychotherapy used to create subconscious change in a patient in the form of new responses, thoughts, attitudes, behaviours, or feelings.

In vitro fertilization (IVF): A type of ART that involves the fertilization of the egg by the sperm in an incubator outside the body, and transfer of the embryo back into the uterus.

Kinesiology: An alternative therapy that uses gentle muscle-monitoring techniques to access the subconscious mind and gain accurate information about the patient's current issues and what is needed to help their body, mind, and spirit to restore balance.

Medicare: The Australian Universal Health Insurance Scheme which covers 85 percent of all medical service costs and hospitalization in the public hospital system. Medicare does not cover the costs associated with CAM, whether medicines or services provided by therapists.

Naturopathy: A form of alternative medicine based on a belief in vitalism, a special energy that guides bodily processes such as metabolism, reproduction, growth, and adaptation.

Pharmaceutical Benefits Scheme (PBS): A program of the national government that provides subsidized prescription drugs to Australians.

Reflexology: Treatment that involves the physical act of applying pressure to the feet, hands, or ears without the use of oil or lotion. It is based on a system of zones/reflex areas that reflect an image of the body on the feet and hands, with the premise that such work affects a physical change to the body.

Traditional Chinese medicine (TCM): A system of primary health care that includes acupuncture, Chinese herbal medicine, remedial massage, exercise and breathing therapy, and diet and lifestyle advice. TCM takes a holistic approach to understanding normal function and disease processes and focuses as much on the prevention of illness as it does on the treatment.

Western herbal medicine: An alternative therapy that involves using plants and plant material to create medicines to help prevent or treat various illnesses.

References

Adams, J., Sibbritt, D., Broom, A., Loxton, D., Pirotta, M., Humphreys, J., & Lui, C.W. (2011). A comparison of complementary and alternative medicine user and use across geographical areas: A national survey of 1,427 women. *BMC Complementary and Alternative Medicine, 11*, 85.

Armstrong, A., Thiebout, S., Brown, L., & Nepal, B. (2011). Australian adults' use of complementary and alternative medicine in the treatment of chronic illness: A national study. *Australian and New Zealand Journal of Public Health, 35*(4), 384–390.

Bishop, J.L., Northstone, K., Green, J.R., & Thompson, E.A. (2011). The use of complementary and alternative medicine in pregnancy: Data from the Avon Longitudinal Study of Parents and Children (ALSPAC). *Complementary Therapies in Medicine, 19*(6), 303–310.

Crawford, R. (2006). Health as a meaningful social practice. *Health: An Interdisciplinary for the Social Study of Health, Illness & Medicine, 10*(4), 401–420.

Dawson, A.A., Diedrich, K., & Felberbaum, R.E. (2005). Why do couples refuse or discontinue ART? *Archives of Gynecology and Obstetrics, 273*, 3–11.

de Lacey, S., Smith, C.A., & Paterson, C. (2009). Building resilience: A preliminary exploration of women's perceptions of the use of acupuncture as an adjunct to In Vitro Fertilisation. *BMC Complementary and Alternative Medicine, 9*, 50.

Dwyer, J.M. (2011). Is it ethical for medical practitioners to prescribe alternative and complementary treatments that may lack evidence?—No. *Medical Journal of Australia, 195*(2), 79.

Esmail, N. (2007). *Complementary and alternative medicine in Canada: Trends in use and public attitudes, 1997–2006* (Public Policy Sources 2007, No. 87). Vancouver: The Fraser Institute.

Frawley, J., Adams, J., Sibbritt, D., Steel, A., Broom, A., & Gallios, C. (2013). Prevalence and determinants of complementary and alternative medicine use during pregnancy: Results from a nationally representative sample of Australian pregnant women. *Australian and New Zealand Journal of Obstetrics & Gynaecology, 53*, 347–352.

Gaffney, L., & Smith, C.A. (2004). The views of pregnant women to complementary therapies and medicines. *Birth Issues, 13*, 43–50.

Gray, M., Qu, L., & Weston, R. (2008). *Fertility and family policy in Australia* (Research Paper No. 41). Melbourne: Australian Institute of Family Studies.

Hall, H.G., Griffiths, D.L., & McKenna, L.G. (2011). The use of complementary and alternative medicine by pregnant women: A literature review. *Midwifery, 27*(6), 817–824.

Harris, P.E., Cooper, K.L., Relton, C., & Thomas, K.J. (2012). Prevalence of complementary and alternative medicine (CAM) use by the general population: A systematic review and update. *International Journal of Clinical Practice, 66*(10), 924–939.

Herbert, D., Lucke, J., & Dobson, A. (2009). Infertility, medical advice and treatment with fertility hormones and/or in vitro fertilization: A population perspective from the Australian Longitudinal Study on Women's Health. *Australian and New Zealand Journal of Public Health, 33*, 353–379.

Hilder, L., Zhichao, Z., Parker, M., Jahan, S., & Chambers, G.M. (2014). *Australia's mothers and babies 2012* (Perinatal statistics series no. 30. Cat. no. PER 69). Canberra: Australian Institute of Health and Welfare.

Li, Z., Zeki, R., Hilder, L., & Sullivan, E.A. (2013). *Australia's mothers and babies 2011* (Perinatal statistics series no. 28. Cat. no. PER 59). Canberra: Australian Institute of Health and Welfare.

Macaldowie, A., Wang, Y.A., Chambers, G.M., & Sullivan, E.A. (2013). *Assisted reproductive technology in Australia and New Zealand 2011*. Sydney: National Perinatal Epidemiology and Statistics Unit, the University of New South Wales.

MacLennan, A., Wilson, D., & Taylor, A. (1996). Prevalence and cost of alternative health in Australia. *Lancet, 347*, 569–573.

Mercer, S.W., & Reilly, D. (2004). A qualitative study of patient's views on the consultation at the Glasgow Homoeopathic Hospital, an NHS integrative complementary and orthodox medical care unit. *Patient Education and Counselling, 53*, 13–18.

O'Reilly, E., Sevigny, M., Sabarre, K. A., & Phillips, K.P. (2014). Perspectives of complementary and alternative medicine (CAM) practitioners in the support and treatment of infertility. *BMC Complementary and Alternative Medicine, 14*, 394.

Pedersen, I.K. (2013). "It can do no harm": Body maintenance and modification in alternative medicine acknowledged as a non-risk health regime. *Social Science & Medicine, 90*, 56–62.

Rayner, J.A., Forster, D., McLachlan, H.L., Kealy, M., & Pirotta, M. (2010). Women's use of complementary medicine to enhance fertility: The views of fertility specialists in Victoria, Australia. *Australian and New Zealand Journal of Obstetrics & Gynaecology, 50*(3), 305.

Rayner, J., McLachlan, H.L., Forster, D.A., & Cramer, R. (2008). [Australian women's use of complementary and alternative medicines to enhance fertility: Exploring the experiences of women and practitioners.] Unpublished data.

Rayner, J., McLachlan, H.L., Forster, D.A., & Cramer, R. (2009). Australian women's use of complementary and alternative medicines to enhance fertility: Exploring the experiences of women and practitioners. *BMC Complementary and Alternative Medicine, 9*, 52.

Rayner, J., Willis, K., & Burgess, R. (2011). Women's use of complementary and alternative medicine for fertility enhancement: A review of the literature. *Journal of Alternative & Complementary Medicine, 17*(8), 685–690.

Rayner, J., Willis, K., & Dennis, C. (2012). Older Australian women use complementary fertility care: A practice audit. *Journal of Alternative & Complementary Medicine, 18*(1), 1–2.

Rayner, J., Willis, K., & Pirotta, M. (2011). What's in a name? Integrative medicine or simply good medical practice? *Family Practice, 28*(6), 655–660.

Rayner, J., Willis, K., & Thorpe, R. (2011). [Women's use of online social networking to keep informed about the use of complementary medicines for fertility enhancement. A study conducted in 2011 with funding from Faculty of Health Sciences, La Trobe University]. Unpublished data.

Read, S.C., Carrier, M.-E., Whitley, R., Gold, I., Tulandi, T., & Zelkowitz, P. (2014). Complementary and alternative medicine use in infertility: Cultural and religious influences in a multicultural Canadian setting. *Journal of Alternative and Complementary Medicine, 20*(9), 686–692.

Reid, K., & Alfred, A. (2013). Quality of life, coping strategies and support needs of women seeking Traditional Chinese Medicine for infertility and viable pregnancy in Australia: A mixed methods approach. *BMC Women's Health, 13*, 17.

Rowe, R., & Calnan, M. (2006). Trust relations in healthcare—the new agenda. *European Journal of Public Health, 16*(1), 4–6.

Sibbritt, D., Adams, J., & Lui, C.W. (2011). Health service utilisation by pregnant women over a seven-year period. *Midwifery, 27*, 474–476.

Sibbritt, D., Catling, C.J., & Adams, J., Shaw, A.J., & Homer, C.S.E. (2014). The self-prescribed use of aromatherapy oils by pregnant women. *Women and Birth, 27*, 41–45.

Sim, T., Hattingh, L.H., Sherriff, J., & Tee, L. (2014). Perspectives and attitudes of breastfeeding women using herbal galactagogues during breastfeeding: A qualitative study. *BMC Complementary and Alternative Medicine, 14*, 216.

Sim, T., Sherriff, J., Hattingh, H., Parsons, R., & Tee, L. (2013). The use of herbal medicines during breastfeeding: A population-based survey in Western Australia. *BMC Complementary and Alternative Medicine, 13*, 317.

Sirois, F.S. (2008). Motivations for consulting complementary and alternative medicine practitioners: A comparison of consumers from 1997–8 and 2005. *BMC Complementary and Alternative Medicine, 8*, 16.

Smith, C.A., Armour, M., & Betts, D. (2014) Treatment of women's reproductive health conditions by Australian and New Zealand acupuncturists. *Complementary Therapies in Medicine, 22*(4), 710–718.

Smith, C.A., Bateson, D.J., & Weisberg, E. (2013). A survey describing the use of complementary therapies and medicines by women attending a family planning clinic. *BMC Complementary and Alternative Medicine, 13*, 224.

Smith, C.A., Ussher, J.M., Perz, J., Carmody, B., & de Lacey, S. (2011). The effect of acupuncture on psychosocial outcomes for women experiencing infertility: A pilot randomized controlled trial. *Journal of Alternative & Complementary Medicine, 17*(10), 923–930.

Smith, J.F., Eisenberg, M.L., Millstein, S.G., Nachtigall, R.D., Shindel, A.W., Wing, H., Cedars, M., Pasch, L., Katz, P.P., & the Infertility Outcomes Program Project Group. (2010). The use of complementary and alternative fertility treatment in couples seeking fertility care: Data from a prospective cohort in the Unites States. *Fertility & Sterility, 93*(7), 2169–2174.

Sointu, E. (2006). The search for wellbeing in alternative and complementary health practices. *Sociology of Health & Illness, 28*(3), 330–349.

Stankiewicz, M., Smith, C., Alvino, H., & Norman, R. (2007). The use of complementary medicine and therapies by patients attending a reproductive medicine unit in South Australian: a prospective survey. *Australian and New Zealand Journal of Obstetrics & Gynaecology, 47*(2), 145–149.

Steel, A., Adams, J., Sibbritt, D., Broom, A., Gallios, C., & Frawley, J. (2014). Determinants of women consulting with a complementary and alternative medicine practitioner for pregnancy related conditions. *Women & Health, 54*(2), 127–144.

Strouss, L., Mackley, A., Guillen, U., Paul, D.A., & Locke, R. (2014). Complementary and alternative medicine use in women during pregnancy: Do their healthcare providers know? *BMC Complementary and Alternative Medicine, 14*, 85.

Swift, W., Stollznow, N., & Pirotta, M. (2007). The use of alcohol and medicines among Australian adults. *Australian and New Zealand Journal of Public Health, 31*(6), 529–532.

Willis, K., & Rayner, J. (2015). The nexus between the social and the medical: How can we understand the proliferation of complementary and alternative medicine for enhancing fertility and treating infertility? In N.K. Gale & J.V. McHale (Eds), *The Routledge handbook of complementary and alternative medicine in social science and law* (pp. 110–125). London: Routledge.

Xue, C., Zhang, A., Lin, V., da Costa, C., & Story, D. (2007). Complementary and alternative medicine use in Australia: A national population-based survey. *Journal of Complementary & Alternative Medicine, 13*(6), 643–650.

Zhang, A.L., Story, D.F., Lin, V., Vitetta, L., & Xue, C. (2008). A population survey on the use of 24 common medicinal herbs in Australia. *Pharmacoepidemiology & Drug Safety, 17*, 1006–1013.

CHAPTER 13

Traditional Chinese Medicine Practitioners' Constructions of "Hard" and "Soft" Evidence in the Treatment of Fertility Issues: Opportunities and Challenges

Ana M. Ning, PhD
Department of Sociology, King's University College, University of Western Ontario, Canada

Learning Objectives

1. To understand how Chinese medical practitioners in British Columbia and Ontario, Canada, construct evidence of the effectiveness and safety of their practices.
2. To appreciate the relevance of ethnographic research for highlighting a broader conceptual framework beyond the emphasis on bioscientific evidence bases to assess the validity of any therapeutic modality.
3. To learn about opportunities and challenges for combining encompassing types of "hard" (bioscientific) and "soft" (experiential) evidence bases in reproductive health care.
4. To consider the possibility of a truly symmetrical and integrative health care system that includes multiple epistemologies to meet diverse health care needs.

Introduction

This chapter is an ethnographic account of traditional Chinese medicine (TCM) practitioners' constructions of appropriate evidence bases of their practices in two Canadian provinces (British Columbia and Ontario), in the context of TCM's unique position as a state-regulated health profession in these settings. This circumstance is unlike that in the rest of Canada—and in most western countries—where TCM remains a complementary and alternative medical (CAM) practice operating outside of the mainstream health care system. The question of appropriate evidence bases, in which bioscientific standards to evaluate the safety and efficacy of any therapeutic modality are privileged, is a major controversy in the integration of CAM practices into the public health care domain (Barry 2006; Daly, 2005; De Bruyn, 2001; Dean, 2004; Denny, 1999; Rappolt, 1997; Villaneuva-Russell, 2005). The concept of evidence itself is highly contested: different stakeholders define and interpret evidence differently for their own purposes of recognizing, legitimating, and regulating health professions. To date, limited ethnographic research has been conducted that clarifies what constitutes "sufficient evidence" to assess complex, multi-factorial, synergistic, and interactive health systems such as TCM in order to support its integration, although significant qualitative research addresses TCM effectiveness in transnational encounters (Baer 2008; Barnes, 2005; Farquhar, 1994; Kelner & Wellman, 2014; Zhan, 2009).

In this chapter, I explore contemporary constructions of TCM evidence as a complex undertaking in which providers, knowledge, experiences, and science intersect in interesting and sometimes contradictory ways. To illustrate how TCM

Box 13.1: "Soft" and "Hard" Evidence

Biomedicine and TCM are foundationally empirical. That is, they use observation to explain or predict nature's phenomena. TCM uses experience to verify knowledge without constructing an ordered scientific system (Scheid, 2002; Unschuld, 1985). Biomedicine deems TCM's empirical approach "soft" because it is not validated by "hard" scientific instruments such as statistical analysis, controlled experiments, and quantifiable data, which are generally characterized as "objective," and "value-free" (Cassell, 2006; Villanueva-Russell, 2005). Academics and the media have long debated the division between "soft" and "hard" sciences (Barry, 2006; Dean, 2004; Rappolt 1997; Waldram, 2000). Feminist scholars critique the hierarchy of "scientific" value, whereby "natural sciences" are more highly valued than social sciences (Cassell, 2006; Keller, 1985; Martin, 1997). However, there is bias in both qualitative and quantitative research, given the researchers' interpretation of data, the selectiveness of the research questions, and the materials to be included or excluded in final knowledge productions.

evidence is used and applied in context, I focus primarily on TCM's cited contributions in reproductive health that rely substantially on empirical/experiential methods rooted within the unique systemic logic of TCM. While the empirical bases of **"soft" evidence** within TCM—experiential, historical, observational, oral—inform TCM practitioners' identities and practices, they also negotiate the dominant **"hard" evidence** of biomedical treatment of fertility issues (see box 13.1).

A focus on TCM's cited contributions in reproductive health is both theoretically and socially relevant. Since the 2000s, for example, interest in acupuncture, a key component of TCM in the treatment of fertility issues in North America, has exploded, prompting many mainstream fertility clinics to offer this alternative option alongside their regular biomedical interventions (Delosantos, 2012; Dooley, 2006; Gurevich, 2010; Hopton, Curnoe, Kanaan & MacPherson, 2012). Paying attention to various types of evidence in TCM practitioners' narratives of fertility treatments also illuminates the potential for a more expanded conceptual framework to assess the validity of any therapeutic modality—one that includes multiple epistemologies (that is, ways of knowing, theories, and methods).

What Is "Evidence"?

Similar to that of other social scientists (Coburn & Biggs, 1986; McClean, 2003; Saks, 1992), my research (Ning, 1997, 2008, 2013) has found that many TCM practitioners have undergone a process of **biomedicalization**—that is, they have adopted the western biomedical model and rejected the more holistic aspects of traditional practice. The biomedicalization of TCM is a result of pressure to gain recognition, legitimacy, and regulation within local and global contexts where the "gold standard" for establishing "scientific" evidence of therapeutic efficacy and safety is mainly **randomized controlled clinical trials (RCTs)** (Ernst, 2000; Saks, 1992).

Interestingly, TCM's popularity in China is declining during the country's 21st-century economic boom, as cosmopolitan consumers now interpret it as a "traditional" practice, less desirable than the "modern" western biomedicine (Karchmer, 2010). The latter's association with the more prestigious symbols of science and technology is valorized over the traditional Chinese diagnostic practices, which rely strongly on sensorial experiences like touching, feeling, observing, smelling, and listening to patients' bodies. The current Chinese government is adopting western biomedical standards for evaluating the safety, efficacy, and educational standards of all medical practice, thus overturning the longstanding prestigious place of TCM in Chinese history (Karchmer, 2010; Qiu, 2007).

In the Canadian settings, my interviews with TCM practitioners reveal more nuanced narratives about the evidence bases of their regular practices. My previous findings, which showed that many practitioners assert the legitimacy of their TCM practices by biomedicalizing their practice, have not fully held. Here, I uncover multiple types of legitimate evidence that TCM practitioners in Canada use to justify their practices in ways that often suggest the higher effectiveness of TCM over biomedicine, especially in reproductive health. Many TCM practitioners resort to what Hobsbawm and Ranger (1983) have called the "invention" of tradition, by highlighting the validity of unique experiential or "soft" types of evidence that are inherent to the original philosophy of TCM, and which they claim are equally compelling or even more reliable than the scientific or "hard" evidence underlying biomedicine.

This chapter aims to explore the following research questions:

1. What constitutes legitimate types of TCM evidence of therapeutic effectiveness and safety?
2. How do TCM practitioners integrate "soft" (experiential) and "hard" (scientific) evidence in reproductive health?
3. What constitutes "sufficient evidence" to validate successful fertility treatments in the absence of hard (scientific) evidence?

Methodology

My research entailed 12 months of fieldwork in two distinct phases (August–December 2010 and December 2011–August 2012) with five TCM practitioners in British Columbia (BC) and five in Ontario (ON).[1] As an "interested researcher" (MacDonald & Bourgeault, 2000), I describe myself as someone who has a long history of research in complementary/alternative and biomedical health care who is also a scholar committed to critical reflection and analysis. My position as an interested researcher ultimately helped me develop solid rapport with the TCM practitioners.

My data collection primarily involved participant observation of simulated TCM treatments on medical mannequins[2] or those performed on me as a TCM patient, as well as in-depth, open-ended interviews with the TCM practitioners. I interviewed three female and two male TCM practitioners in each province, all of whom were already known to me from previous personal and professional connections. Prior to meeting the practitioners individually in their homes, offices, or public venues (restaurants, coffee shops), I sent them a detailed copy of my research protocol, including its ethical clearance from my university, as well as a tentative list of research questions in three main areas: background training and experience; individual descriptions and meanings of "evidence"; and types of scientific and non-scientific evidence used in TCM practices.

All of the practitioners in my research were ethnically Chinese, ranged in age from early 40s to mid-50s, were originally trained in mainland China, and had been in Canada between 10 and 20 years. They were selected for their extensive knowledge of and experience in TCM so that they could address complex questions about TCM evidence. Such questions may not have been possible to elicit from locally trained TCM practitioners whose training remains more limited in both scope and practice in comparison to those trained overseas. Because some of the participants are very well known in their respective TCM communities, their names have been changed to protect their identity. The stories that follow are compiled from information gathered over several interviews.

Narratives of TCM Evidence

Martha[3] is a TCM practitioner with nearly 30 years of experience practising TCM in both her home and host countries. She was part of the first group of students to enter university in 1977 following the Cultural Revolution in China. After graduating from a five-year program in TCM, she found employment in a prestigious department of internal medicine at a local TCM university where she held teaching, research, and clinical responsibilities for four years prior to immigrating to Canada in the mid-1980s. In Canada, she furthered her studies in reproductive biology, earning a Master's of Science which enabled her to work as a researcher on gene therapy. She later left this position to develop her own school of TCM in Toronto, offering the first comprehensive TCM program of its kind in Ontario. Despite many successful patient testimonials about her TCM treatments, she doesn't feel her skills are recognized in Canada due to the fact that TCM is perceived as an alternative treatment rather than being fully integrated in the public health care system. She claims to have faced much criticism, skepticism, and disrespect about her work from biomedical practitioners who questioned the legitimacy of her treatment outcomes due to the absence of appropriate evidence bases. Below, she expresses candidly her second-class treatment as a TCM practitioner in Canada for being unable to demonstrate "hard" scientific evidence in her successful fertility treatments:

> Last week I gave a talk at a fertility clinic in downtown Toronto. I shared many successful stories of patient testimonials about their TCM treatments for fertility issues. I have several patients who got pregnant after many years of trying conventional methods, and they were more surprised when they found out they

got pregnant the second time! They didn't think they could get pregnant so fast the second time! The fertility specialists however, were very skeptical about TCM. They kept asking me, "Where's your proof? Where are your articles? Where's your hard evidence? Where are your clinical trials?" Regardless of patient testimonials, and detailed philosophical explanations of ***yin/yang***, they still dismissed me by claiming that my results were a mere coincidence, they were individual cases, and basically their question was "where are your evidence bases?" I know there's some proof regarding acupuncture for fertility, which has been published in some articles, but I didn't want to argue with them.... Everything is evidence based, double-blinded clinical trials; you can't change people's mentality. I have a lot of patient testimonials—why not consider this as evidence? Even in biomedical journals, there are single case reports, why not TCM? It's unfair, these double standards, we're treated as second class.

Martha's story exemplifies TCM practitioners' marginal position in mainstream health care (see box 13.2). Notably, this marginality is a direct reflection of TCM's use of "soft" evidence.

Sam and Teresa are a husband and wife team of TCM practitioners who run their own TCM clinic in downtown Vancouver, BC, which they opened after immigrating

Box 13.2: Legitimacy of Traditional Medicine Cross-Culturally

In China and India, indigenous healing systems have long co-existed with western biomedicine, sharing legitimacy and popularity. In China, TCM—including acupuncture, herbal therapies, **moxibustion**, massage therapy (***tui na***), and relaxation techniques such as ***tai chi*** and ***qi gong***—still provides significant health care for much of the population, especially in rural areas. East Indian Ayurvedic medicine and western biomedicine are part of the mainstream health care system in India, just as in British, French, German, and Italian medicine, where homeopathy, humoralism, and western biomedicine co-exist (Hogle, 1999; Janzen, 2002; Payer, 1990; Whitaker, 2003). In Canada, only a few CAM modalities—acupuncture/TCM, chiropractic care, midwifery, and naturopathy—are regulated health professions in some provinces, and only some extended health benefit plans cover them, which reflects the subordination of CAM within the health care system.

to Canada about 10 years ago. Both were trained as (biomedical) physicians and TCM practitioners in China, but they specialized in TCM. By the time they arrived in BC in the early 2000s, TCM had become a regulated health profession, which meant that they were required to pass written and practical tests before practising TCM in that province. Both Sam and Teresa noted that being allowed to practice TCM only has proved beneficial because it enabled them to improve their skills, treating mostly chronic cases after patients turned to them as a last resort, but also because, as Teresa put it, "we saw how Chinese medicine is better than western medicine … Chinese medicine has a perfect foundation."

In contrast, Wayne, who was primarily trained as a clinician in TCM and was also a researcher in molecular biology and physiology in China, is comfortable with combining both modalities of care in his research at a Toronto public hospital that focuses on identifying active ingredients in Chinese herbs to treat cystic fibrosis. Below, he shares observations gained in 20 years of research in Toronto that merges biomedical and TCM types of evidence to evaluate treatment efficacy:

> There are many mechanisms that TCM can use to compensate for a defective gene like in cystic fibrosis, by adjusting the body holistically. Western medicine discovered the defective gene in 1989, and after 20 years of research, there is still no cure, no way to correct the defective gene. So, patients are only offered antibiotics and physio[therapy]. We can compensate for the defective gene by using existing TCM treatments for asthma … cystic fibrosis is a very severe form of asthma. By using acupuncture, herbal treatments, we can improve symptoms, patients become more comfortable, their asthma is not as severe, they live all right, and their life span is prolonged. The usual life span for a cystic fibrosis patient is 20 years, but now we have patients who are 50 and still alive. We can't say we have the cure for the disease because of the defective gene, but we can help patients become a carrier of a mutant gene.[4] This is very good evidence that TCM is effective.

Wayne's insights and familiarity with TCM and biomedicine demonstrate his ability to comfortably navigate in both medical worlds, appreciating what each approach can offer, unlike Sam and Teresa who are clearly partial to TCM. Nonetheless, these three practitioners' narratives imply that TCM's higher effectiveness is based on its unique foundation.

All 10 TCM practitioners whom I interviewed acknowledged that TCM has its own epistemology, which may not befit the biomedical standards of evaluation based on RCTs. In their view, TCM is more inductive rather than deductive—that is, more experiential than scientific—and linked to ancient observations of individuals' trial-and-error experiences with food consumption and dealing with ailments and natural disasters in different environments. Such empirical knowledge has been modified and adjusted over generations through case studies. As Martha explains:

> You have to understand, TCM did not come from test tubes, labs, molecular biology, chemistry, cell research—it was empirical, experimental, based on daily lives. It was the way people found out about medicine when they were searching for food, finding ways to fight against natural disasters, finding ways to fight against diseases, then TCM was discovered. TCM is empirical—do you believe in that or not? When people searched for food, they came across food that gave diarrhea, yet some thought it might stimulate bowel movement in others. When it was too cold, you could take spicy food. When you press in certain points, it alleviates headaches, toothache—that's how meridians were discovered.

By declaring TCM's reliance on experiential, "soft" evidence as a reflection of its unique philosophy and practice, three TCM practitioners specifically highlighted the positive attributes of what biomedical practitioners discount as "non-scientific" evidence. One of them—Joanne, trained in both TCM and biomedicine in China—uses primarily acupuncture in her Vancouver-based practice. Acupuncture is compatible with most of her Canadian patients' preference to avoid potential hazardous interactions with biomedical interventions. It is generally believed to have no side effects if practised competently, and is also one of the few TCM components that has successfully undergone RCTs for various conditions including infertility (Ernst, 2000; Huang & Chen, 2008; Isoyama et al., 2012; Rubin, Opsahl & Ackerman, 2012). Hence, western audiences seem more inclined to use it. As Joanne maintains, "not everything can show—spirit, energy.... [l]ike religion, you cannot show which one is good or better. But you can show that people are getting better. Isn't this enough evidence?"

In turn, Sam's explanation of TCM's experiential evidence clearly expresses his conviction that TCM is more effective than biomedicine given its preventative value:

> What is evidence? It's a good question. We can't see but feel the patients' pulse. Ultrasounds, CT scans, MRIs, blood tests say this person is okay. Five or 10 years later, they come back when the problem arises, but it may be too late. Western medicine treats diseases. In Chinese medicine, when you have a disease, it's already too late. It's better to treat someone before they get sick. In Chinese medicine, you can feel it, and we can do something from an early stage. Pulse reading tells clearly about a person's condition, and not just through a patient's report of feelings. It takes years to learn and to meet the right masters to learn from.

His wife and TCM partner Teresa insists that TCM was a very successful medical system that preceded western biomedicine. In her words, "Chinese medicine has a perfect foundation, diagnosis and perfect treatment, but you can't see the energy when you do pulse readings, or apply acupuncture needles, it is hard to learn to feel it [energy]." By emphasizing TCM's "perfect foundation" and its focus on energy, Teresa is suggesting that TCM's effectiveness is rooted in its longer history and experiential basis.

In so doing, I contend that Teresa is using tradition as a symbolic device to legitimate a health profession with deeper historical roots than biomedicine. Anthropological theory has shown that a group's identification with tradition is often used in political struggles of the present (Hanson, 1989) or as a "political symbol" (Keesing, 1982) because calling something a tradition creates a sense of authenticity and ownership for the group making that claim. To understand tradition as (re)invented (Hobsbawm & Ranger, 1983) does not invalidate its authenticity or the right of a group or culture to claim it; rather, it draws analytical attention to the processes of its production and use (MacDonald, 2008).

In contrast, James and Marilyn, another husband and wife TCM team, specializing in the treatment of fertility issues in their two private TCM clinics in Vancouver and Richmond, BC, are skeptical about TCM's reliance on "non-scientific" evidence. Both were primarily trained in biomedicine in China and subsequently obtained Master's degrees in clinical immunology and molecular biology overseas.[5] Because they were unable to find research work in Canada due to language barriers and limited local experience, friends encouraged them to practise TCM without a licence, given that it was an unregulated profession in BC in the mid-1990s. James began refreshing his limited TCM training by working in a local Chinese herbal store, and by observing his friends practising TCM. Meanwhile, Marilyn returned to China to sharpen her TCM skills and after four years in Canada they opened their first TCM clinic in Vancouver. Despite their successful use of TCM in the treatment of male and female infertility in their Canadian clinics, James argues that the exclusive use of TCM in health care is insufficient because of its lack of "scientific" evidence:

> Purely Chinese medical diagnosis is insufficient because it's not scientific. Sixty percent of my mind follows the western medical model. When a patient comes with a problem, I still want to know the western diagnosis. I ask them, did you see your family physician, what kind of lab work have you done? All this is very helpful. Even in purely TCM hospitals in China, they still use CT scans, ultrasounds to diagnose problems. There's a lot of intersection in China. There, TCM relies on western diagnostic tools to establish the best diagnosis.

Asked what constitutes "enough evidence" of effectiveness in their TCM practices in the absence of scientific evidence, Marilyn responded:

> Patients' feelings—for example, if pain has improved after two or three [TCM] treatments. In the case of infertility, it is easy to demonstrate how our treatments are effective.... We check if sexual activity has improved ... let's say, previously a patient only had sex once a week, but after treatments, it increased to three times a week. We also do a pulse reading to check the ***qi*** rating, look at the colour of tongue, use acupuncture points to improve irregular menstrual periods.

Although James and Marilyn point to TCM's lack of scientific validity in diagnosis and treatment, they have successfully used TCM to treat fertility issues (see box 13.3). Just as conventional biomedical practitioners' skepticism of alternative health practices is shaped by the cultural lens of their bioscientific training (Helman, 2002), as Canadian TCM practitioners and Chinese biomedical physicians, James' and Marilyn's practice of TCM is also influenced by western scientific discourse. This tension between legitimizing health practices through science ("hard evidence") or traditional medicine ("soft evidence") is continually played out in many TCM practitioners' interpretations of their work in the pursuit of professional recognition.

Applying "Soft" and "Hard" Evidence to Reproductive Health

All practitioners in my study use the following six types of "soft" evidence to establish effectiveness and safety standards of their TCM practices:

1. Experiential, such as pulse diagnosis to feel the flow of energy, along a patient's body meridians, known as an elusive entity named *qi* in TCM.
2. Observational, by paying attention to one's physical complexion and vitality as expressed through the colour of one's tongue, face, eyes, and ears.
3. Tactile, by palpating different body parts such as arms, legs, ears, stomach, etc.
4. Historical, by referring to, and interpreting ancient TCM texts.
5. Foundational knowledge, by following the eight guiding principles of syndrome differentiation.[6]
6. By considering patient reports of symptoms, and testimonials of treatment outcomes.

Box 13.3: Fertility and Infertility Cross-Culturally

Fertility is a universal human concern and so is anguish over infertility. When a woman fails to conceive, various cultural interpretations are used to explain and address her infertility. Lay explanations focus on personal responsibility, supernatural forces, or others' malevolence. Professional explanations rely on expert knowledge of specific disease etiologies such as hormonal imbalances, sexually transmitted diseases, nutritional deficiencies, and energy blockages. Generally, different explanations for infertility lead to different interventions including self-help, folk healing, or professional treatment, depending on individuals' values, beliefs, education, and material capital (e.g., income, accessibility/affordability of health care services). Broader structural factors such as liability issues, insurance plans, and state sanctions may also influence the choice of health care modalities.

The following narratives illustrate my participants' application of "soft" evidence independently or concurrently with biomedical "hard" evidence to establish effective fertility treatments. The TCM practitioners who have successfully treated various types of male and female infertility acknowledge the relevance of including both "soft" and "hard" types of evidence. They believe equally that integrating both TCM and biomedical interventions is the most successful approach in reproductive health. In their practices, James and Marilyn prefer to include only certain TCM components such as acupuncture, massage therapy (*tui na*), and moxibustion, excluding Chinese herbs to treat fertility issues. As James explains:

> Many of our patients are already in IVF [in vitro fertilization] procedures or in hormonal treatments, so we don't give them herbs, only acupuncture. I don't want to be blamed by the fertility specialists. ... IVF is very expensive; it costs over $10,000. If success is achieved [with Chinese herbs], then no problem, but if there's no success, they may say, it might have been the herbs! So, I tell my patients the truth—that I don't use herbs, and even if they don't mind [taking Chinese herbs], I still don't give them the herbs.

In turn, Martha, despite being a strong advocate of TCM's unique philosophy and experiential basis, agrees that combining biomedicine and TCM provides the most reliable methods to achieve proper diagnosis and treatment for any condition, but especially for women's health issues:

> Western diagnosis is very important, especially through regular physicals, scans. TCM is essential not to diagnose diseases, but to differentiate syndromes, to find the nature of the conditions, whether they are caused by heat, cold, dampness, dryness, and then which organ or meridian is obstructing the flow of energy.... Differentiation is very important because individuals are different, constitutions are different, signs and symptoms are manifested differently ... I wouldn't say that certain conditions are better treated by TCM alone, because people are different, there are many options, but some conditions can be better addressed with TCM because it's natural, less invasive, and these can be menstrual problems, menopause, and fertility issues.

James, Marilyn, and Martha strongly emphasize the importance of learning about the biomedical diagnosis prior to using TCM in the treatment of fertility issues. As Martha reasons:

> Western diagnosis is very important especially for some conditions such as early stages of cancer and fertility issues. For infertility patients, I'd like to know if patients have hormonal problems, if they have been diagnosed with PCOS [polycystic ovarian syndrome], if they have blocked tubes, or if males have some issues like lower sperm count, lazy, or inactive sperm. I'd like to know the western diagnosis, but I don't necessarily have to have patients' full records.

In addition to considering the biomedical diagnosis for any fertility issues prior to administering TCM, James thinks that biomedical criteria are also helpful to measure the effectiveness of TCM fertility treatments:

> It's easy to say how effective TCM is for fertility treatments. For male infertility, all patients already had a sperm analysis before they came to see us. After three months of acupuncture treatment, we ask them to get another sperm analysis to check on the morphology and morbidity. If there's sperm improvement, then this shows our treatment was effective. We also do a pulse rating to check on the *qi*, energy level, and we touch on certain points, paying attention to kidney functioning. If the energy level is not strong enough in certain points, we increase the energy level with acupuncture. When the energy is stronger, one's libido is higher and lasts longer.... For women, we ask about their hormonal levels, whether they are high or low, whether they have endometriosis, or irregular periods. After we do the pulse rating, we do the acupuncture to balance the energy. If one's period was irregular and it becomes more regular, this is one measure of success.

> If someone used to have major PMS, and symptoms are improved, and if they used to have hormonal over-function, and after two or three cycles of acupuncture treatment, their hormonal level is down, these are signs of effectiveness.

Practitioners acknowledged that it is challenging to measure the success rates of their TCM fertility treatments that result in live births because patients often integrate biomedicine or, many quit after one or two months of TCM treatments because the treatments are costly and not covered by public or even most private insurance plans. They also pointed out that patients' age may influence the overall pregnancy rates, recognizing that older patients (aged 45 and above), especially women, have lower success rates.

According to biomedical literature, the outcome measures of acupuncture in fertility treatments are inconclusive. In studies that demonstrate the positive effects of acupuncture when applied independently or concurrently with biomedicine, health improvements are cited in several areas: higher pregnancy rates during IVF treatment cycles; increased blood flow to the uterus leading to improved endometrial lining; increased sperm count and quality; improved ovulation frequency; and reduced stress and anxiety levels (Delosantos, 2012; Huang & Chen, 2008; Isoyama et al., 2012; Manca di Villahermosa et al., 2013; Rubin, Opsahl & Ackerman, 2012). In contrast, in studies that discredit acupuncture by demonstrating no improvement in ovulation, reduction in anxiety and stress, or increase in successful IVF rates, acupuncture is often administered in short terms (less than four weeks), or applied just prior to embryo transfers during IVF procedures (El-Toukhy & Khalaf, 2009; Madaschi et al., 2010; Pastore, Williams, Jenkins & Patrie, 2011). In other words, the conditions under which acupuncture is used in these studies are inappropriate for evaluating its efficacy.

When asked about these mixed results, most TCM practitioners responded by asserting that each individual has a different constitution, and for successful conception to occur there must be a total balance of mind, body, and lifestyle. As Rhonda, a well-known Toronto-based TCM practitioner explains:

> In TCM, the kidney system is responsible for human reproduction, growth, and development. The kidneys are where we store our essence, which is the foundation of the body and its functions, and can be transformed into *qi*. If we plan to have children, it is important that we support our kidney essence, by avoiding overwork and excessive physical exertion, irregular dietary habits, inadequate rest, and chronic illness. We must also avoid exposure to cold and damp conditions, deal with our stress and emotions appropriately, abstain from or reduce consumption

> of coffee, tobacco, and alcohol. Conception and proper growth of the fetus all depend on strong kidneys. So for us, the issue is not whether a patient has hormonal problems, or other morphological problems, but how strong their kidney energy is. This makes sense since some of our patients have been diagnosed with "unexplained infertility"—biomedicine cannot find anything wrong with them but can't understand why they can't get pregnant.

In short, biomedical reports of unsuccessful acupuncture treatments often omit factors that extend beyond the singular applications of acupuncture prior to conventional fertility interventions. TCM, like many other CAM treatments, does not consider a therapeutic effect such as successful conception to rest on a single remedy (e.g., herb) or technique (e.g., acupuncture), but in an energetic system that comprises the patient, the prescribed treatment, the healer, and the treatment setting (Barry, 2006, p. 2647). By relying on "soft" evidence, TCM practitioners like Rhonda account for broader factors beyond the physical body (e.g., lifestyle, vital energies, diet, environment) to address reproductive health.

Conclusion

Most of the TCM practitioners whom I interviewed maintain the relevance of TCM's unique types of "soft" evidence to address different health issues successfully, including infertility. They advance monolithic interpretations of TCM evidence as if it has remained unchanged over time. This sense of historical legitimacy occurs within the discourse of tradition by inferring an uninterrupted link to the original foundations of TCM. In fact, scholars of TCM have maintained that TCM itself has undergone numerous changes, from an exclusively experiential to an increasingly biomedicalized practice, following different political, economic, and social upheavals throughout Chinese history (Farquhar, 1994; Scheid, 2002; Unschuld, 1985, 1992; Zhan, 2009). While there appears to be justification for the biomedicalization of contemporary TCM in local and global settings—namely, legal recognition and adherence to dominant scientific evidence bases (Ning, 2008, 2013; Saks, 1992; Scheid, 2002)—the conversations in this chapter paint a more complex picture. As these conversations illustrate, the reinterpretation of tradition to demonstrate TCM's effectiveness is juxtaposed with rejection and accommodation of biomedicine to explain the successful outcomes of TCM.

In reproductive health, there was a general consensus among those whom I interviewed that both TCM and biomedicine offer equally reliable diagnostic and treatment evidence, including opportunities for collaboration. This finding raises two critical issues that have major implications for continuing fruitful discussion about what constitutes legitimate evidence bases necessary to assess the validity of any therapeutic modality, and for whom—patients, biomedical practitioners, or policy makers. On the one hand, by according importance to both "soft" TCM and "hard" biomedical evidence to establish successful fertility treatments, TCM practitioners revealed possible areas of intersection between "alternative" (TCM) and "conventional" (biomedical) health care. In other words, their experiences confirm my previous theorization that CAM and biomedical systems are homologous rather than dichotomous symbolic systems (Ning, 2013), operating in a continuum of overlapping and diverse values and symbols.

On the other hand, by disclosing opportunities to integrate TCM and biomedicine in reproductive health, my findings also highlight the potential for a broader conceptual framework encompassing multiple epistemologies (ways of knowing, theories, and methods) beyond a single (bioscientific) evidence base to evaluate the effectiveness, safety, and educational standards of any health modality. Unquestionably, since state-regulated health care in Canada remains the exclusive domain of biomedicine with the exception of some CAM modalities in some provinces,[7] the Canadian health care system illustrates the position of asymmetrical medical pluralism (Janzen, 2002). In other words, the dominance of biomedicine and the subordination of CAM are reflected in their differential incorporation into mainstream health care. An expanded framework to evaluate any therapeutic modality could facilitate interdisciplinary dialogue toward coordinating a potentially symmetrical integrative health care system in which the contributions of different epistemologies meet diverse health care needs.

Acknowledgements

This research was supported by funding from the King's University College's Faculty Research Grant. I wish to thank the editors of this volume (Jennie Hornosty and Costanza Torri) for reading earlier drafts of this manuscript and for providing very useful comments, which helped strengthen this chapter. My deepest gratitude goes to the individuals who participated in this study but who, for reasons of confidentiality, remain anonymous.

Notes

1. Fieldwork occurred in two distinct phases to accommodate my parental leave.
2. Given ethical concerns raised by the Research Ethics Committee at my university during

approval for my research protocol regarding potential conflicts of interest associated with eliciting permission from the TCM practitioners' patients to observe actual clinical interactions, I decided to focus on simulated rather than actual demonstrations of treatments.

3. All the real names of the participants have been altered with pseudonyms to maintain their anonymity and confidentiality.
4. According to biomedicine, cystic fibrosis (CF) is caused by two copies of a mutated gene that a patient has inherited from both parents. In principle, a CF carrier does not have the disease but can pass it on to their offspring, if their partner is also a CF carrier. By citing the benefits of TCM treatment for CF, Wayne is suggesting that CF patients can potentially live long enough to be carriers of the disease, although they may not be cured from it.
5. James received Master's of Science degrees in clinical immunology and molecular biology and Marilyn received a Master's of Science in molecular biology.
6. Syndrome differentiation represents a TCM classificatory system for disease causation beyond organic pathologies. It is allegedly different from the biomedical classification of disease etiology that explains disease causation in terms of organic agents such as bacteria, germs, viruses, tumours, or genetic defects. Syndrome differentiation is based on eight guiding principles to identify syndromes or energy imbalances in terms of interior/exterior, heat/cold, *yin/yang*, and deficiency/excess. Once syndromes are identified, the next step involves determining which organ (heart, lung, kidneys, bladder, stomach, spleen, gall bladder, intestines, or liver) is responsible for a particular syndrome. After syndrome and organ differentiations are established, pathogenic cosmic factors such as wind, fire, dampness, dryness, heat, cold, etc. are also considered to complete TCM diagnosis.
7. Acupuncture, TCM, chiropractic care, midwifery, and naturopathy are regulated health professions in some Canadian provinces, and some extended health benefit plans cover them (Achilles et al., 1999; Boon, 2002; De Bruyn, 2001; Tataryn & Verhoef, 2001).

Critical Thinking Questions

1. What assumptions underlie the division between "soft" and "hard" evidence bases, and why do you think "hard" evidence is increasingly privileged in today's world?
2. What do you think are the opportunities and challenges for combining different types of evidence bases to assess the effectiveness, safety, and educational standards of any health care modality?
3. Do you think a truly symmetrical, integrative health care system is possible or desirable in Canada? Why or why not?

Glossary

Biomedicalization: The process in which complementary and alternative medical practices accommodate with the biomedical model in order to gain legitimacy, recognition, and regulation in biomedically dominant arenas.

"Hard" evidence: A term applied to biomedical constructions of therapeutic efficacy and safety based on "scientific" instruments, e.g., statistical analysis, controlled experiments, quantifiable data, which are presumed to be more "objective" and "value-free."

Moxibustion: A TCM technique involving the burning of mugwort, a small spongy herb, close to the human body to facilitate healing.

Qi: Vital force or bioenergy as designated in Chinese medicine and philosophy.

Qi gong: A component of TCM involving meditation and coordinating slow flowing movements with deep rhythmic breathing.

Randomized controlled clinical trials (RCTs): These are specific types of scientific experiment to test the efficacy of medical interventions and to collect information about adverse drug reactions within a patient population. Study subjects are randomly allocated into experimental (receiving treatment) and control (non-receiving or placebo treatment) groups to provide comparisons.

"Soft" evidence: A term applied to knowledge derived from direct observations and trial and error sensorial experiences without being verified by "scientific" instruments, yet adjusted and modified over time through case studies.

Tai chi: Often used in TCM as a preventative health strategy involving relaxation physical exercises.

Tui na: A component of TCM that involves massaging specific points in the human body as a form of therapeutic intervention.

Yin/yang: A Chinese philosophical conceptualization of apparently oppositional forces or tangible dualities that are actually complementary or interdependent, such as light and dark, hot and cold, life and death, male and female, sun and moon, etc.

References

Achilles, R., Adelson, N., Antze P., Biggs, C.L., Chabot, P., Gilmour, J., & Muldoon, J. (1999). *Complementary and alternative health practices and therapies: A Canadian overview*. Toronto: York University Centre for Health Studies.

Baer, H. (2008). The emergence of integrative medicine in Australia: The growing interest of biomedicine and nursing in complementary medicine in southern developed society. *Medical Anthropology Quarterly, 22*(1), 52–66.

Barnes, L. (2005). American acupuncture and efficacy: Meanings and their points of intersection. *Medical Anthropology Quarterly, 19*(3), 239–266.

Barry, C. (2006). The role of evidence in alternative medicine: Contrasting biomedical anthropological approaches. *Social Science and Medicine, 62*(11), 2646–2657.

Boon, H. (2002). Regulation of complementary/alternative medicine: A Canadian perspective. *Complementary Therapies in Medicine, 10*, 14–19.

Cassell, J. (2006). Perturbing the system: "Hard science," "soft science," and social science, the anxiety and madness of method. In E. Whitaker (Ed.), *Health and healing in comparative perspective* (pp. 74–84). New Jersey: Pearson Prentice Hall.

Coburn, D., & Biggs, C.L. (1986). Limits to medical dominance: The case of chiropractic. *Social Science and Medicine, 22*(10), 1035–1046.

Daly, J. (2005). *Evidence-based medicine and the search for a science of clinical care*. Berkeley: University of California Press.

De Bruyn, T. (2001). Taking stock: Policy issues associated with complementary and alternative health Care. In *Perspectives on complementary and alternative health care: A collection of papers prepared for Health Canada* (pp. 17–29). Ottawa: Health Canada.

Dean, K. (2004). The role of methods in maintaining orthodox beliefs in health research. *Social Science and Medicine, 58*, 675–685.

Delosantos, M. (2012). *The use of TCM as an adjunct to western fertility treatments for the management of female infertility* (Capstone project). Retrieved from Pacific University Common Knowledge (School of Physician Assistant Studies, Paper 294).

Denny, K. (1999). Evidence-based medicine and medical authority. *Journal of Medical Humanities, 20*(4), 247–263.

Dooley, M. (2006). Complementary therapy and obstetrics and gynaecology: A time to integrate. *Current Opinion in Obstetrics and Gynaecology, 18*(6), 648–652.

El-Toukhy, T., & Khalaf, Y. (2009). The impact of acupuncture on assisted reproductive technology outcome. *Current Opinion in Obstetrics and Gynaecology, 21*(3), 240–246.

Ernst, E. (2000). *Herbal medicine: A concise overview for professionals.* Oxford: Butterworth-Heineman.

Farquhar, J. (1994). *Knowing practice: The clinical encounter in Chinese medicine.* Boulder, CO: Westview Press.

Gurevich, R. (2010, June 6). *What does medical research say about acupuncture and infertility?* Retrieved from http://infertility.about.com/

Hanson, A. (1989). The making of the Maori: Cultural invention and its logic. *American Anthropologist, 91*(4), 890–902.

Helman, C. (2002). *Culture, health, and illness* (5th ed.). Oxford: Butterworth-Heineman.

Hobsbawm, E. & Ranger, T. (1983). *The invention of tradition.* Cambridge: Cambridge University Press.

Hogle, L. (1999). *Recovering the nation's body: Cultural memory, medicine and the politics of redemption.* New Jersey: Rutgers University Press.

Hopton, A., Curnoe, S., Kanaan, M., & MacPherson, H. (2012). Acupuncture in practice: Mapping the providers, the patients, and the settings in a national cross-sectional survey. *British Medical Journal Open, 2*(1), 1–10.

Huang, S., & Chen, A. (2008). Traditional Chinese medicine and infertility. *Current Opinion in Obstetrics and Gynaecology, 20*(3), 211–215.

Isoyama, D., Cordts, E., van Niewegen, A., Carvalho, W., Matsumura, S., & Barbosa, C. (2012). Effect of acupuncture on symptoms of anxiety in women undergoing in vitro fertilization: A prospective randomized controlled study. *Acupuncture in Medicine, 30*(2), 85–88.

Janzen, J. (2002). *The social fabric of health: An introduction to medical anthropology.* Boston: McGraw-Hill.

Karchmer, E. (2010). Chinese medicine in action: On the postcoloniality of medical practice in China. *Medical Anthropology, 29*(3), 226–252.

Keesing, R. (1982). Kastom and anticolonialism on Malaita: "Culture" as political symbol. *Mankind, 13*(4), 357–373.

Keller, E. (1985). *Reflections on gender and science.* New Haven: Yale University Press.

Kelner, M., & Wellman, B. (2014). *Complementary and alternative medicine: Challenge and change.* New York: Routledge, Taylor and Francis.

MacDonald, M. (2008). *At work in the field of birth: Midwifery narratives of nature, tradition and home.* Nashville: Vanderbilt University Press.

MacDonald, M., & Bourgeault, I. (2000). The politics of representation: Doing and writing interested research on midwifery. *Resources for Feminist Research, 28*(1–2), 151–168.

Madaschi, C., Braga, D., Figueira, R., Iacorelli, A., & Borges Jr., E. (2010). Effect of acupuncture on assisted reproductive treatment outcomes. *Acupuncture in Medicine, 28*(4), 180–184.

Manca di Villahermosa, D., Santos, L., Nogueira, M., Vilarino, F., & Barbosa, C. (2013). Influence of acupuncture on the outcomes of in vitro fertilization when embryo implantation has failed: A prospective randomized controlled clinical trial. *Acupuncture in Medicine, 31*(2), 157–161.

Martin, E. (1997). How science has constructed a romance based on stereotypical male-female roles. In L. Lamphere, H. Ragone & P. Zavella (Eds), *Situated lives: Gender and culture in everyday life* (pp. 85–98). New York: Routledge.

McClean, S. (2003). Doctoring the spirit: Exploring the use and meaning of mimicry and parody at a healing centre in the north of England. *Health, 7*(4), 483–500.

Ning, A. (1997). Regulating health professions and Chinese medicine in Ontario. In J.K. Crellin, R.R. Andersen & J.T.H. Connor (Eds.), *Alternative health care in Canada: Nineteenth and twentieth-century perspectives* (pp. 231–241). Toronto: Canadian Scholars' Press.

Ning, A. (2008). Paradoxes of integrative health care: The question of legitimate evidence bases. *International Journal of Diversity in Organizations, Communities and Nations, 7*(6), 237–248.

Ning, A. (2013). How "alternative" is CAM? Rethinking conventional dichotomies between biomedicine and complementary/alternative medicine. *Health, 17*(2), 135–158.

Pastore, L., Williams, C., Jenkins, J., & Patrie, J. (2011). True and sham acupuncture produced similar frequency of ovulation and improved LH to FSH ratio in women with polycystic ovary syndrome. *The Journal of Clinical Endocrinology and Metabolism, 96*(10), 3143.

Payer, L. (1990). Borderline cases: How medical practices reflects national culture. *The Sciences, 30*, 38–42.

Qiu, J. (2007). China plans to modernize traditional medicine. *Nature, 446*, 590–591.

Rappolt, S. (1997). Clinical guidelines and the fate of medical autonomy in Ontario. *Social Science and Medicine, 44*, 957–987.

Rubin, L., Opsahl, M., & Ackerman, D. (2012). P02.15. Acupuncture improves in vitro fertilization live birth outcomes: A retrospective chart review. *BMC Complementary and Alternative Medicine, 12*(Suppl. 1), 71.

Saks, M. (1992). The paradox of incorporation: Acupuncture and the medical profession in modern Britain. In M. Saks (Ed.), *Alternative medicine in Britain* (pp. 183–200). Oxford: Clarendon Press.

Scheid, V. (2002). *Chinese medicine in contemporary China: Plurality and synthesis*. Durham, NC & London: Duke University Press.

Tataryn, D., & Verhoef, M. (2001). Combining conventional, complementary and alternative health care: A vision of integration. In *Perspectives on complementary and alternative health care: A collection of papers prepared for Health Canada* (pp. 87–109). Ottawa: Health Canada.

Unschuld, P. (1985). *Medicine in China: A history of ideas*. Berkeley: University of California Press.

Unschuld, P. (1992). Epistemological issues and changing legitimation: Traditional Chinese medicine in the 20th century. In C. Leslie & A. Young (Eds), *Paths to Asian medical knowledge* (pp. 44–62). Berkeley: University of California Press.

Villanueva-Russell, Y. (2005). Evidence-based medicine and its implications for the profession of chiropractic. *Social Science and Medicine, 60*(3), 545–561.

Waldram, J. (2000). The efficacy of traditional medicine: Current theoretical and methodological issues. *Medical Anthropology Quarterly, 14*(4), 603–625.

Whitaker, E. (2003). The idea of health: History, medical pluralism, and the management of the body in Emilia-Romagna, Italy. *Medical Anthropology Quarterly, 17*(3), 348–375.

Zhan, M. (2009). *Other-worldly: Making Chinese medicine through transnational frames.* Durham, NC: Duke University Press.

CHAPTER 14

The Value of Complementary and Alternative Medicine for Breast Cancer Survivorship

Ausanee Wanchai, RN, PhD
Boromarajonani College of Nursing, Thailand

Jane M. Armer, RN, PhD, FAAN, CLT
Sinclair School of Nursing, University of Missouri; Ellis Fischel Cancer Center, United States

Bob R. Stewart, EdD
Sinclair School of Nursing, University of Missouri, United States

Learning Objectives

1. To understand the value of complementary and alternative medicine as perceived by women with breast cancer.
2. To gain awareness about the complexity of the decision-making process for complementary and alternative medicine use among women with breast cancer.
3. To recognize the types of complementary and alternative medicine most widely used by women with breast cancer.
4. To recognize sources of complementary and alternative medicine information for women with breast cancer.

Introduction

Breast cancer is the most common cancer and the leading cause of cancer death among women in both developed and developing countries. Worldwide, breast cancer accounted for 1.7 million of all new cancer cases in 2012 and it is also the most common cause of death among cancer deaths in women (522,000 deaths in 2012)

(World Health Organization [WHO], 2013). In 2013, the American Cancer Society (ACS) reported that it was expected that an estimated 232,340 women in the US would be diagnosed with invasive breast cancer and 39,620 women would die of breast cancer. However, early detection and advances in treatment of breast cancer have increased the number of **breast cancer survivors**. The ACS reported that, in 2013, the five-year survival rate for invasive breast cancer patients is 90 percent, and 98 percent for those with localized breast cancer (see box 14.1).

Box 14.1: Stages of Cancer Survivorship

According to Mullan (1985), there are three stages of cancer survival:

1. Acute survival begins with the initial cancer diagnosis and continues to initial treatment completion.
2. Extended survival is the stage in which patients deal with aggressive treatments and uncertain prognosis.
3. Permanent survival evolves from extended disease-free survival when the likelihood of recurrence is sufficiently low.

Previous studies have shown that survivors face many problems, both physical and psychosocial, after completion of treatment. The physical problems from treatment side effects include lymphedema, fatigue, weight gain, sleep disturbance, and osteoporosis (Mayer et al., 2007). Meanwhile, fear of recurrence, normative mood changes, uncertainty, an increased sense of vulnerability, feeling of loss, concern about body image, negative self-concept, emotional distress related to role adjustments and family response, and concern about finances and employment are psychosocial problems that are experienced by many breast cancer survivors (Knobf, 2007). Consequently, it is not surprising that, even though there is a lack of rigorous clinical evidence about the efficacy of complementary and alternative medicine (CAM) to alter disease progression of breast cancer, some breast cancer survivors choose to use options outside mainstream medicine, such as CAM, to increase their self-care abilities and to maintain physical and emotional well-being following cancer and the side effects of treatment (Wanchai, Armer & Stewart, 2010).

Based on the National Center for Complementary and Integrative Medicine (NCCIM) (2012), CAM refers to a group of health care systems, practices, and products that exist outside **western medicine**, which can be categorized into four types, including (1) natural products, such as herbal medicines, minerals, vitamins, and probiotics; (2) mind-body medicine, including meditation, acupuncture, yoga, and *tai chi*; (3) manipulative and body-based practices such as osteopathy, massage, or chiropractic; and (4) other CAM practices such as traditional healers, *qi gong*, or healing touch.

Worldwide, breast cancer survivors have been reported as a group of patients who used CAM more often than people diagnosed with other types of cancer, such as colorectal, prostate, or gynecological cancer. Boon, Olatunde, and Zick (2007) reported that the rate of CAM use has significantly increased in breast cancer survivors. More importantly, while women with breast cancer use CAM for their health and well-being, only half of them discuss CAM practices with their health care providers, mostly their oncologists (Navo et al., 2004). This needs to be taken into account by health care providers to prevent CAM-related problems, such as delay in seeking medical treatment or even more serious problems, such as interaction between CAM and conventional treatment. It is essential for health care providers to understand the following questions: How valuable is CAM for breast cancer survivors? How do breast cancer survivors make decisions to use CAM? What is the most common type of CAM used by breast cancer survivors? What are factors influencing the use of CAM among breast cancer survivors?

The purpose of this chapter is to gain awareness of the decision-making process regarding CAM use among women with breast cancer and to analyze the CAM types most commonly used by women with breast cancer according to the categories identified by NCCIM. Finally, sources of CAM information, such as family, friends, and media, will also be described in this chapter.

The Value of CAM for Women with Breast Cancer

Leininger (2006) pointed out that people in different cultures have their own meanings of care, which is dependent on factors such as spirituality, language, ethnohistory, and environmental context. This is also confirmed by two published qualitative studies regarding the meaning of CAM as perceived by breast cancer survivors (Wanchai, Armer & Stewart, 2010, 2012). The participants in the former study were Caucasian American breast cancer survivors (n = 9) and the latter participants were Thai breast cancer survivors living in Thailand (n = 17). The goal of the two studies was to explore how breast cancer survivors perceived the value of CAM. The results of the two studies were similar: while the American breast cancer survivors described the value of CAM in terms of (1) coping with disease and treatment, (2) holistic care, and (3) emotional support, the Thai breast cancer survivors reported the meaning of CAM as (1) an additional beneficial choice for health, (2) an emotional and psychological healing, and (3) a powerful physical healing.

In addition, many scholars also reported the perceived value of CAM among breast cancer survivors in terms of reasons for using CAM (Boon, Olatunde & Zick, 2007; Buettner et al., 2006; Matthews et al., 2007). Numerous reasons are cited in their findings, but the primary perceived values of CAM among women with breast cancer can be summarized in two categories, namely CAM as a choice for promoting physical health (e.g., to boost the immune system, stabilize the current condition, and promote general wellness) and CAM as a means of supporting emotional and psychological health (e.g., for stress management, psychological support, a more holistic health care approach, and increased quality of life) (Boon, Olatunde & Zick, 2007).

CAM as a Choice for Promoting Physical Health

Breast cancer survivors perceive CAM as a choice for promoting physical health in dealing with disease, managing side effects of conventional treatment, and improving their health and well-being. With regard to the first of these benefits, a previous study has shown that many breast cancer survivors used CAM because they felt unsatisfied with western medicine (Lengacher et al., 2006). In other words, they felt that western medicine alone would not be able to alleviate signs and symptoms of cancer or side effects of cancer treatment. Consequently, they sought out CAM, in addition to conventional cancer treatment.

It is the case that treatment methods such as surgery, chemotherapy, and radiation are the accepted conventional ways to treat breast cancer. However, some treatment methods, such as chemotherapy, may lead to feelings of distress for women with breast cancer. Many women complain of severe side effects from those treatments, such as fatigue, nausea, vomiting, sleep disturbance, and hot flashes. More importantly, these side effects can affect the quality of life in breast cancer survivors on both physical and psychological levels. Previous studies reported that among women diagnosed with breast cancer who used CAM, most viewed CAM as an aid to mitigate the unpleasant side effects of conventional treatments (Chen et al., 2008; Hann, Baker, Denniston & Entrekin, 2005).

In addition to reducing these side effects, CAM is perceived by breast cancer survivors as a valuable additional option for improving health and well-being. This is because breast cancer survivors believe that CAM can enhance their health by increasing the body's inner strength and helping to boost their immune system (Ernst & Hung, 2011).

CAM as a Resource for Emotional and Psychological Health

Although advances in breast cancer diagnosis and treatment mean that survivors are living longer, many survivors continue to experience both physical and psychological problems resulting from their cancer. Therefore, it is not surprising that they seek a way to recover their mental and physical well-being by, following a holistic approach provided by CAM. For breast cancer survivors, CAM has been valued as an important resource for improving their emotional and psychological health. The appeal of this effect should be considered in relation to the substantial short- and long-term stresses associated with the diagnosis of breast cancer. Holzner and colleagues (2001) reported that in the early phase following initial treatment (within one to two years), the quality of life of breast cancer survivors had been reduced both in terms of their emotional well-being (e.g., depression and fear of recurrence) and social identity (e.g., being unable to do housework by themselves, changing from an active role in the family to a passive one). Holzner and colleagues (2001) also found that in the intermediate remission period (two to five years after initial treatment), although most breast cancer survivors reported good quality of life, some experienced psychological problems (e.g., existential worries, depression) that impacted their emotional well-being, ability to resume social and family roles, cognitive functions, and sexuality. In addition, even after the completion of treatment, many survivors continued to suffer from emotional stresses related to their cancer diagnosis and treatment, even feeling more emotional than during the time when they were receiving treatment (Schnipper, 2001). One study has shown that breast cancer survivors are more likely to have higher rates of depressive symptoms and greater impairment to their quality of life at this time than those who have not had cancer (Deshields, Tibbs, Fan & Taylor, 2006).

It has also been reported that some breast cancer survivors chose to use CAM precisely because they viewed it as compatible with a holistic approach and thus more psychologically appealing than conventional medicines. This can be attributed to the personal attention provided and a more well-rounded approach to health provided by CAM (Eliott, Kealey & Olver, 2008). Additionally, some breast cancer survivors also reported using CAM as a way of increasing their sense of control over their well-being, or reducing physical and psychological distress (Lengacher et al., 2006).

In summary, both physical and psychological health play important roles in breast cancer survivors' choice to use CAM. Additionally, CAM can be valuable for women living with breast cancer from the time of diagnosis throughout the course of cancer survivorship.

Decision-Making Process for CAM Use Among Women with Breast Cancer

Balneaves, Weeks, and Seely (2008) reported that decision making for CAM use is very individualized and multifaceted, dependent on individual beliefs and social context. However, the main phases of the CAM decision-making process by cancer patients fall into four stages: (1) taking stock of treatment options, (2) gathering and evaluating CAM information, (3) making CAM decisions, and (4) revising CAM decisions.

Balneaves and colleagues (2008) stated that the first step of CAM decision making begins at the time of cancer diagnosis because patients want to find other methods that might enhance the effectiveness of conventional treatment and mitigate unpleasant side effects. During the initial phase of the CAM decision, cancer patients also begin to gather and evaluate the possible role of CAM in their health care by balancing the potential risks and benefits of CAM use. However, as they seek out CAM information from various sources, either from personal experience or from professional advice, they sometimes feel overwhelmed by information about CAM and may become distressed. For the third phase of the CAM decision, Balneaves and colleagues identified three decision pathways that applied in some form to most cancer patients. Patients in the midst of conventional treatment who had high levels of anxiety and were conflicted about adding CAM to their treatment regimen frequently delayed their decision to use CAM. Patients who wanted to prioritize conventional treatment in their care plan tended only to adopt CAM practices that could be easily combined with conventional treatment. Finally, patients who were already attracted to CAM as a natural and holistic approach to their cancer treatment generally did incorporate CAM into their treatment.

All of the phases of CAM decision making mentioned above occurred after their cancer diagnosis and during conventional treatment. However, at the end of conventional treatment, some cancer patients re-evaluated their CAM decision in response to new information regarding their disease progression and prognosis and new data on the efficacy of specific CAM therapies. In addition, this is the time when many survivors become interested in increasing their physical and emotional energy using methods such as CAM.

A few studies have explored the decision-making pathways for CAM use among breast cancer survivors. For example, in a qualitative study conducted by Boon and colleagues (1999), the researchers used focus groups to understand the decision-making process for possible CAM use by Canadian breast cancer survivors. The results of the study showed similar process of CAM decision making used by breast cancer survivors as mentioned above. However, this study reported that breast cancer survivors would make a decision as to whether or not to use CAM by comparing its perceived advantages and disadvantages. Advantages reported by the participants included enhanced chances of survival, mitigating negative experiences with conventional medicine, and the opportunity to be proactive and prevent further illness. However, important disadvantages were also reported, including the high cost of CAM treatment, limited access to CAM therapy, and the large amount of time required to complete CAM therapy.

Recently, we (Wanchai et al., 2012) conducted an ethno-nursing qualitative research study to explore how Thai breast cancer survivors living in Thailand seek out and access CAM therapies. We found a two-part process consisting of an initial stage of seeking and gathering CAM information followed by a final stage of trying out many types of CAM. In the former stage, we found that Thai breast cancer survivors began to seek out and gather CAM information from various sources immediately upon their diagnosis with breast cancer, before making a decision to include CAM in their care practices. Examples of CAM information sources were people around them and media resources, rather than health care providers. After gathering information about CAM, Thai breast cancer survivors would try many types of CAM, rather than use only one specific type.

In summary, it can be concluded that the CAM decision-making process is nuanced and individualized. The decision may change at any time during the course of treatment and survivorship, depending on the cancer patient's satisfaction with their treatment and their access to and attitude toward CAM. Therefore, continuous assessment and re-evaluation about CAM decision making throughout patient's cancer journey are important tasks.

Types of CAM Used by Women with Breast Cancer

Based on the four categories of CAM identified by NCCIM (2012), previous studies reported that natural products (e.g., herbs, vitamins, foods) were the types of CAM most frequently used, followed by mind-body medicine (e.g., meditation, prayer, mental healing), other CAM practices (e.g., homeopathic medicine, naturopathic medicine, traditional Chinese medicine, *qi gong*, reiki, therapeutic touch), and manipulative and body-based practices (e.g., osteopathy, massage, chiropractic) (Owens, Jackson & Berndt, 2009).

Interestingly, previous studies also reported differentiation in the types of CAM preferred by breast cancer survivors based on ethnic and cultural backgrounds. For example, in western countries, Owens and colleagues (2009) found that black,

Latino, and Hispanic women were more likely to use CAM for spiritual healing, followed by herbal remedies or diet therapies, whereas Caucasian women were more likely to use dietary methods, spiritual healing, and physical methods such as massage and acupuncture. In Asian countries, Chen and colleagues (2008) reported that Chinese women with breast cancer were more likely to use supplements such as *Ganoderma lucidum* capsules, vitamins, or ginseng, than Chinese herbal medicine, along with physical activities such as *qi gong*, *tai chi*, or dancing. Similarly, a study by Wonghongkul, Dechaprom, Phumvichuvate, and Kertsang (2002) reported that herbal medicines were the type of CAM most used by Thai breast cancer survivors, followed by changing their nutrition or lifestyle and practising prayer.

In other words, cultural factors, such as country of origin and ethnicity, influence breast cancer survivors' decisions about CAM use. Leininger draws attention to the specific influences of family systems, health status, socio-cultural orientation, spirituality, language, and ethno-history (Leininger, 2006). However, more research is needed to determine whether and how these factors along with factors such as, socio-economic status, education, and family income may influence CAM use among women living with breast cancer.

Sources of CAM Information for Women with Breast Cancer

Studies have shown that breast cancer survivors seek out information about CAM from various sources before making a decision to use it as mentioned earlier (Abdullah, Lau & Chow, 2003; Fasching et al., 2007; Gulluoglu, Cingi, Cakir & Barlas, 2008; Kremser et al., 2008; Molassiotis et al., 2006). However, among these sources, family and friends were the most frequently consulted sources, followed by media (including the Internet), magazines, books, newspapers, or journals (Kremser et al., 2008). In addition, some studies also reported that women with breast cancer tend to consult their physicians before using CAM (Fasching et al., 2007; Molassiotis et al., 2006). CAM providers were also identified as sources of CAM information for women with breast cancer (Kremser et al., 2008). Finally, self-help groups and health insurance companies were the least common source of CAM information mentioned by women with breast cancer (Fasching et al., 2007).

The challenge is that not all breast cancer survivors disclose their CAM use to their physicians. A previous study by Shen and colleagues (2002) reported that among women with advanced-stage breast cancer, the decision to discuss CAM use with their physician was influenced by the type of CAM therapy being used. For example, women using herbal medicines were likely to disclose this to their physician, but were less likely to mention the use of therapies such as chiropractic, imagery, spiritual healing, hypnosis, acupuncture, or energy healing. Future research to investigate this relationship is needed, as are further studies on breast cancer survivors' reasons for concealing CAM use from their health care providers.

Conclusion

Use of CAM among women with breast cancer is increasingly popular because they perceive it as a choice for promoting their physical health and their emotional and psychological health. Decision making for CAM use among women with breast cancer is dependent on individual beliefs and social context. The types of CAM most used by these women are natural products, mind-body medicine, and manipulative and body-based practices. Finally, common sources of CAM information are family, friends, and media. Health care professionals who wish to integrate CAM into western medicine need to be concerned with all of these issues.

Critical Thinking Questions

1. What is the most important consideration when choosing CAM for breast cancer survivors' care practices?
2. Why do breast cancer survivors from different cultural backgrounds choose to use different types of CAM?
3. What methods may be used to help health care providers (e.g., physicians or nurses) become better informed about CAM practices used by breast cancer survivors?
4. How might health care providers collaborate with patients who choose to add CAM to their treatments?

Glossary

Breast cancer survivor: A person diagnosed with breast cancer from the time of initial diagnosis until death.

Western medicine: A health care system whose approach to breast cancer treatment is characterized by the use of pharmaceutical drugs, radiation therapy, and/or surgery.

References

Abdullah, A.S., Lau, Y., & Chow, L.W. (2003). Pattern of alternative medicine usage among the Chinese breast cancer patients: Implication for service integration. *American Journal of Chinese Medicine, 31*, 649–658.

American Cancer Society. (2013). *Global cancer facts & figures 2013*. Retrieved June 1, 2013, from www.cancer.org/acs/groups/content/@epidemiologysurveilance/documents/document/acspc-036845.pdf

Balneaves, L.G., Weeks, L., & Seely, D. (2008). Patient decision-making about complementary and alternative medicine in cancer management: Context and process. *Current Oncology, 15*(Suppl. 2), S94–S100.

Boon, H., Brown, J.B., Gavin, A., Kennard, M.A., & Stewart, M. (1999). Breast cancer survivors' perceptions of complementary/alternative medicine (CAM): Making the decision to use or not to use. *Qualitative Health Research, 9*, 639–653.

Boon, H.S., Olatunde, F., & Zick, S.M. (2007). Trends in complementary/alternative medicine use by breast cancer survivors: Comparing survey data from 1998 and 2005. *BMC Women's Health, 7*. doi: 10.1186/1472-6874-7-4

Buettner, C., Kroenke, C.H., Phillips, R.S., Davis, R.B., Eisenberg, D.M., & Holmes, M.D. (2006).

Correlates of use of different types of complementary and alternative medicine by breast cancer survivors in the nurses' health study. *Breast Cancer Research and Treatment, 100*, 219–227. doi: 10.1007/s10549-006-9239-3

Chen, Z., Gu, K., Zheng, Y., Zheng, W., Lu, W., & Shu, X.O. (2008). The use of complementary and alternative medicine among Chinese women with breast cancer. *Journal of Alternative and Complementary Medicine 14*, 1049–1055. doi: 10.1089/acm.2008.0039

Deshields, T., Tibbs, T., Fan, M.Y., & Taylor, M. (2006). Differences in patterns of depression after treatment for breast cancer. *Psycho-Oncology, 15*, 398–406. doi: 10.1002/pon.962

Eliott, J.A., Kealey, C.P., & Olver, I.N. (2008). (Using) complementary and alternative medicine: The perceptions of palliative patients with cancer. *Journal of Palliative Medicine, 11*, 58–67. doi: 10.1089/jpm.2007.0102

Ernst, E., & Hung, S.K. (2011). Great expectations: What do patients using complementary and alternative medicine hope for? *Patient, 4*, 89–101. doi: 10.2165/11586490-000000000-00000

Fasching, P.A., Thiel, F., Nicolaisen-Murmann, K., Rauh, C., Engel, J., Lux, M.P., Bani, M.R. (2007). Association of complementary methods with quality of life and life satisfaction in patients with gynecologic and breast malignancies. *Supportive Care in Cancer, 15*, 1277–1284. doi: 10.1007/s00520-007-0231-1

Gulluoglu, B. M., Cingi, A., Cakir, T., & Barlas, A. (2008). Patients in northwestern Turkey prefer herbs as complementary medicine after breast cancer diagnosis. *Breast Care, 3*, 269–273. doi: 10.1159/000144045

Hann, D., Baker, F., Denniston, M., & Entrekin, N. (2005). Long-term breast cancer survivors' use of complementary therapies: Perceived impact on recovery and prevention of recurrence. *Integrative Cancer Therapies, 4*, 14–20. doi: 10.1177/1534735404273723

Holzner, B., Kemmler, G., Kopp, M., Moschen, R., Schweigkofler, H., Dünser, M., Sperner-Unterweger, B. (2001). Quality of life in breast cancer patients—not enough attention for long-term survivors? *Psychosomatics, 42*, 117–123.

Knobf, M.T. (2007). Psychosocial responses in breast cancer survivors. *Seminars in Oncology Nursing Forum, 23*, 71–83. doi: 10.1016/j.soncn.2006.11.009

Kremser, T., Evans, A., Moore, A., Luxford , K., Begbie, S., Bensoussan, A., & Zorbas, H. (2008). Use of complementary therapies by Australian women with breast cancer. *Breast, 17*, 387–394. doi: 10.1016/j.breast.2007.12.006

Leininger, M.M. (2006). Culture care diversity and universality theory and evolution of the ethnonursing method. In M.M. Leininger & M.R. McFarland (Eds), *Culture care diversity and universality: A worldwide nursing theory* (2nd ed.) (pp. 1–41). Sudbury, MA: Jones and Bartlett Publishers.

Lengacher, C.A., Bennett, M.P., Kip, K.E., Gonzalez, L., Jacobsen, P., & Cox, C.E. (2006). Relief of symptoms, side effects, and psychological distress through use of complementary and alternative medicine in women with breast cancer. *Oncology Nursing Forum, 33*, 97–104. doi: 10.1188/06.ONF.97-104

Matthews, A.K., Sellergren, S.A., Huo, D., List, M., & Fleming, G. (2007). Complementary and alternative medicine use among breast cancer survivors. *Journal of Alternative and Complementary Medicine, 13*, 555–562. doi: 10.1089/acm.2007.03-9040

Mayer, D.K., Terrin, N.C., Menon, U., Kreps, G.L., McCance, K., Parsons, S.K., & Mooney, K.H. (2007). Health behaviors in cancer survivors. *Oncology Nursing Forum, 34*, 643–651. doi: 10.1188/07.ONF.643-651

Molassiotis, A., Scott, J.A., Kearney, N., Pud, D., Magri, M., Selvekerova, S., & Patiraki, E. (2006). Complementary and alternative medicine use in breast cancer in Europe. *Supportive Care in Cancer, 14*, 260–267. doi: 10.1007/s00520-005-0883-7

Mullan, F. (1985). Seasons of survival: Reflections of a cancer physician. *New England Journal of Medicine, 313*, 270–273.

National Center for Complementary and Integrative Medicine (NCCIM). (2012). *What is complementary and alternative medicine?* Retrieved May 1, 2013 from http://nccam.nih.gov/health/whatiscam

Navo, M.A., Phan, J., Vaughan, C., Palmer, J.L., Michaud, L., Jones, K.L., & Smith, J.A. (2004). An assessment of the utilization of complementary and alternative medication in women with gynecologic or breast malignancies. *Journal of Clinical Oncology, 15*, 671–677. doi: 10.1200/JCO.2004.04.162

Owens, B., Jackson, M., & Berndt, A. (2009). Complementary therapy used by Hispanic women during treatment for breast cancer. *Journal of Holistic Nursing, 27*. doi: 10.1177/0898010108330801

Schnipper, H.H. (2001). Life after breast cancer. *Journal of Clinical Oncology, 19*, 3581–3584.

Shen, J., Andersen, R., Albert, P.S., Wenger, N., Glaspy, J., Cole, M., & Shekelle, P. (2002). Use of complementary/alternative therapies by women with advanced-stage breast cancer. *BMC Complementary and Alternative Medicine, 2*. doi: 10.1186/1472-6882-2-8

Wanchai, A., Armer, J.M., & Stewart, B.R. (2010). Breast cancer survivors' perspectives of care practices in western and alternative medicine. *Oncology Nursing Forum, 37*, 495–500. doi: 10.1188/10.ONF.494-500

Wanchai, A., Armer, J.M., & Stewart, B.R. (2012). Performance care practices in complementary and alternative medicine by Thai breast cancer survivors: An ethnonursing study. *Nursing & Health Sciences, 14*, 339–344. doi: 10.1111/j.1442-2018.2012.00730.x

Wonghongkul, T., Dechaprom, N., Phumvichuvate, L., & Kertsang, S. (2002). *Quality of life and alternative therapy used in long-term breast cancer survivors*. Symposium conducted at the meeting of the Fifth Nursing Academic International Congress: Cultural Diversity in Alternative Health Care and Nursing Therapeutics. Khon Kean, Thailand.

World Health Organization. (2013). *Latest world cancer statistics global cancer burden rises to 14.1 million new cases in 2012: Marked increase in breast cancers must be addressed* [media release]. Retrieved July 13, 2014 from www.iarc.fr/en/media-centre/pr/2013/pdfs/pr223_E.pdf

CONCLUSION

Jennie M. Hornosty, PhD
Retired Professor, Sociology, University of New Brunswick; Adjunct Research Professor in Sociology, Carleton University; and Senior Fellow, Centre on Governance, University of Ottawa

Concluding Overview

Traditional medicine (TM) and traditional healing practices have existed for millennia. While in large parts of the western, industrialized world,[1] biomedicine is the accepted primary model for health care delivery, traditional medicine remains the chosen mode of health care for many in parts of Asia, Africa, and Latin America.[2] However, this seeming dichotomy between users of TM and biomedicine is neither precise nor unequivocal. As various contributors to this book have shown, there is some fluidity between TM and biomedicine in both the Global South and the Global North. In Ecuador, for example, traditional midwives are being integrated into biomedical health services; in Indonesia, lactating women may question the efficacy of a traditional medicine for increasing the supply of breast milk because it lacks scientific evidence. On the other hand, women in Australia and Canada are increasingly searching out complementary and alternative medicine (CAM)[3] to address their reproductive health and fertility issues. In other words, it could be argued that the hegemonic status of each of these two primary health care systems is being contested, albeit in different locations, for different reasons and in different degrees.

In compiling the contributions for this book, our intent was to illustrate the breadth of TM as used by women in relation to their reproductive health in the Global South, and to understand how cultural context shapes women's decisions to rely on traditional medicine or therapies. At the same time, we wanted to highlight some of the research on CAM use by women in the Global North. As a number of the contributors have shown, the affinity between TM and cultural beliefs is an important factor in women's motivations to use TM for their reproductive health concerns in the Global South. By contrast, in the Global North, women—who are the predominant users (Keshet & Simchai, 2014; Kristoffersen et al., 2014; Park, 2005)—turn to CAM because of its holistic approach and the presumption that CAM is more "natural," and hence safer. A number of explanations have been advanced for the increased popularity of CAM in the Global North, including people's growing dissatisfaction with biomedicine and concerns about the safety of pharmaceuticals. Hall and colleagues (2011) note that pregnant women use CAM therapies because these are considered "safe" alternatives to pharmaceuticals. Others attribute the difference to gendered patterns of health behaviour more generally, whereby females are socialized to be more health-conscious and are likely to be consumers of health care magazines where natural health products and CAM therapies are discussed (Keshet & Simchai, 2014). In their examination of why women tend to favour CAM, Keshet and Simchai (2014) suggest, "engagement with holistic spiritualities validates women's traditional work of relational care, and legitimates the work of emotional care" (p. 81). A holistic approach also means that patients are encouraged to take an active role in managing their illness and healing process that facilitates "feelings of trust, acceptance, empowerment" and promotes self-development (Williams-Piehota et al., 2011, p. 28).

In the Global South, as we saw in various contributions, women choose TM for primary care over biomedicine (when both are available) because it aligns more with their cultural and traditional values, because of skepticism of and cultural insensitivity on the part of biomedical health professionals, and because of the affordability and general proximity of TM. Other reasons for not seeking health services from biomedical health care providers, especially among women with an indigenous background, are lack of accessibility and transportation costs, time constraints, language and cultural barriers, and opposition from their husbands or family to biomedical health care.

In the Global North, CAM is used as a complement to biomedicine and is viewed as a means to have greater control over one's life. This desire to have more control over one's life can be interpreted as a response to post-modernity and the fragmentary nature of modern life, as well as to what Beck (1992) refers to as the "risk society" (Hornosty, Easthope & Broom, 2016). At the same time, the individualized and subjective understandings of health and disease that are characteristics of CAM are congruent with neoliberalism and the emphasis on individual responsibility for health. The emphasis in CAM on self-care—and what some have termed "healthism"—is consistent, Fries (2014, p. 9) argues, with neoliberal strategies for the governance of population health. In the same way, the growing popularity of CAM can be viewed as a response to social marketing strategies in many western countries that promote individual responsibility for health outcomes in keeping with the market-oriented neoliberal mode of social organization (Crawshaw, 2013). However, it is important to remember that this emphasis on individual responsibility and the need to make healthy lifestyle choices both ignores the social determinants of health and can encourage "victim blaming."

A historical perspective—presented in the first part of the book—points to the central role women have always played in providing care related to reproductive health issues. It also highlights the continuity of certain traditional medicine practices and the fluidity in our understanding in the western world of complementary and alternative medicine. From the chapters in this section, we see that midwifery, now more "mainstream" in the Canadian and American landscape, has a long and rich tradition in Indigenous societies that sustained a complex set of social relationships. Similarly, traditional lay midwives played a central role in settler immigrant communities until the late 19th century when licensed male physicians increasingly gained the monopoly over maternity care and childbirth. Today, according to the Canadian Association of Midwives, there are over 1,300 registered midwives in Canada, and midwifery is a legal and regulated profession in most provinces and territories (Canadian Association of Midwives, 2014; Canadian Midwifery Regulators Consortium, 2013). It is also interesting to note that, while today various herbal medicines are considered as CAM, in Colonial North America (1492–1899) various botanical medicines were used to support fertility as well as deal with other gynecological problems; early Americans also integrated medicinal plants into a pharmacopoeia based on common European herbal remedies.

The contributors to this collection have also illustrated how CAM/TM therapies involve a diverse set of practices and beliefs, thus making comparisons between different social and cultural contexts challenging. It is clear that how we conceive of CAM/TM varies in time and place. Broom (2014, p. 425) sums up this challenge well when he explains that CAM "is ultimately a socially constructed and dynamic entity that is historically and culturally variable ... that helps us ascribe meanings to practices that are hugely diverse." Health Canada, for example, included 4,000 different practices in its catalogue of CAM health care approaches (Smith & Simpson, 2003, p. 3). In speaking of TM, the World Health Organization (WHO) similarly points to the diversity of practices, beliefs, approaches, and medicines that fall under the umbrella of TM. However, a distinguishing feature of TM is that it is "part of a wider belief system, and considered integral to everyday life and well-being" (WHO, May

2002a, p. 1). A cross-cultural perspective provides greater depth to our understanding of the continuities and differences between TM and CAM.

Rather than health practices being categorized dichotomously as biomedical or traditional medicine, there is a shift globally toward a merging of different modalities into a more hybrid "integrative health care" (IHC) (Boon & Kachan, 2008; Possamai-Inesedy & Cochrane, 2013). However, this development is not without challenges. Various contributors to this book have shown us that different epistemological assumptions are at the root of biomedicine and CAM/TM, thus making integration of the two somewhat difficult and problematic. The holistic approach of TM, which focuses on the whole person in his or her total environment, is radically different from biomedicine, which approaches the body as a machine comprised of different parts that can be analyzed and treated separately (see Armstrong & Armstrong, 2003, pp. 18–42 for a good critical analysis of biomedicine). Such differences, for example, are evident in the case study examining the choice of birthing practices among Quechua women living in Bolivia. Despite epistemological incompatibilities, there are examples of integrative primary health care in both the Global North and the Global South. Boon & Kachan (2008) argue the success of integrative medicine depends on a number of institutional factors: "champions" for such programs, staff members receptive to new approaches, and trust and respect between practitioners. The importance of such factors is illustrated in the case studies from Ghana, Ecuador, and the experiences of traditional Chinese medicine practitioners in Canada. Besides epistemological incompatibilities, contributors also raised questions about appropriation and marginalization of traditional medicine by biomedicine.

Future Directions and Research

This edited collection has provided the reader with a cross-section of primary and secondary research that looks at some of the current issues pertaining to how women use TM and CAM modalities to address various reproductive health concerns broadly defined—whether in giving birth, breast feeding, enhancing fertility, or promoting their general well-being—as well as giving some recent examples of integrative medicine. This is a burgeoning and critical area of research and we have a lot more to learn. Indicated below are some research topics and questions that need further exploration.

The move toward integrative health care, which is especially strong in Canada, the United States, and United Kingdom, particularly within oncology services (Hilbers & Lewis, 2013), raises important questions about how integration in fact occurs. Are certain "knowledges" and paradigms devalued or co-opted, and how are decisions made when there are competing worldviews, especially given the hegemony of biomedicine in large parts of the world? In their compelling argument, Hollenberg and Muzzin (2010) suggest that what is happening in integrative medicine is paradigm appropriation and assimilation of TM by biomedicine. They suggest that CAM modalities are adopted in piecemeal ways without an understanding of the traditions and healing systems of which they are a part. Similarly, Possamai-Inesedy and Cochrane (2013) raise questions about "the achievability of a more true form of integration in the presence of the hegemonic influence of the biomedical paradigm within the IHC setting" (p. 67). At the same time they note that CAM practitioners are themselves pushing for integration where there is biomedical dominance, as this has the potential to demonstrate the efficacy of their treatments through randomized control trials and to legitimize their knowledge. A number of contributors to this collection touched on some of the challenges raised by integrative health care; much more research is needed in this regard, especially in the Global South where TM has been dominant. Particular attention needs to be paid to epistemological differences between CAM/TM and biomedicine and how these get negotiated in different cultural and social contexts. What are the pre-conditions and challenges for integrative medicine to work in practice? One interesting example is that of the Anishnawbe Health Toronto Community Centre, that combines traditional Indigenous practices, naturopathic medicine, and conventional practices with physicians and nurses to provide health services to Indigenous peoples (Walji, Weeks, Cooley & Seely, 2010). Many more case studies of working models of IHC in different cultural and social contexts globally are needed, including in the area of women's reproductive health.

Additional research is also needed on the users of CAM/TM. How do factors such as gender, class, ethnicity, "race," and age—and the intersection of these—shape peoples' experiences of CAM/TM? Research using a range of theoretical perspectives to examine both the role of structure and agency in explaining CAM use is needed (Stratton & McGivern-Snofsky, 2008). We know that some biomedically trained professionals are incorporating alternative treatment modalities into their practices. However, there is limited research on why this is happening. Are certain health care professionals more likely to incorporate CAM—and if so, why? The recent creation of the Canadian Interdisciplinary Network for Complementary and Alternative Medicine Research (IN-CAM), funded by the Canadian Institutes for Health Research, is one important avenue for coordinating research that uses a variety of disciplinary perspectives and methods to study CAM.

We need to know a lot more about what factors influence women in the Global South to prioritize traditional medicines over biomedicine as well as explore reasons why some women put their faith in biomedicine. Is there a class difference, for example, between those who choose TM compared to those who opt for biomedicine? Are there structural impediments or religious beliefs that play a significant role in the choices that women make? We need to know more of how patriarchy, which is still strong in many communities, influences women's health care choices, especially of concern in the case of reproductive health. Given that previous experiences influence future choices, more research is needed on how biomedical health care providers see their role in areas where women prefer traditional health care practitioners. Are they receptive or hostile to delivering their services in a culturally appropriate way? Are they qualified and trained in the cultural norms in which they are working?

As we see from the collections in this book, there is interesting and diverse research going on in the area of CAM/TM and women's reproductive health. However, there are also many significant gaps in our knowledge. While we know that in the Global North women are more likely to use complementary and alternative medicine than men, there is little information on how gender intersects with other social identities such as "race" or indigeneity or ethnic identity in influencing such use. Or how do any of these identities intersect with others, such as sexual identity, class, age, or immigrant status? Do lesbian, transgender, or bisexual women differ in their approach to CAM for their reproductive health needs? How do women construct reproductive health in different communities and cultures that might favour CAM use?

Similarly, in the Global South, we need to more fully understand how cultural and religious beliefs systems impact on women's decision to use traditional therapies for reproductive health concerns. Also, how important are factors such as age, class, religiosity, patriarchy, and indigeneity in influencing women's use of TM practices as opposed to biomedical options? Conversely we need to know what factors influence women to reject traditional health care practices.

In both the Global North and Global South, research is needed to understand better which women choose to use CAM for reproductive health concerns and how they make their decisions. What are their subjective experiences of CAM? Are there certain reproductive health issues for which CAM or TM is more effective than others? And, are there particular modalities that are more safe and efficacious than others? To answer such questions, a population-based survey that examined women's reasons for using CAM/TM in different cultural contexts in both the Global North and Global South would be extremely informative. As well, a cross-sectional study would help in this regard. Are women who use CAM/TM for reproductive health different from women who do not and, if yes, in what ways? Is the use of CAM/TM in one situation, such as during pregnancy and childbirth, a predictor of future use for other reasons? A longitudinal study of CAM/TM users would be most informative and would provide a more comprehensive picture of how and why CAM/TM usage changes over time.

In her address to the WHO Congress on Traditional Medicine in 2008, the Director-General, Dr. Margaret Chan, stressed the important role TM plays in the daily lives in peoples of Asia, Africa, and Latin America. While acknowledging the importance of modern drugs and measures that can have critical life and death impacts on peoples' lives, she emphasized that TM must be considered a "precious resource" that should be "respected and supported as a valuable source of leads for therapeutic advances and the discovery of new classes of drugs" (Chan, 2008, p.5). Some of the challenges currently posed by CAM/TM are the lack of adequate research on indigenous TM knowledge and products, an inadequate evidence base as to efficacy and safety, the absence of international and national standards for training of practitioners, and the limited information related to access and affordability (Bodeker & Kronenberg, 2002; WHO, 2002a).

To harness the potential contribution of TM to health in both the Global South and Global North, the WHO has implemented a global strategy that supports research and development in TM (WHO, 2013). Of concern is to understand the safety and efficacy and quality of traditional medicines and products. Such research would expand the knowledge base of TM and provide guidance on regulatory and quality assurance standards. At the same time, one needs to be sensitive to the possible misappropriation of TM. This knowledge is important to ensure proper use and effectiveness of TM and would assist in regulating products and practices and the training of practitioners (WHO, 2013). However, as Abdullahi (2011) has argued, given the "ethnocentric tendencies in modern medicine," there is a danger that TM could be co-opted in a way that would jeopardize its identity and integrity. This is a vast and important area of research that can be best explored from a multiplicity of perspectives and by using different methodologies. Bodeker & Kronenberg (2002, p. 1583) caution, furthermore, that such research must be sensitive to social, cultural, and economic contexts, both to help shape research questions and to establish action priorities. Questions of accessibility and equity, for example, differ in industrialized societies from those in developing countries where "inadequate and expensive conventional medical services are factors in ... reliance on traditional medicine" (Bodeker & Kronenberg, 2002, p. 1585). In the Global North, access to CAM is generally restricted to those with the economic means to pay for it. Given that CAM/TM and biomedicine are premised on different approaches to the body and different understandings of health and healing, much more research is also needed on how to appropriately evaluate the effectiveness of CAM/TM. Are randomized control trials, the current "gold standard" for assessing efficacy, appropriate measurement tools in all situations?

The WHO's 2014–2023 global strategy promotes the integration of CAM/TM services into national health systems and encourages member states to develop their own national policies in this regard (WHO, 2013). Hence, another important research question would be to explore the degree to which CAM/TM are incorporated into different national health policies. To what degree is this happening and what are the implications of such for population and public health in the respective countries? To what extent is CAM/TM integrated into curricula at medical schools and nursing programs, and how is this done? In Canada, for example, most medical schools include education about CAM in their curriculum; however, there is limited knowledge on the specifics. We also know that some biomedically trained doctors work with CAM practitioners or refer patients to them (Hornosty et al., 2016). Again, empirical information on this is scarce.

Final Thoughts

As the brief discussion above has indicated, there are numerous research areas that need further exploration with respect to CAM/TM as well as integrative health care, both with respect to women's reproductive health needs as well as health and well-being more generally. This is a critical research area, given the continuing widespread use of CAM/TM throughout the world. According to a WHO media release, up to 80 percent of people in the Global South use traditional medicine for primary health care (WHO, 2002b). One estimate is that over their lifetime, 73 percent of Canadians will use CAM (Deveau, 2010). Clearly this is an area of great interest and concern. Culturally sensitive and accurate and reliable information is needed to assist consumers, biomedical health care providers, traditional practitioners, and policy makers. We hope that the issues raised by the contributors to this book—with their multidisciplinary approaches and international perspectives—will stimulate debate and point the way toward promising avenues for future research.

Notes

1. Often referred to as the Global North.
2. Generally considered to be part of the Global South.
3. As explained in the General Introduction, the World Health Organization (WHO) describes CAM as adaptations of TM that are used in industrialized countries.

References

Abdullahi, A. (2011). Trends and challenges of traditional medicine in Africa. *African Journal of Traditional, Complementary and Alternative Medicines, 8*(5 Suppl.), 115–123.

Armstrong, P., & Armstrong, H. (2003). *Wasting away: The undermining of Canadian health care* (2nd ed.). Don Mills, ON: Oxford University Press.

Beck, U. (1992). *Risk society: Towards a new modernity.* London, UK: Sage.

Bodeker, G., & Kronenberg, F. (2002). Public health matters. A public health agenda for traditional, complementary, and alternative medicine. *American Journal of Public Health, 92*(10), 1582–1591.

Boon, H., & Kachan, M. (2008). Integrative medicine: A tale of two clinics. *BMC Complementary and Alternative Medicine, 8*(32). doi:10.1186/1472-6882-8-32

Broom, A. (2014). The sociology of complementary and alternative medicine. In J. Germov (Ed.) *Second opinion. An introduction to health sociology* (5th ed.). South Melbourne, Australia: Oxford University Press.

Canadian Association of Midwives. (2014, November 20). *News & announcement—The Canadian Association of Midwives celebrates the unanimous support to establish a National Day of the Midwife in Canada* [media release]. Retrieved from www.canadianmidwives.org/80-news/The-Canadian-Association-of-Midwives-celebrates-the-unanimous-support-to-establish-a-National-Day-of-the-Midwife-in-Canada.html

Canadian Midwifery Regulators Consortium. (2013, December). *Legal status of midwifery in Canada.* Retrieved from http://cmrc-ccosf.ca/node/19

Chan, M. (2008, November). *Address at the WHO congress on traditional medicine.* Speech presented at the WHO Congress on Traditional Medicine, Beijing, China. Transcript available from www.who.int/dg/speeches/2008/20081107/en/

Crawshaw, P. (2013). Public health policy and the behavioural turn: The case of social marketing. *Critical Social Policy, 33*(4), 616–637.

Deveau, D. (2010, March 12). Integrated health services crossing the divide. *The Vancouver Sun.* Retrieved from www.vancouversun.com/sunrun/Integrated+health+services+crossing+divide/2676343/story.html?__lsa=240a-decd

Fries, C. (2014). Older adults' use of complementary and alternative medical therapies to resist biomedicalization of aging. *Journal of Aging Studies, 28*, 1–10.

Hall, H., Griffiths, D., & McKenna, L. (2011). The use of complementary and alternative medicine by pregnant women: A literature review. *Midwifery, 27*, 817–824.

Hilbers, J., & Lewis, C. (2013). Complementary health therapies: Moving towards an integrated health model. *Collegian, 20*, 51–60.

Hollenberg, D., & Muzzin, L. (2010). Epistemological challenges to integrative medicine: An anti-colonial perspective on the combination of complementary/alternative medicine with biomedicine. *Health Sociology Review, 19*(1), 34–56.

Hornosty, J., Easthope, G., & Broom, A. (2016). Complementary and alternative health care. In J. Germov & J. Hornosty (Eds), *Second opinion: An introduction to health sociology* (2nd Canadian ed.). Toronto: Oxford University Press.

Keshet, Y., & Simchai, D. (2014). The "gender puzzle" of alternative medicine and holistic spirituality: A literature review. *Social Science & Medicine, 113*, 77–86.

Kristoffersen, A., Stub, T., Salamonsen, A., Musial, F., & Hamberg, K. (2014). Gender differences in prevalence and associations for use of CAM in a large population study. *BMC Complementary and Alternative Medicine, 14*, 463.

Park, J. (2005, March). *Use of Alternative Health Care* (Health Reports 16.2). Ottawa: Statistics Canada.

Possamai-Inesedy, A., & Cochrane, S. (2013). The consequences of integrating complementary and alternative medicine: An analysis of impacts on practice. *Health Sociology Review, 22*(1), 65–74.

Smith, M., & Simpson, J. (2003). Alternative practices and products: A survival guide. *Health Policy Research Bulletin, 7.* Ottawa: Health Canada.

Stratton, T., & McGivern-Snofsky, J. (2008). Toward a sociological understanding of complementary and alternative medicine use. *The Journal of Alternative and Complementary Medicine, 14*(6), 777–783.

Walji, R., Weeks, L., Cooley, K., & Seely, D. (2010). Naturopathic medicine and aboriginal health: An exploratory study at Anishnawbe Health Toronto. *Canadian Journal of Public Health, 101*(6), 475–480.

Williams-Piehota, P., Sirois, F., Bann, C., Isenberg, K., & Walsh, E. (2011). Agents of change: How do complementary and alternative medicine providers play a role in health behavior change? *Alternative Therapies in Health and Medicine, 17*(1), 22–30.

World Health Organization (WHO). (2002a, May). *Traditional medicine growing needs and potential—WHO policy perspectives on medicines* (No. 002). Geneva, Switzerland: Author. Retrieved from: http://apps.who.int/medicinedocs/en/d/Js2293e/

WHO. (2002b, May 16). *WHO launches the first global strategy on traditional and alternative medicine* [media release]. Retrieved from www.who.int/mediacentre/news/releases/release38/en/#

WHO. (2013). *WHO traditional medicine strategy 2014–2023*. Geneva, Switzerland: Author. Retrieved from http://apps.who.int/iris/bitstream/10665/92455/1/9789241506090_eng.pdf

CONTRIBUTORS

Jane M. Armer is a Professor at Sinclair School of Nursing, University of Missouri; Director of Nursing Research, Ellis Fischel Cancer Center; and Director of the American Lymphedema Framework Project in Columbia, Missouri, USA. She specializes in breast cancer-related lymphedema and survivorship. She has conducted extensive research in the area of lymphedema measurement, prevalence, signs and symptoms, and self-management among breast cancer survivors. She has authored and co-authored numerous book chapters. She also has published more than 100 scholarly articles in professional journals and presented hundreds of scientific papers at professional conferences.

Cecilia Benoit was born and raised in Newfoundland, with ancestry of Mi'kmaw, French, and Irish. She is a Professor in the Department of Sociology at the University of Victoria, Canada and scientist at the Centre for Addictions Research of British Columbia. In addition to research focused on the historically-suppressed occupation of midwifery and the organization of maternity care, she has been involved in a variety of projects that employ mixed methodologies to investigate the social determinants of health inequities of marginalized groups, including Indigenous women in Vancouver's Downtown Eastside, young people confronting health stigmas linked to obesity and asthma, workers in lower-prestige service occupations, adults in the sex industry, street-involved youth in transition to adulthood and pregnant women and their families dealing with poverty, substance use, and other challenges.

Dena Carroll is a member of the Chippewa of Nawash Unceded First Nations, located in Neyaashiinigmiing (Cape Croker), Ontario, Canada. She recently retired from the British Columbia Provincial Government as Director, Aboriginal Policy with the Ministry of Children and Family Development in British Columbia. Throughout her 15+ year career with the BC Government she worked on Aboriginal policy, treaty and services/programs areas related to Aboriginal health including consultation on Aboriginal midwifery legislation in BC, early childhood development, disability, women's and senior's issues, and post-secondary education. She has partnered with Cecilia Benoit to co-author a number of articles including narratives on Aboriginal midwifery in British Columbia and other women's health issues. She has a BA in Sociology and a MBA from the University of Victoria, Canada.

Tamer Edirne is the director of the Family Medicine Department in Pamukkale University, Medical School, Denizli, Turkey. He is involved in undergraduate and postgraduate medical education, research, and clinical practice. He is an Associate Professor and head of the family medicine residency program. His lectures contain several topics about family practice philosophy, primary care research basics and patient-centred primary care. His research has included papers, abstracts and book chapters concerning family medicine, domestic violence, complementary and alternative medicine, and adolescent motherhood.

Daniel Hollenberg received his doctorate in Community Health from the University of Toronto, Canada, where he conducted a pioneering study of integrative medicine settings in Canada. His postdoctoral work at McMaster University and the University of Ottawa explored the introduction of CAM in Canadian hospital settings with comparative research in Shanghai, China. As Research Associate with the Office of Health Policy, Royal College of Physicians and Surgeons of Canada, Ottawa, he led the first in-depth study of traditional, complementary and alternative medicine use in rural/remote areas of Ontario, Canada, including First Nations/Aboriginal healing; and was a co-investigator for the first national, in-depth study of physician underemployment and unemployment in Canada. With a strong background in Medical Anthropology and Medical Sociology, he maintains broad research interests related to integrative medicine including clinics and hospital settings, interprofessional education and collaboration amongst CAM and biomedical professions, and traditional medicine and international/global health. He continues to publish numerous peer-reviewed articles and book chapters related to these research areas. Currently, he is also linking research with practice by completing clinical training as an Integrative Health Coach at Mount Royal University, Calgary.

Jennie M. Hornosty is a recently retired Professor of Sociology from the University of New Brunswick, and is an Adjunct Research Professor in Sociology at Carleton University and a Senior Fellow, School of Governance, University of Ottawa. She is a feminist and critical sociologist, passionate about issues of social justice and inequality. She has an academic interest in health and illness, the Canadian health care system, gender issues, the corporatization of the academy and Marxist theory. Her more recent interest in complementary and alternative medicine stems from both personal experience and her scholarly reading in the field. Dr. Hornosty's primary research areas have focused on violence against women within a rural and farm context, and examining the links between family violence and animal abuse. She is the

Canadian editor of *Second Opinion: An Introduction to Health Sociology*, Canadian Edition, 1st and 2nd editions, published by Oxford University Press.

Nadine E. Ijaz is a critical qualitative health researcher whose substantive interests converge at the intersect between social justice, state policy, epistemology, and traditional/Indigenous, complementary, and integrative medicine. She is also a trained medical herbalist, clinical nutritionist, and shiatsu therapist with more than 15 years of clinical and teaching experience.

Cheryl Lans is a Senior Staff member of the Institute for Ethnobotany & Zoopharmacognosy in the Netherlands. She holds a Master's and PhD from Wageningen University, the Netherlands. She conducted postdoctoral research on medicinal plants used for animal health at the University of Victoria, British Columbia. This was a follow up to similar research conducted in Trinidad and Tobago. Her published papers include the research topic of women's reproductive health.

Julie Laplante is Associate Professor of Anthropology in the School of Sociological and Anthropological Studies at the University of Ottawa. Senior research fellow at the Max Planck Institute for Social Anthropology (2006-2010) she has published in numerous journals and is the author of Healing Roots (2015) and Pouvoir guérir (2004). Her work in Brazilian Amazonia and at two extremes of the Indian Ocean (Cape Town in South Africa and Jogja in Java Indonesia) revolves around the question of the plant, the molecule, knowledge, clinical trials, and bodily abilities in healing.

Ana M. Ning is a medical anthropologist, and Associate Professor in the Department of Sociology at King's University College at The University of Western Ontario. Her research expertise and interests are in the areas of addiction and mental health, biomedicine, and complementary and alternative medicine, with wider application in public policy and clinical settings. While her published research has focused on health-related issues, her interests and perspectives are also relevant to diverse anthropological and sociological concerns, including social theory, crime, and social control, as well as culture, gender, and ethnicity.

John Paul Nyonator is a PhD candidate and a student fellow of the Global Strategy Lab of the University of Ottawa. He has academic experience in sociology and population health with a focus on maternal and child health and health systems. He has worked and travelled in Africa and South East Asia dealing with the feeding of infants, the health of mothers, and integration of traditional medicine into formal health care systems. He currently serves as a student representative on the advisory board of the Canadian Society for the Sociology of Health.

Jo-Anne Rayner is a Senior Research Fellow at the Australian Centre for Evidence Based Aged Care, La Trobe University. She is a qualitative researcher with extensive experience in public health research and has particular interest in the use of complementary medicines as a health care option. In addition to her research on women's use of complementary medicine to enhance fertility, she is undertaking research into older people's use of CAM to manage the symptoms of chronic illnesses.

Natália Rejane Salim was an undergraduate in Midwifery at the University of São Paulo. She holds a PhD in Midwifery from the School of Nursing at the University of São Paulo. She is a board member of São Paulo Midwives Association. She was a visiting scholar at the Faculty of Social Sciences at University of Ottawa in Canada between 2012 and 2013. She works on care practices, birth contexts, and the humanization of health care of women in Brazil. She is currently an Associate Professor at the School of Nursing, Women's Health Area, at the Federal University of São Carlos-Sao Paulo, Brazil.

Bob R. Stewart is a Professor Emeritus in the College of Education and an Adjunct Clinical Instructor at Sinclair School of Nursing, University of Missouri, Columbia, USA. He specializes in research design and breast cancer survivorship. He recently co-authored a chapter in the book *Lymphedema: Complete medical and surgical treatment.* He has also published extensively in various professional journals.

Costanza Torri holds a degree in Economics at Ancona University, Italy, and completed a Master's degree at IAMM-CIHEAM, Montpellier, France. Subsequently, she completed a DEA (Diploma of Specialised Studies) in Sociology and a PhD in Sociology at Paris 1 Panthéon-Sorbonne. Prior to her appointment at the University of New Brunswick, she was a post-doctoral fellow at the University of Montreal, Centre for International Studies, and a research fellow at the Human Rights Research Centre, University of Ottawa. She has worked extensively in Asia and Latin America on a number of research projects concerning gender entrepreneurship and development, traditional health, intercultural health practices, and indigenous communities.

Ausanee Wanchai is deputy director for research and academic services and nursing instructor at Boromarajonani College of Nursing Buddhachinaraj, Phitsanulok province, Thailand. She specializes in complementary and alternative medicine use by breast cancer survivors. She recently co-authored a chapter in the book *Lymphedema: Complete medical and surgical management* (CRC Press, 2015). She also has published more than 20 peer-reviewed articles in various professional journals.

Rachel Westfall was born and raised in British Columbia, Canada. She has Bachelor's and Master's degrees in Botany and a PhD in Interdisciplinary Studies, with a focus on herbal medicine, midwifery care, and out-of-system childbirth. She is the lead social researcher and methodologist for the Yukon government's Bureau of Statistics. She specializes in mixed methods research, working with hard-to-reach populations, and evidence-based policy development. In addition to her academic publications, she has written and published young adult fiction and poetry.

Karen Willis is a health sociologist and qualitative research methodologist. Her research examines how people make choices about heath care. This work has covered complementary and alternative therapies, private versus public care, mammography screening, and how farmers and fishers stay healthy in difficult times. Her current research examines the disconnect between health care professionals and their patients in goal setting for chronic condition self-management. She is currently Associate Dean, Learning and Teaching, at Australian Catholic University, Melbourne, Australia.

INDEX

www.ingramcontent.com/pod-product-compliance
Lightning Source LLC
LaVergne TN
LVHW080036210926
848481LV00011B/3206
* 9 7 8 1 5 5 1 3 0 9 1 8 7 *